# Preventing Birth

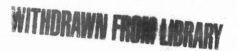

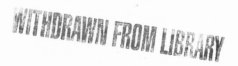

ETHICS IN A CHANGING WORLD
is a series that responds to issues
dealing with the ethical implications
of developments in science and technology.
Publications in this series present technically reliable accounts
of such development and an extended examination
of the ethical issues they raise.

VOLUME 3 • ETHICS IN A CHANGING WORLD

# Preventing Birth
## Contemporary Methods
## and Related Moral Controversies

*James W. Knight*

and

*Joan C. Callahan*

*University of Utah Press*
*Salt Lake City*
*1989*

ETHICS IN A CHANGING WORLD
Margaret P. Battin and Leslie P. Francis, Editors

**Library of Congress Cataloging-in-Publication Data**

Knight, James W., 1948–
    Preventing birth.

    (Ethics in a changing world ; v. 3)
    Bibliography: p.
    Includes index.
    1. Contraception.    2. Contraception—Moral and
ethical aspects.    I. Callahan, Joan C., 1946–
II. Title.    III. Series.
RG136.K595   1989         176         88-28053
ISBN 0-87480-319-5

FOR OUR PARENTS: Theda Slaughter
and, in loving memory,
L. C. Knight, Mary Callahan, and Joseph Callahan

# Contents

# Preface

The purpose of this book is to contribute to the general understanding of the scientific and social aspects of contemporary birth control methods and to the public discussion of a number of the moral issues that are related to those methods. It is a book we hope might be of interest to a heterogeneous audience, including general readers interested in reproduction and concerned about questions of reproductive rights, policymakers, political activists, legal commentators, reproductive scientists, moral philosophers, and members of groups working in the area of family planning. We realize all too well that writing a book for such an audience is not an easy task. We hope, however, that the book is clear enough and its topics important enough for it to be of use to such a varied audience.

Reproductive capacities play an extremely important role throughout most of the lifetime of each person. Yet, it is surprising how little some of us actually know about the details of reproduction. Further, billions of us, particularly women, practice some form of birth control. Yet, without a relatively clear understanding of human reproductive structures and processes, it is difficult to understand how the birth control technologies we use actually work. Knowing how they work is important, not only for prudential reasons, but for moral reasons as well. For example, it is not commonly realized that a number of contemporary methods function, primarily or secondarily, as measures which act after conception has taken place rather than acting to prevent conception. Thus, some methods commonly referred to as "contraceptives" (meaning against conception) may in fact allow conception and effect birth control by acting in ways which preclude maintenance and continued development of a conceptus. Commonly used oral contraceptives are an example. Although these preparations are appropriately understood as contraceptives—because their primary mode of acting involves preventing ovulation—they cause changes in a woman's reproductive system which interfere with implantation of a conceptus should breakthrough ovulation and fertilization occur. Other commonly used technologies and technologies in various stages of development routinely allow fertilization and act primarily by interfering with successful implantation and maintenance of the conceptus. Since many people hold that human rights, including a right to life, commence with human conception, these facts about the action of a number of contemporary birth control methods are morally relevant and need to be known by individuals adopting these methods. This is one of the reasons these methods raise the moral issue of informed consent to medical interventions, since many of the methods we shall discuss are available only through health care practitioners.

The facts we have just sketched show, too, how a number of contemporary birth control technologies quite directly raise the question of the morality of elective abortion. An implication of the position that human beings must be recognized as persons from the moment of conception onward is that elective use of those technologies which involve, primarily or secondarily, abortifacient action is as morally unacceptable as elective use of induced surgical abortion. We address this question in detail, giving particular attention to the central secular argument for the claim that a right to life must be recognized from the moment of human conception onward. Our conclusion is that this argument is seriously flawed and that the elective use of birth control technologies with abortifacient action and the elective use of induced surgical abortion are morally permissible and should not be proscribed by restrictive public policies.

Another moral concern raised by contemporary birth control technologies is respect for the right of individuals to decide what risks they will assume in adopting a method of birth control. This is also directly connected to the question of informed consent to medical interventions. If an individual's genuinely informed consent to the use of a birth control technology is to be obtained, it is important that individuals be in a position to evaluate claims made about the various risks purported to be associated with the use of various methods. Some risks are commonly overestimated while others are commonly underestimated. Thus, another object of the book is to explain clearly the nature and extent of risks associated with these methods.

We believe that issues like those just pointed out will make this book of interest to general readers as well as to readers in the other categories mentioned. Policymakers and political activists, in particular, should find it noteworthy that the moral concerns raised by contemporary birth control methods actually press in two directions. For example, the testing and use of some contemporary birth control methods in developing nations and in certain populations in developed nations raise special concerns about harm, exploitation, and informed consent. On the other hand, certain public policies raise concerns about paternalistic preclusions of birth control options for women who might, after making a rational assessment of the potential risks, find these options best suited to their needs. Some of these preclusions have been supported by feminists. But it is not clear that depriving women of some of these choices is really in the best interests of women. Thus, contemporary birth control methods raise important questions about what public policies best serve women's interests and needs. Another issue of particular relevance to policymakers and political activists has already been touched upon, namely, the preclusion of the availability of some promising new birth control technologies because of their potential use as abortifacients.

Legal commentators, moral philosophers, scientists engaged in various areas of research on reproduction, and those working in family planning services should be aware that analysts often do not know enough about the facts involved when writing on so-called applied ethics and public policy. We hope that this book might serve as a good example of how careful teamwork between an analyst and a scientist can avoid the kinds of questionable empirical assumptions that analysts are sometimes inclined to make and the kinds of questionable assumptions about what counts as knowledge and what is morally acceptable that practitioners are sometimes inclined to make. We hope, in short, that this book is an example of good work in practical ethics and that we have lived up to what we believe is the analyst's responsibility to know the facts and the practitioner's responsibility to scrutinize the philosophical assumptions that inform and the moral consequences that follow from his or her practice.

We begin, in Chapter 1, with an historical overview of male and female birth control methods. This look at the history of attempts to manage fertility reveals a consistent desire on the part of individuals to control when they will and will not reproduce and a glance at the tensions that can arise between individuals and their societies as a result of that desire.

In Chapter 2, we address the question of societal interest in controlling individual reproduction, whether that control is expressed in pronatalist or antinatalist societal policies and practices. We offer an account of some of the kinds of political and philosophical reasons which give rise to a societal interest in controlling reproduction and sexual behavior generally. Chapters 1 and 2 introduce both the general methods and moral controversies that are discussed in greater detail later on.

In Chapters 3 and 4, we offer an overview of human reproductive anatomy, physiology, and endocrinology, which is necessary as background for understanding the birth control measures discussed in Chapters 5 and 6. Although Chapters 3 and 4 are primarily scientific, we discuss here some historical and lingering myths and other phenomena which have had and continue to have important effects on attitudes toward social equality of men and women and sexual self-image, for example, myths associated with menstruation, contemporary accounts of so-called premenstrual syndrome, and the belief that a larger penis is "better" than a smaller one.

In Chapters 5 and 6, we distinguish between birth control methods that are properly considered contraceptive (i.e., their primary action is to prevent conception) from others that are properly considered abortifacient (i.e., they routinely allow fertilization and their primary action is to interfere with the establishment of the conceptus). We describe the former methods in Chapter 5, and the latter, as well as current surgical methods of inducing abortion, in Chapter 6. Chapters 5 and 6 also point out the potential hazards to women attending the adoption of the techniques discussed there, and in Chapter 6 we briefly address the question of the right of women to have available potentially harmful products no longer obtainable through the American market and other products unlikely to receive Food and Drug Administration approval in the foreseeable future.

The material in Chapters 5 and 6 makes it clear that one of the most morally controversial aspects of a number of contemporary birth control methods is their abortifacient capacity. Having already seen in Chapter 2 some significant relationships between attitudes toward readily available, effective contraception and abortion, in Chapter 7 we turn to a detailed discussion of the morality of a social policy permitting women to elect abortion as a way of exercising reproductive choice.

Chapter 8 concerns the potential of contemporary birth control methods to harm ova, conceptuses, embryos, or fetuses. This discussion raises the questions of moral responsibility and of legal liability for mutagenic and teratogenic harms which result in prenatal death or in the birth of damaged infants. We take up these questions in Chapter 9.

There is a growing body of legal, medical, and philosophical literature proposing that the state has not only a right but a duty to protect gametes and prenatal human beings from certain avoidable harms. One question of significant social concern raised by this position pertains to the moral responsibility and legal liability of women who cause prenatal harm by acting or failing to act in certain ways during their pregnancies. Since questions regarding moral responsibility and legal liability for prenatal harms resulting from the use of birth control methods can only be adequately addressed in the light of a broader discussion of responsibility and liability for mutagenic and teratogenic harm and the state's right to protect the interests of future persons, we concentrate on this more general question in Chapter 9. On the issue of maternal liability for prenatal harm, we draw a conclusion which builds on our discussion and coheres with our conclusion in Chapter 7 on the question of elective abortion. We also address the questions of employer liability for mutagenic and teratogenic harms in the workplace and the moral justifiability of so-called fetal protection policies, which exclude fertile women from certain jobs unless they are willing to be sterilized. Here, we draw a conclusion which coheres with our discussion in Chapter 6 on the question of the autonomy of women in regard to the availability of certain contraceptive or abortifacient products. Finally, we discuss informed consent to the assumption of various risks associated with birth control technologies, and we end the chapter with some reflections on the problem of getting genuinely informed consent to such risks in certain populations.

Chapter 10 focuses on some questions about the possible future of birth control technologies, in particular, possible developments in male contraception. Here, we explain the problems with developing contraceptives for men that are analogous to oral contraceptives for women, but we point out that some of the research currently under way holds out hope for the emergence of more

contraceptive options for men in the not-too-distant future. We conclude the chapter and book with some reflections on the future prospects of birth control technologies more generally.

JCC
Lexington, Kentucky
June 1988

JWK
Blacksburg, Virginia
June 1988

# Acknowledgments

The excellent illustrations which appear in this book were drawn by K. June Mullins.

We are grateful to Gwen Linkous, Lisa Massoudi, and Jean Eaton, not only for typing several drafts of large portions of the manuscript, but also for their extraordinary attention to details that we sometimes managed to overlook. Jean Eaton deserves special thanks for what amounted to a genuinely heroic effort in helping JCC bring the final version of the manuscript to press while JWK was out of the country.

Although copy editors generally go without acknowledgment, Christian Milord deserves special mention in thanks for his diligent work on the manuscript and for a number of helpful substantive suggestions. The book has also been improved by the comments and probing questions of our reviewers, Margaret Pabst Battin, Leslie Francis, Bonnie Steinbock, and Richard Worley. Peggy Battin and Leslie Francis have also served as our editors at the University of Utah Press. We are deeply grateful to them and to David Catron, Director of the University of Utah Press, for their constant enthusiasm for the project, their unwavering faith in our completing the book despite several unforeseeable delays, and their support of our going forward with a book more than twice the size we originally projected. We owe David Catron additional thanks for consistently making himself personally available to us and for making the journey from first draft to print a remarkably easy one. And we are particularly grateful to Peggy Battin for giving us the opportunity to work together on a project combining scientific and humanistic questions. Our very different backgrounds and sometimes different perspectives combined to make the task of writing a unified work a rich and rewarding experience for us both.

We are also grateful to Carolyn Bratt, Deborah Mathieu, and Patricia Smith for their helpful comments on Chapter 9.

To Ronnie Sheehy and to David and Jennifer Crossen, JCC owes special thanks for all their loving support and for providing the space and time to work. Checking the proofs would have been an ordeal without Jennifer's cheerful, generous, and astute help, which she gave enthusiastically despite enormous demands on her time from other quarters.

Finally, we acknowledge with deep appreciation not only her loving encouragement and support of the project but also the constructive suggestions for the book's improvement given by JWK's wife, Mänette Monroe, irreplaceable friend to us both.

# 1
# Birth Control Techniques: An Historical Overview

## INTRODUCTION

In many ways, human history can be viewed as one species' continuing attempt to fully bridle nature. This endless struggle is well exemplified in the history of human reproduction. Our attempts to control when we will and when we will not reproduce seem clearly to stretch back into prehistory (Carr-Saunders 1922; Reuter 1923; Sumner, Keller, and Davie 1927; Duncan 1929; Thompson 1935; Himes 1936). Yet, despite the constancy of this desire to control our reproductive capacities, human reproduction has been, and continues to be, the locus of some of our most interesting and most difficult moral, legal, and political struggles. As this book goes to press, reproductive issues (including sex education in public schools; availability of contraceptives to minors; mass media advertising of contraceptives; availability of sexually explicit literature; the development and use of conception-enhancing technologies, such as artificial insemination by a donor, in vitro fertilization, and surrogate motherhood; and, more generally, the rights of women to control their own reproductive destinies) remain matters of serious dispute both within society and within the courts. At the same time, there is a tremendous effort in most developing nations to severely limit population growth as a matter deemed crucial to national survival. Indeed, some nations (China, for example) have strict government policies that determine family size rather than leave it up to the decision of individuals.

—— During the past century, women in many societies have achieved greater and greater social freedom. This freedom cannot be separated from, and in significant measure is due to, the stunning advancements that have been made in birth control technology. New, progressively reliable methods have allowed women to control their fertility with increasing effectiveness. This reproductive freedom, in turn, has contributed to women's liberty to choose societal roles other than mother and homemaking. In addition, effective birth control technologies have given women the freedom to engage in sexual activity without the previous fear of pregnancy. Possessing this freedom, which historically belonged chiefly to men, has brought to women much greater equality within heterosexual relationships. In addition, the development of antiseptic techniques has made the early termination of a pregnancy safer for a woman than carrying a fetus to term (see Chapter 7). This, coupled with the enormous improvements in abortion methods, has made abortion early in pregnancy a safe, relatively accessible, and widely elected option for women confronted with unwanted pregnancies.[1] But despite the wide use of various forms of contraception and abortion, both practices continue to cause intense moral disagreement.

Even a cursory examination of customs and laws governing sexual interactions and birth control reveals that there is a great variety of attitudes toward sexual interaction among different cultures and that attitudes within a single culture often shift. For example, prostitution was often tied to religion in the ancient West and Near East, where intercourse with temple prostitutes was viewed as an act of respect for the temple deity. Greek *hetaerae* ("companions") were frequently women of high social status. Roman *meretrices*, on the other hand, were low on the social register and were required to dress in ways that made their occupation clear to all. Still, prostitution was accepted in Rome and flourished in the Middle Ages, when licensed brothels served as a source of income for a number of municipalities. Indeed, it was only when venereal disease reached epidemic proportions in Western and Central Europe during the sixteenth century that serious efforts to control prostitution were undertaken. In contrast, the Jews rejected temple prostitution, along

---

[1] Abortion is not readily available to all women. Elective abortion remains illegal in a number of countries, particularly in African, Latin American, and Islamic countries. Even in countries where elective abortion is a right protected by law, access is often limited as a result of public policies. In the United States, for example, the Hyde amendment to health appropriation legislation (which went into effect in 1977) prohibits use of public funds for elective abortion, putting the procedure (which generally costs several hundred dollars) out of reach for many poor American women who do not wish to continue their pregnancies.

with the sexual practices that tended to accompany the fertility-based religions, and they developed the view that procreation is the primary purpose of sexual interaction, an attitude which carried over into Christianity (Williams 1958; Sussman 1976).

Population control was frequently discussed by the Greeks. Infanticide was legalized by Solon in the sixth century B.C. Plato (c. 347–266 B.C.) favored a legal prohibition on procreation by those prior to the age of 20 and after the age of 40. But other authors, Aristotle (384–322 B.C.) among them, preferred not to enforce abstinence, and favored regulating family size by using contraception, abortion, and infanticide (in the case of deformed infants).

The ancient Greeks accepted sexual interaction as a normal pleasure. Homosexual relationships were accepted, perhaps partially because of their "sterile" nature (Kisch 1910). Homosexuality was also accepted in ancient Rome, as were marriage to eunuchs, abortion, and infanticide. Galen (c. 199–129 B.C.), Lucretius (c. 99–55 B.C.), Pliny the Elder (23–79), and Soranus of Ephesus (98–138) all discussed birth control (some had better ideas than others). There is a tendency among some contemporary authors writing on developments in reproductive technology to think that the recent advances in birth control methods and in techniques which aid reproduction in infertile and subfertile couples were responsible for first separating the procreational and "recreational" aspects of sexual interaction. But the works of these early authors clearly indicate that this distinction has been with us at least since the beginnings of Western civilization.

Without a true understanding of reproductive science, our earliest ancestors were most reliant on abortion and infanticide to limit reproduction. But even though contraception as such was relatively ineffective in limiting births until quite recently, the desire for reproductive control encouraged men and women to try what were often astounding measures to prevent pregnancies or births. The earliest known techniques were primarily the responsibility of men.

TRADITIONAL MALE TECHNIQUES

*Coitus Reservatus* Confucius said that failure to have sons is unfilial, for sons must carry a family forward to preserve the worship of ancestors. As we shall see in more detail in Chapter 2, contemporary Chinese families are strenuously encouraged by their government to limit family size to one child. But that is a very recent trend, and the traditional need for children to help work the land, high child mortality rates, the Chinese emphasis on familial piety, the sharing of child-rearing responsibilities within extended families, and the Confucian mandate to produce sons have led to a staggering population in China (currently at one billion). Despite the past emphasis on proliferation among Chinese peasants, however, literate Chinese are said to have practiced coitus reservatus (withholding ejaculation) rather extensively. The belief was that a man could save his *yang* essence and gain strength from the female *ying* essence if he had intercourse with as many women as possible without ejaculating. By doing this, his sperm would grow stronger and stronger, resulting in fine offspring when he ejaculated with the wife chosen to bear his children (Green 1971).

Far more recently, coitus reservatus was championed by John Humphrey Noyes. The founder of a nineteenth-century religious, communistic community, Noyes might have been speaking for the contemporary women's movement rather than the Oneida Perfectionists when he wrote: "We are not opposed to procreation. But we are opposed to involuntary procreation. We are opposed to excessive and, of course, oppressive procreation" (Noyes 1849). Given that Noyes seems to have rejected the use of other available contraceptive techniques as "unnatural, unhealthy, . . . indecent, and . . . destructive to love," he promulgated coitus reservatus (Noyes 1870).

Because coitus reservatus requires tremendous self-control, it has never been a popular or widely successful contraceptive technique. And even without a "true" ejaculation, some sperm may be emitted in pre-ejaculate fluid; this could lead to pregnancy despite admirable control on the man's part. Although the technique was eloquently defended in the late nineteenth century by those who practiced it, it was also condemned (along with masturbation and coitus interruptus) as being responsible for disorders as diverse as "sexual enfeeblement" and tumors in the female reproductive tract.

*Coitus Interruptus*   Coitus interruptus (withdrawal before ejaculation) is somewhat less demanding than coitus reservatus and is still used extensively, particularly in developing nations, among the poor in developed nations, and among sexually active teenagers who are afraid or embarrassed to seek contraceptive aids.

Despite the wide use of coitus interruptus, the influence of the Judeo-Christian tradition has often led to its moral condemnation in Western societies. The condemnation rests on the story of Onan (Gen. 38:6–10), son of Judah, who was commanded by his father to take Tamar, the widow of Onan's brother in a levirate marriage (i.e., a marriage required of Jewish brothers when the brothers had lived together and the deceased brother was childless). Onan withdrew during intercourse with Tamar, spilling his "seed" on the ground. This, the story says, "displeased the Lord," and Onan was slain. Following early rabbinical interpretation, the story has been held in some Christian sects (including Roman Catholicism) to condemn coitus interruptus. But Onan's sin seems far more clearly to have been his refusal to fulfill the duty of the levirate, which required that he give his sister-in-law children who would bear his brother's name. Such a violation of established filial duty struck at the heart of the solidarity necessary to protect the family, clan, and tribe in biblical nomadic life (McKenzie 1965).[2]

Like coitus reservatus, coitus interruptus is not as effective a contraceptive measure as might be thought, since sperm may be emitted in pre-ejaculate fluid. And like coitus reservatus, coitus interruptus has also been condemned for purported medical reasons. Eighteenth-century French physicians, for example, railed against the practice, contending not only that it leaves women without sexual satisfaction but also that it leads to a physical deterioration of men which could ultimately result in death. Part of this view seems to have been tied to a quasi-magical belief that male semen is a vital fluid. Practicing coitus interruptus encouraged more frequent intercourse and therefore increased the loss of vital fluid (McLaren 1983).

The contemporary term *onanism* has two meanings: withdrawal during intercourse and masturbation. This is not surprising, since both involve the "spilling of seed." The fact that condoms involve

---

[2]Though many seem to know the story of Onan, few seem to know what occurred later. Judah, who promised to send his third son, Shelah, to Tamar when he was grown, failed to do so. Tamar subsequently disguised herself as a harlot, and seduced Judah, who impregnated her. When Judah discovered her trick, he acknowledged her twins as his, and declared Tamar more righteous than he, since he had failed to keep his promise to send Shelah to her to fulfill the duty of the levirate (Gen. 38:11–26). Interestingly, the story shows far more tolerance for fornication than for breach of the levirate.

the same "waste" of spermatazoa partially accounts for religious prohibitions on their use. Indeed, the use of a condom simply amounts to providing an intravaginal sac to catch the semen that would otherwise have to be spilled outside the woman. Although we might think of the condom as a quite modern invention, the idea is an ancient one.

*Condoms*   The earliest uses of sheaths to cover the penis seem to have been for purposes of decoration and identification of social rank and to protect the penis from certain transmissible parasitic diseases as well as from insect bites. Himes (1936) suggests that it was but a short step to the use of sheaths to prevent the spread of venereal disease and that many of the earliest penile sheaths were utilized for that purpose. The legend of King Minos of Crete and his wife, Paisiphae, suggests that sheaths may have been used in Imperial Rome — but ironically to promote conception. According to the legend, the semen of Minos was full of serpents and scorpions, which caused injury to the women with whom Minos had intercourse. Prokris, who was living under the protection of Minos, set out to help solve his problem. Prokris taught Minos to use the bladder of a goat to cast off his treacherous semen; this then allowed him to impregnate Paisiphae, who bore him many children. It is unclear whether the sheath was worn by Minos or was a female sheath placed intravaginally. Whichever, the story clearly suggests that sheaths of some sort were used in Imperial Rome to prevent infection and to promote conception.

The Italian anatomist Gabriello Fallopius (1523–1562) is perhaps most widely recognized for his description of the Fallopian tubes (oviducts of the female), which bear his name (see Chapter 3). But in addition to being a well-versed general anatomist, Fallopius was a recognized early authority on syphilis, and he has been credited with the first published description of the condom. His *De Morbo Gallico Liber Absolutismus* (published posthumously in 1564) contains a description of a linen sheath purportedly invented by Fallopius to prevent the spread of syphilis. By 1738, the condom was described as a sac of fine animal membrane. The term *condum* came into use after appearing in a 1706 poem ("A Scot's Answer to a British Vision") and in a 1717 treatise on syphilis by Daniel Turner (Turner 1717; Astruc 1738; Himes 1936; Green 1971). By the 1720s, condoms were clearly being used for contraception in Europe. They were called

"French letters" by the British, because they washed up on the beaches and were said to have drifted in from France. Not to be outdone, the French called the condom "the English riding coat." But the attributions were not fully in jest. The condom was associated with sexual promiscuity and the love of pleasure, "vices" which, as we shall see, were held to be antithetical to societal good. Neither country, then, was anxious to be associated with its invention or wide use (see, e.g., Bernstein 1940; McLaren 1983).

A genuine revolution in condom use came in the mid-1880s with the vulcanization of rubber, which allowed for the mass production of condoms. Currently the rising fear of AIDS (Acquired Immune Deficiency Syndrome) in both the heterosexual and homosexual populations is causing an ever-increasing number of people to advocate and use condoms for one of their earliest purposes — prevention of the spread of a deadly infectious disease. Commercial television networks in the United States are now airing condom advertisements, and the public is debating whether minors should be instructed in school on condom use and whether condoms should be made available in high school infirmaries.

*Sterilization* Historically, mutilation of the male genitals has not been uncommon. But contraception has not generally been the explicit motivation for such mutilation. Himes (1936) reports that subincision (an operation which involves permanently splitting and sometimes removing parts of the male urethra; see Chapters 3 and 10) was commonly practiced among preliterate Australian natives, and at least in some tribes it seems to have been an extension of the rite of circumcision that completes the ceremonial transition from boyhood to manhood. One result of subincision is that urination must be accomplished in a squatting position. Another consequence is that during ejaculation, semen is deviated from its normal course and dribbles out over the testicles (see Chapter 3). There seems to be no evidence that subincision was practiced for explicitly contraceptive reasons. But, as Himes points out, since the operation clearly interferes with the optimal conditions for fertilization, the practice of subincising may well have been adopted initially for controlling fertility. Awareness of the original motive may have been lost and the practice may have been continued merely as a ritual, like so many other societal practices (as well as beliefs and taboos) that originated for certain practical reasons but were continued after the original motivation became lost in the misty past (cf. MacIntyre 1981).

As recently as the early part of this century, various forms of interference with male genitalia were used to prevent masturbation in England and the United States, where it was thought that masturbation caused "genital weakness, impotence, dysury, vertigo, epilepsy, hypochondriasis, loss of memory, manalgia, fatuity," and even death (Green 1971). Circumcision was commonly used as a "cure" for mild "cases." But for recalcitrant masturbators, infibulation was preferred.

Infibulation involves pulling the foreskin (see Chapter 3) well over the tip of the penis, piercing two holes in it, and inserting a silver ring or fibula to hold it in place. Use of infibulation dates back at least to Imperial Rome, where it was used by comic actors and musicians, who associated deepening of the voice with penile erections and who used the ghastly method to prevent them — an erection with a fibula in place would be excruciating. Green (1971) notes that Karl August Weinhold, a professor of surgery and medicine at the University of Halle, suggested early in the nineteenth century that infibulation be used for contraceptive purposes. Birth control champions ignored the suggestion, but, as has been noted, infibulation was adopted by the medical profession to "cure" intractable masturbators.

Historically, full-scale castration has not commonly been used for contraceptive purposes either. Occasionally, castration has been employed for unambiguously medical purposes, for example, to treat tuberculosis of the testicles and to retard the spread of prostate cancer (e.g., Peschel and Peschel 1987). More often, castration has been used as a way of making amenable slaves of the vanquished in war, as a form of punishment for sexual offenses (including adultery), and as a way of qualifying men to perform certain tasks open only to eunuchs, such as care of palatial quarters for women in China.

Castration has also been voluntarily undertaken by some Christians in order to make themselves "eunuchs for the kingdom of heaven's sake" (see Matt. 19:12). Also, as is well known, castration was carried out in Italy from at least the early seventeenth century until late into the nineteenth century (and perhaps even into the twentieth century) on potential opera singers and choirboys to preserve their high-pitched prepuberal voices (e.g., Green 1971; Guttmacher 1973; Peschel and Peschel 1987). For example, castrati (boys emasculated before puberty) were apparently utilized in the Sistine choir until they were expelled from the Sistine Chapel by Pope Leo XIII, who was pontiff from 1878 to 1903. Also known as *evirati* (emasculated men) and *musici* (musicians), the castrati were commonly held to have voices even sweeter than those of women and their ornamental operatic style, known as *bel canto* (beautiful song), included arpeggios, runs, roulades, cadenzas, and trills. Since prepuberal emasculation involves depriving the male body of the increased production of androgen hormones in the interstitial Leydig cells of the testes (see Chapter 3) and thus prevents the rapid growth of male vocal chords resulting from androgen stimulation during puberty, it is not surprising that the voices of the castrati were often claimed to be especially sweet. By preventing elongation of the male vocal chords, prepuberal castration may well have kept the vocal chords of the castrati at their prepuberal length (7–8 mm), which is shorter than the average mature woman's vocal chords (8–12 mm). Pope Clement VIII (pontiff from 1592 to 1605) was apparently quite taken with the voices of the castrati, and declared that producing castrati for church choirs was to be recognized as *ad honorem Dei* (to the honor of God) (e.g., Peschel and Peschel 1987).

Such honor, as well as the impressive payments made to the most talented castrati in opera, led many of Italy's impoverished parents to have their sons castrated. A number of these boys, however, had no musical gifts, and apparently it was not uncommon for these castrati to become priests. Further, despite the honor and wealth achieved by a few castrati, many others led tragic lives. Prepuberal emasculation causes primary hypogonadism, a condition characterized by a number of physical abnormalities in adulthood, including an infantile penis, lack of the usual distribution of male axillary hair, distribution of pubic hair in a female pattern, lack of beard growth, elevated amounts of subcutaneuous fat in a characteristically female distribution (i.e., in the hips, buttocks, and breasts), certain facial distortions (in some cases) and disproportionately long arms and legs. Their physical appearance made castrati common objects of public jokes and ridicule, and the autobiography of one castrato, Filippo Balatri, suggests that being "neuter" beings may have been a source of torment for many castrati (Peschel and Peschel 1987).

Although these examples suggest that explicit contraceptive motives for rendering men partially or fully, temporarily or permanently incapable of impregnation have not been common, the idea of rendering a man infertile without rendering him impotent goes back at least to Hippocrates (c. 460–370 B.C.), who, following Aristotle, believed that male "seed" flows from the brain and that cutting the veins behind the ears would block its downward passage and make a man sterile. Galen also believed this, but (thankfully) the stratagem seems not to have been put into practice (Green 1971). More recently, however, the development of an effective male sterilization operation which does not involve the maiming of full castration — vasectomy (see Chapters 3 and 10) — helped to engender a tide of eugenic sterilization laws in the United States early in this century.

Indiana was the first state to enact a compulsory sterilization law. A prison physician, Harry Sharp, used the population at the Indiana State Reformatory to develop the vasectomy, erroneously believing that it would prevent the "feeble-minded" boys in his charge from masturbating. Sharp perfected the technique during the last decade of the nineteenth century, and Indiana passed its compulsory sterilization law in 1907 (Robitscher 1973a). Subsequently, all the compulsory sterilization laws passed prior to 1925 were declared unconstitutional. However, in 1925, statutes in Michigan and Virginia were upheld by the highest courts in those states, and in 1927, the U.S. Supreme Court upheld Virginia's law in the famous case of Carrie Buck, a "feeble-minded" patient at the Virginia State Colony of Epileptics and Feeble-Minded who was the daughter of a woman in the same institution and the mother of an illegitimate, purportedly feeble-minded child (*Buck v. Bell* 1927). Justice Oliver Wendell Holmes immortalized the decision to uphold Virginia's sterilization statute by declaring that "three generations of imbeciles [were] enough." In the wake of this support, the 1930s saw as many as 25,000 eugenic sterilizations of persons classified as insane, feeble-minded, idiots, imbeciles, and epileptics as well as those classified as rapists, habitual criminals, persons with criminal tendencies, drunkards, drug fiends, syphilitics, moral and sexual perverts, moral degenerates, and "other degenerate persons" (Paul 1973). By 1943, eugenic sterilizations in the United States totalled nearly 41,000 men and women, and by 1963, nearly 63,000 men and women had been sterilized for eugenic purposes (Robitscher 1973b). After 1963, eugenic sterilizations declined dramatically, and few are performed in this country today, although nearly all states do have statutes which

permit sterilization of the mentally incompetent under clearly circumscribed conditions. Virtually all existing statutes and contemporary court decisions require that sterilization be in the best interest of the person to be sterilized. And since incompetent women
(rather than incompetent men) sometimes do get pregnant and give
birth and are likely to suffer as a result, the most common sterilizations of the incompetent today are performed on women.

Most recently, vasectomy has slowly been gaining in popularity as a voluntary method of birth control, although voluntary female
sterilization (see Chapter 5) is by far more common in the United
States and in other countries (see, e.g., the discussion of China in
Chapter 2). We shall return to the topic of male sterilization in Chapter 10.

## TRADITIONAL FEMALE TECHNIQUES

*The Concentration on Methods for Women*   Without question, greater
attention and scientific research has been focused on female, rather
than on male, methods of birth control. It is sometimes claimed that
the concentration on developing methods for women is rooted in
sexism and men's unwillingness to share the burdens of controlling
fertility. For example, in discussing "the pill," Margaret Mead once
suggested that the concentration on developing female contraception is to be explained by the reluctance of men to experiment on
their own bodies (Mead 1971). It is also well known that societies
have often adopted the Aristotelian view that women are congenitally defective and that medical practitioners have sometimes adopted
the Platonic view that women's physical complaints are linked to
their biological capacity for reproduction. Historically, this bias significantly contributed to the medical profession's interest in learning about the female reproductive system (e.g., McLaren 1983; see
also the discussion of the menstrual cycle and premenstrual syndrome in Chapter 4). It is surely true that men are, in general, less
interested in controlling their fertility than are women (Djerassi 1981)
and that they are less willing than are women to volunteer for fertility control clinical trials (Hartmann 1987). But citing sexism as
the explanation for the concentration on the development of birth
control methods for women is too simplistic, since there are many
significant social and scientific reasons for concentrating on methods for women.

Among the social reasons for concentration on techniques for women is that women must assume the serious physical dangers and discomforts associated with pregnancy. Further, high child mortality rates can be devastating to women, and in the past have led some women to seek a means of avoiding pregnancy, often without the knowledge of their male partners, in societies where such avoidance would be condemned (Himes 1936). Moreover, the burden of primary responsibility for child rearing has traditionally (fairly or not) fallen on women. Since women have the most at stake when it comes to matters of reproductive control, it is not surprising that women have been far more anxious to effectively control their fertility than men have been. And since they have the most at stake, it is crucial to the well-being of women that safe and effective means of fertility control be readily available to them.

Foremost among the scientific reasons for concentrating on birth control methods for women is that the probability of successfully controlling the fate of a single ovum (egg) released once a month in a cyclical manner is obviously much greater than the probability of destroying or rendering inactive the millions of spermatozoa present in each ejaculate of a fertile man. Additionally, a fertile ovum will be present in a narrow window of time (see the discussion of the "safe period" in the next section) while spermatozoa are in continuous production, making their numbers virtually infinite and making them far less amenable to management without interfering with sperm production itself. Interference with sperm production involves interference with stem cells (see Chapter 3), which cannot currently be done without inducing irreversible sterility. Thus, the basic differences in human gametogenesis (see Chapters 3 and 4) unquestionably make concentration on female techniques considerably more promising than concentration on male techniques.

Differences in male and female neuroendocrine control also suggest that methods which will not induce permanent infertility are more likely to be possible for women than for men. In brief, there are two neuroendocrine control centers in women, the tonic and the cyclic, and interference with the cyclic is possible (via the use of exogenous steriods, e.g., the pill) without interfering with the tonic (see Chapter 4). In men, this is not possible because there is only one center of control. Thus, attempts to develop a male pill similar to preparations available for women hold out virtually no promise of success (see Chapter 10). Given that science tends to proceed most rapidly by selecting to control that which seems most amenable to control, modern scientific efforts have focused on the female cycle and how the usually single ovum per monthly cycle might be kept from being fertilized or, if fertilized, from continuing to develop.

The importance to women of having control over their fertility and the biological facts mentioned above make it reasonable to concentrate on developing female birth control methods. It cannot be emphasized strongly enough, however, that modern high-quality condoms combined with effective spermicides create a mutually safe and (when properly used) highly effective contraceptive method which is cheap and readily available to men. Vasectomy is also readily available to men. Thus, men already have available to them effective birth control techniques, and hence they cannot rely on the social and scientific arguments for the concentration on techniques for women to excuse them for failure to help shoulder the burdens of reproductive responsibility. We shall return to the topic of male contraception in Chapter 10, where we shall explore some of the possibilities for expanding the availability of male birth control methods.

Like male sterilization, female contraception has a long, sometimes sordid past. Ancient techniques included violent jerking to set the semen off course, leaping about to rid the vagina of semen, vaginal plugs, and a host of concoctions swallowed or placed in the vagina. Many of these were based solely on magic, but those that involved placing an object or substance in the vagina did create a barrier or kill sperm, and in principle at least they may have had some contraceptive efficacy (Himes 1936). Although abortion and infanticide were commonly used to control population in Greece, the physicians Hippocrates and Soranus disapproved of them. Because of this disapproval, Soranus (who was followed in the sixth century by Aëtios of Amida) attempted to provide effective contraceptive advice. Although Soranus occasionally recommended a magical solution (e.g., drinking the water in which blacksmiths cool hot metals, a measure still used in some parts of the world today), he generally rejected the use of magical potions and magical devices (e.g., amulets) and his various recommendations for pessaries (vaginal depositories) such as soft wool, avoiding intercourse during times in a woman's cycle when she was thought to be most likely to conceive (although he was mistaken about when this is), cleaning the vagina immediately after intercourse, and introducing astringents into the vagina prior to intercourse, all reveal general insight into how to prevent conception, even if the particular stratagems were unlikely to be very successful in practice. Of the ancients, Soranus has probably had the most influence on the development of contraceptive methods for women.

*The "Safe" Period*   Throughout history, many cultures have restricted insemination for various periods. Although some of these restrictions in early societies (and in modern preliterate societies) seem to have been for magical or religious reasons or for reasons pertaining to the protection of a developing fetus, it is often clear that prohibitions against intercourse (or, at least, against insemination, which was to be prevented by coitus interruptus) have been for contraceptive purposes.

Unfortunately, guesses about a woman's safe or sterile period have often been mistaken. Soranus and Aëtios recommended avoidance of coitus just before and just after menstruation. They were joined by Avicenna (980–1037), Islam's great medieval scientist and philosopher, who recommended avoidance just after menstruation (e.g., Himes 1936; Green 1971). Other explicitly contraceptive traditions and recommendations include abstinence or coitus interruptus during menstruation, during pregnancy, or for months or even years following childbirth, all of which are relatively safe periods (the last mentioned if a women is breast-feeding). As we shall see in Chapter 4, menstruation, pregnancy, and lactation are all associated with an endocrine status which inhibits follicular growth and ovulation.

Before the nineteenth century, it was generally believed that ovulation and menstruation coincided; thus, there are numerous suggestions in the literature that coitus was safe during the midperiod—that is, during the middle of a woman's cycle—which is precisely when she is most likely to conceive (e.g., Himes 1936; Loebl 1974). Indeed, it was not until the 1930s that scientists really began to understand the true sequence of hormonal changes during the menstrual cycle. As we shall see in Chapter 4, a woman ovulates (releases an egg) approximately fourteen days prior to the onset of the next menses, or on day fourteen for a woman with a typical cycle of twenty-eight days. While the expected fertile life span of spermatozoa in the female tract is approximately 48 hours, there have been reports that some sperm may survive for twice that duration (Edwards 1980), and motile sperm have been found in the cervix as long as 205 hours after insemination (Insler et al. 1980). The expected fertile life span of an ovum is approximately one-half that of spermatozoa. Thus, it follows that in general the "fertile period" occurs approximately from day ten to day eighteen for a woman with a regular twenty-eight-day cycle and the "safe period" comprises the remaining days. The problem with relying on the traditional calendar or "rhythm" method to avoid conception is that the days mentioned are averages based on the total population and the days of each period vary among women. Further, even women with "normal" cycles may have their cycles disrupted by any number of factors, including illness, physical or emotional stress, use of various medications, climatic changes, and aging. Hence the old joke: What do you call women who practice rhythm? The answer: Mothers.

Considerably more promising than the traditional rhythm method is the recently developed symptothermal method, which combines the basal body temperature method and the vaginal mucus (or Billings) method. The technique is highly individualistic, utilizing precise charting of a woman's basal body temperature (i.e., temperature immediately after awakening in the morning when the body is at rest) and charting of the presence and characteristics of a woman's vaginal mucus. Temperature rises slightly after ovulation, and vaginal mucus becomes clear and slippery just prior to ovulation (see Chapters 3 and 4). Diligent tracking of such changes during her cycle can substantially help a woman avoid (or achieve) pregnancy. Success, however, depends on consistency and accuracy in observation, and the failure rate in the first year of using this method is said to be between 24 and 30 percent (i.e., 24 to 30 births per 100 users), though effectiveness is significantly enhanced when combined with condom use (Planned Parenthood Federation of America 1985, 1986; Hartmann 1987). Although it is cumbersome and imprecise, one of the most attractive features of this method of birth control is that it involves no hormonal alterations or physically invasive interventions, and it therefore avoids the side effects and risks associated with oral contraceptives, intrauterine devices, and other methods discussed in detail in Chapters 5 and 6.

It has also been suggested that using the safe period can have some other interesting advantages for some people in continuing relationships. For example, it makes intercourse a relatively "scarce resource" rather than something which can simply be taken for granted. Since coitus disappears from the relationship for regular periods of time, other forms of intimacy must be developed to replace it. Further, since contraceptive control is less automatic and not just quietly seen to by the woman, it is among the methods that make contraceptive achievement a shared project (see, e.g., Luker 1984; Hartmann 1987).

*Vaginal Pessaries*  The oldest vaginal depositories recorded are Egyptian and are described in the Petrie Papyrus, found at Kahum in 1889. The papyrus dates back to the reign of Amenemhat III of the Twelfth Dynasty (c. 1850 B.C.). The recommendations include inserting a pint of honey, natron (native sodium carbonate), auyt gum, or crocodile dung cut up in auyt paste. Pessaries containing gumlike substances were common in the ancient world, and prescriptions containing dung occur in the contraceptive literature for over 3,000 years, including in the Islamic literature, where elephant dung was recommended (e.g., Himes 1936; Green 1971). While the inherent spermicidal properties of dung are more than a little doubtful, the insertion of dung in a paste would have provided some physical obstruction to sperm transport (as would dense mixtures in honey) and reduced the number of spermatozoa reaching the potential site of fertilization in the oviduct (see Chapter 3). Thus, such pessaries are among the oldest of the barrier techniques of female contraception.

Among other substances recommended over the centuries were cedar gum and olive oil (Aristotle had recommended that these be smeared on the penis); pepper; unripe gallnut; pomegranate pith; ginger; dry figs and naton; pomegranate skins with gum and rose oil (all the preceding recommended by Dioscorides in the first century A.D.); ground-up cabbage blossoms; pitch; ox gall; animal ear wax and whitewash; sesame oil; leek seeds; spindle oil with honey and pitch; crushed crocus or mint; jelly made of glycerine, starch, and chinosol; tobacco juice; and quinine and coconut butter mixed with borax and salicylic acid (this last was recommended by British birth control champion, Marie Stopes). The list of concoctions goes on and on (see, e.g., Himes 1936; Green 1971). Some recipes hold out virtually no hope of contraceptive effectiveness while others, the ones which would markedly affect the intravaginal environment, hold out some promise as spermicides (e.g., those containing vinegar, lemon, and other astringents and those, like spindle oil, containing various acids). As might be guessed, many of these mixtures were hard on their users.

In addition to gummy substances and chemical substances placed intravaginally, a great variety of physical objects have been used as pessaries, some with deadly results. The Djukas (a bush tribe) of Dutch Guiana are known to have placed okralike seed pods into the vagina (with one end snipped to allow entry of the penis) to create a female sheath. The West African Dahomeys crush a root and apply it as a vaginal plug, and several tribes in central Africa are known to use rags and chopped grass. The natives of Easter Island have made occluders of seaweed and algae. Such plugs, not always easily recovered, have led to horrible infections and an untold number of painful deaths for women intent on preventing conception (Himes 1936).

A less life-threatening (though not innocuous) female barrier contraceptive is the sponge, which is among the oldest contraceptive inserts recorded. Sponges were generally dipped in solutions, such as the ones already mentioned. Interestingly, sponges were probably in common use in certain groups of Jewish women in biblical times. The Hebrew mandate to "increase and multiply" was understood to apply to Jewish men; Jewish women were not formally bound by Hebraic law to avoid taking contraceptive measures (e.g., Biale 1984). Hence, even though the early rabbis almost universally condemned coitus interruptus (Rabbi Eliezer [c. 100 A.D.] seems to have been to sole exception to this), the Talmudic tradition seems not only to have allowed but to have required that women in certain groups (viz., minors, pregnant women, and nursing mothers) "cohabit with the sponge."

The recommendation to use sponges as contraceptives seems not to have been passed along, however, since their mention re-emerges only much later with the discovery of a sponge among the "tools of the trade" found by French satirist Mathurin Regnier in a French prostitute's room at the beginning of the seventeenth century (Regnier 1609; Green 1971). By 1778, sponges were extremely popular in France, and by 1786, silk cords were being attached to them for their easy removal. In 1797, the English utilitarian philosopher, political economist, and social critic Jeremy Bentham (1748–1832) guardedly recommended the sponge in his *Situation and Relief of the Poor.*

It was, however, Francis Place (1771–1854), an English tailor and friend of Bentham, who, in language more accessible than Bentham's, promulgated the use of the sponge by cleverly distributing handbills among the British working classes in 1823. By doing so, Place began the real birth control movement in Europe and set the stage for the American birth control movement, which we shall discuss in Chapter 2.

It is interesting to note that, over the past decade, the only new American entry into the set of contraceptives available over the counter is the Today Vaginal Contraceptive Sponge, introduced in June 1983 by Vorhauer Laboratories. Although not marketed as a barrier aid, the product nonetheless resurrects the ancient idea of combining a barrier and a spermicide.[3] This disposable, one-size-fits-all, polyurethane sponge contains a high dose of the spermicide nonoxynol-9, which is active for twenty-four hours. The product is limited in effectiveness, however, having a 10–20 percent failure rate among American users. Between 1983 and March 1987, nineteen users of the product were affected by toxic shock syndrome, although no such cases occurred during the seven years of clinical trials.[4] Because it may take many years to recognize an exogenous agent as a carcinogen, some have expressed a concern that the product's high dose of spermicide may have carcinogenic potential (see, e.g., Hartmann 1987). The u.s. Food and Drug Administration (FDA), however, has classified the product as a Category 1 safe and effective drug (category 1 products require the most extensive testing for approval). In theory, virtually any exogenous agent might

---

[3] Sponges are not reliable barriers, since they can be pushed about during intercourse. More reliable barriers for women, such as the diaphragm (to be discussed in a moment), require individual fitting. Consequently, Vorhauer Laboratories (VLI) does not market its sponge as a barrier contraceptive. Its primary action is to deliver a spermicide; thus, it is classified by the FDA as a drug. Secondarily, it may have some barrier properties if in place over the cervix and it may absorb some of the ejaculate.

[4] This information is from a telephone conversation with VLI's "Talkline" on 7 August 1987. Eighty percent of cases of toxic shock syndrome are associated with menstruation and the use of tampons. Women who have had toxic shock syndrome are at known risk, and should use *no* vaginal depositories whatever.

function as a carcinogen, but there is no evidence suggesting that nonoxynol-9, even in high doses, is carcinogenic. The Today Sponge is currently the leading nonprescription female contraceptive aid in the United States (Hartmann 1987), and the interest in such a product is well-taken. Combining a condom and a noginal spermicide, such as that delivered by the Today Sponge, creates the most effective kind of nonprescription contraceptive, and a recent study in the *New England Journal of Medicine* suggests that of assisted forms of contraception, the combination of a true mechanical barrier (a condom or diaphragm) and a chemical spermicide provides women the clearest protection against tubal damage leading to infertility (Cramer et al. 1987).

Returning to less recent history, the nineteenth century saw, in addition to the popularization of the sponge, the development of the modern diaphragm, a much more effective barrier than the sponge. Cassanova (1725–1798) had suggested using a dejuiced half lemon as a cervical cap. Some European peasants used and even still use caps of beeswax, and Japanese and Chinese prostitutes are thought to have used disks of oiled paper to cap the cervix. The use of a rubber cervical cap was first recommended in 1838 by the German gynecologist Friedrich Wilde. The cervical cap enjoyed some popularity in England and America until it was replaced by the Mensinga diaphragm, a considerably larger cap which fits into the vagina much like the diaphragms in wide use today. Although it was invented by a German, the Mensinga came to be known as the "Dutch cap," because it was popularized in Holland by Dr. Aletta Jacobs, who opened the world's first birth control clinic there in the early 1880s. It took several decades for the Mensinga diaphragm to reach England and America, but when it did arrive, the English and American birth control movements were well under way (e.g., Green 1971).

By the sixteenth century, contraceptive advice in Islam and Europe had degenerated into a reliance on magic, and it wasn't until the nineteenth century, with the revival of pessaries, that scientifically valid (if less than fully effective) measures reappeared. The re-emergence of the pessary was followed quickly by suggestions for douching (rinsing the vagina by use of a stream of fluid) and the introduction of syringes to make thorough douching more possible.

*Douching*   Although there is evidence that French prostitutes had been using syringes to douche since at least 1600 (Regnier 1609; Green 1971), credit for the invention was claimed by the Massachusetts physician Charles Knowlton in 1832. Himes (1936) contends that it is no exaggeration to say that Knowlton's *Fruits of Philosophy* (1832) was the first genuinely important treatment of contraceptive methods since those of Soranus and Aëtios. Knowlton attempted to publish information on effective contraceptive measures because he was moved by the plight of his poorer patients, who were driven ever deeper into poverty by their continually expanding families. He advocated douching with a syringe, and his general prescriptions for douches included vinegar and solutions of alum and astringent vegetables (e.g., white oak bark, hemlock bark, red rose leaves, green tea, raspberry leaves, and roots). For special conditions, Knowlton recommended solutions containing zinc, baking soda, or sugar and lead. (If none of these was readily available, he advised a thorough douching with cold water.) Knowlton, like Soranus and Aëtios, had struck upon a variety of solutions which create a hostile environment for sperm and may therefore be spermicidal.

The primary problem with postcoital douches, however, is that they have *very* limited effectiveness, since the transport of sperm from the site of ejaculation to the site of fertilization (or at least beyond the reach of the douche) is rapid (see Chapter 4). Besides being generally ineffective, douches which do have spermicidal properties (including soapsuds) tend to be caustic agents which can seriously irritate the epithelial lining of the female reproductive tract. In short, douches should *not* be relied on for contraception.

*Intrauterine Devices*   Although there are stories of Arabs using intrauterine placement of pebbles to prevent pregnancy in their camels during long desert trips, it is ironic that the first modern medical uses of depositories in the human uterus (as opposed to the vagina) were for the promotion of fertility (e.g., Green 1971). It was not until the late nineteenth century that physicians generally began to realize that placing a foreign body in the womb could prevent pregnancy. By 1909, Paul Richter had invented a thread pessary for placement in the uterus, and by 1923, Karl Pust had invented a stem pessary that consisted of a button that protruded into the vagina and a stem that blocked the cervical canal. Pust added several loops of catgut to the stem, which went into the uterus. Although Pust believed that his pessary prevented conception by sealing off the cervix, another German, Ernst Graefenberg, had an experience with a patient which led him to another theory.

Among Graefenberg's patients was a young woman who came to see him about her difficulty conceiving. Graefenberg began treatment with a dilation and curettage (or D and C), a procedure involving dilating the cervical canal through a series of probes, then "scraping" the interior of the uterus with an instrument called a curette (see Chapter 6). Upon examination of the material taken from the woman's uterus, Graefenberg discovered some pieces of catgut and realized that these must have originally been attached to a Pust button pessary. After the D and C, the woman was able to conceive, and Graefenberg began experimenting with intrauterine strings of various sorts. Eventually, he discovered that coiled gold or silver seemed to be most effective and to best stay in place. He presented his findings at the Congress of the German Gynecological Society in Frankfort in 1931. Although physicians had experimented extensively with intrauterine depositories during the nineteenth century (see, e.g., Green 1971), by the early twentieth century, intrauterine devices were taboo. Graefenberg's paper met with outrage, and the IUD went underground until the late 1950s, when several papers suggesting the use of such devices began to appear in the international gynecological literature (see Chapter 6). By 1964, forty countries were testing various kinds of IUDs, and Korea, Japan, and Pakistan had national programs using them (Loebl 1974). By the mid-1970s, dozens of versions were in use around the world, including the Zipper Ring, the Margulies Spiral, the Lippes Loop, the Birnberg Bow, the Ota Ring, Majzlin's Springs, the Robinson Saf-T-Coil, the Butterfly, and the Shamrock. By the late 1970s, it was estimated that forty to fifty million women were using IUDs. Some forty million of these women were in the People's Republic of China (Piotrow, Rinehart, and Schmidt 1979), and currently over sixty million use IUDs there today (Hartmann 1987). However, when G. D. Searle and Company withdrew the Cu-7 and Tatum-T IUDs on January 31, 1986, they were nearly the final manufacturer of IUDs to withdraw their products from the American market (see Chapter 6).

The early unpopularity of IUDs was not misguided. As Corea (1985) points out, IUDs were always associated with infection. This is not surprising, since they must be passed through the cervix, which contains bacteria, into the uterus, which is a virtually sterile field. What is more, when U.S. researchers set out to mass-produce IUDs, they added tails, making it easier for paramedical personnel in the third world to insert and remove the devices and easier for women to see that they were in place and had not been expelled. In some designs (e.g., the Dalkon Shield), the tails, which extend out of the uterus, can act as wicks, drawing bacteria into the uterus. It took some time for scientists to understand how IUDs work; but we now know that one of their actions is to inflame the uterus, thereby making embryonic implantation in the uterus highly improbable (see Chapter 6). By the early 1980s, a number of physicians were acknowledging that IUDs had caused irreversible sterility in some women (Rowe 1981), and by the mid-1980s, it became clear that some IUDs were responsible for an alarming number of raging infections, including a significant number that led to death. Faulty insertion can cause an IUD to perforate and become imbedded in the uterine wall or occasionally to escape into the abdominal cavity, resulting in a fatal infection. Women using IUDs run increased risks of ectopic pregnancies and septic abortions (see Chapter 6). Thus, as Hartmann (1987) points out, an IUD failure is not only a contraceptive failure, it may produce life-threatening medical complications as well.

   At this writing, one company alone (A. H. Robins) faces over 300,000 lawsuits resulting from the use of just one type of IUD, the now infamous Dalkon Shield. Of the suits, roughly 280,000 have been brought by American women. But the Dalkon Shield has had worldwide distribution, and many women in developing countries are unaware that they had the device inserted (either because they were never informed of the intrauterine insertion at all or because they were not given complete information on the precise device used). Many others have not been contacted in enough time to file a claim against Robins (Women's Global Network on Reproductive Rights 1986b).

   The most common as well as the most serious and controversial health risk associated with the IUD is pelvic inflammatory disease (PID), an infection which can cause permanent sterility. As of this writing, the poorly designed Dalkon Shield is associated with the hightest PID rate of all IUDs, the Cu-7 (or Copper-7) with the lowest (Cramer et al. 1985). The removal of IUDs from the American market was primarily the result of a business decision, not a legal mandate. The increase in liability insurance and legal expenses which all IUD manufacturers faced as a result of the Dalkon Shield lawsuits made the continuation of IUD production and marketing unprofitable for multiproduct companies, even those, like Searle, which were producing far safer products.

Despite the risks associated with IUDs, they are highly effective, and an IUD may well be the ideal birth control aid for certain women. We shall return to IUDs and the issue of their availability to women in Chapter 6.

*Oral Contraceptives* Many of the authors we have already referred to prescribed various contraceptive "potions" in addition to sheaths, topical solutions, and solid pessaries. The list of oral prescriptions is virtually endless, including innocuous mixtures of roots, grains, leaves, seeds, vegetables, natural oils, and fruits. Others are more ominous, including mixtures of various urines, concoctions with insect and animal parts (including spider eggs), and poisons, such as arsenic and strychnine. A number of these were taken as abortifacients. And, as might be expected, they sometimes proved as lethal to their users as infections resulting from pessaries and attempts to self-abort were to other women.

The real breakthrough in oral contraception is quite recent. By the 1920s, reproductive physiology was coming of age, and the search for the hormones governing reproduction was well under way. By the early 1930s, estrogen (the hormone responsible for the development of female secondary sex characteristics, among other things), progesterone (the hormone which fosters gestation of the fertilized egg), and testosterone (the hormone responsible for development of male internal genitalia and some male secondary sex characteristics) had been isolated. Insulin (a protein hormone produced by the beta cells of the pancreas) had already been proven to be a life-saving drug for diabetics, and scientists hoped to be able to use the hormones governing sexual development and reproduction to solve a variety of sex-related problems, for example, to cure infertility and impotence and to help women avoid miscarriages. However, because of their biochemical nature as steroid hormones, their low molecular weight, and their short half-lives, these hormones proved to be more difficult to isolate, extract, and purify than others. It was here that a brilliant and fascinating scientist, Russell Marker, entered the picture.

Marker (who mysteriously left the University of Maryland without finishing his degree) apparently had a genius for finding, synthesizing, and altering complex organic molecules. By the mid-1930s, Marker, who was then teaching at Pennsylvania State University, had become interested in steroids. Steroids are chemicals that contain the basic cyclopentophenanthrene ring, four interconnected carbon ring structures, and the sex hormones belong to that group. Marker was aware that hormones and hormonelike substances are found not only in animals but also in plants, and he thought that the sapogenins (a family of chemicals containing steroid structures and occurring in plants) might be used to manufacture steroid hormones. He experimented and found that he was able to produce progesterone through a five-stage transformation of some sapogenins, particularly diosgenin. In the summer of 1940, Marker set out for Mexico with a group of students. They were joined by several Mexican botanists. The group explored the American southwest and Mexico, looking for plants with high sapogenin secretions. The result was that over 100,000 pounds of plants and roots (involving over 400 species) were shipped back to Penn State, where Marker and his students set out to analyze their sapogenin content. Eventually, they found that the root of a particular wild yam growing in the southern Mexican wilderness was rich in diosgenin (the dioscorea or *cabeza de negro* [black head]). Marker knew that the discovery would make progesterone readily available (as well as testosterone and estrogen, which can be manufactured from it; see Chapter 3, Figure 8). He took the information to Parke-Davis Laboratories, where he worked as a consultant. Unsuccessful after two years of attempting to persuade the company to finance the project, Marker suddenly left Penn State at midterm and reappeared in Mexico. He set up a small laboratory in an abandoned pottery shed, hired a few workers to help him collect the roots, and began extracting and transforming the steroids alone. Several months later, Marker appeared in a Mexico City drug firm (Laboratories Hermona) with two glass jars containing roughly 4.5 pounds of a white crystalline powder. It was pure progesterone, worth some $160,000 — a genuine fortune in 1944. Marker made his manufacturing process public in 1949, and several years later he simply disappeared. It is unlikely that anyone will ever discover whether Marker knew that by making progesterone readily available, he made the pill possible.

We shall describe the action of contemporary oral contraceptives in more detail in Chapter 5. For now, it is enough to point out that following release of an ovum from the ovary, a solid structure, the corpus luteum, forms at the site of ovulation. It is the corpus luteum which is the primary source of progesterone secretion in the female. If the released egg is not fertilized, the corpus luteum will regress and the secretion of progesterone (meaning that which promotes gestation) will decrease, triggering the onset of menstruation. If the egg is fertilized, secretion of progesterone is maintained, the uterine lining (which is shed in menstruation) is maintained for implantation of the embryo, and the neuroendocrine events necessary for growth and development of new follicles on the ovary and for ovulation are inhibited by progesterone (see Chapters 3 and 4). By 1897, it was known that no ovulation takes place during pregnancy, and by 1937, that administration of progesterone prevents ovulation in rabbits (Diczfalusy 1979, 1982). But it was Gregory Pincus who realized that since the secretion of progesterone stopped ovulation in the pregnant woman, introducing progesterone should similarly stop ovulation in the nonpregnant woman.

Pincus was one of the world's leading experts on hormones, ovulation, and mammalian gestation when he was persuaded by Margaret Sanger to shift the focus of his research to contraception. Sanger, who founded the American birth control movement (see Chapter 2), was discouraged when she discovered that the best contraceptive that had been developed in Europe was the diaphragm, which, because of availability, problems in fitting and forgetting, failure rates, cultural prohibitions on touching one's genitals or on practicing contraception, lack of privacy for insertion or storage, lack of cooperation from male partners, and so on, was not an appropriate contraceptive for all women. Abraham Stone, a friend of Sanger, arranged a meeting between Sanger and Pincus, and she immediately won him to the cause of finding an effective oral contraceptive for women. Once he turned his attention to the question, Pincus quicky realized that maintaining a woman in a state of pseudo-pregnancy by introducing progesterone would "fool" the ovaries into failure to ovulate. Eventually, the first pill emerged from Searle Laboratories — Enovid. After some field trials, it was approved by the FDA in 1959, and versions of the pill have been the most widely used contraceptives ever since. As we shall see in Chapters 5 and 6, innovations in the basic science associated with oral contraception have recently led to the development of preparations designed to act as abortifacients, such as "morning after pills," which interfere with implantation of the blastocyst (early embryo); oral preparations which induce menstruation and the elimination of the implanted embryo with the shedding of the uterine lining; and subcutaneous implants which release contraceptive chemicals for periods of months or years. All of these methods raise special ethical problems, which we shall touch on in the chapters to come.

.    .    .    .    .    .

So far, we have looked briefly at the main methods of preventing birth that have an established history. We turn next to the social history of birth control. As we shall see, despite the enduring desire of men and women to exercise individual reproductive control so obviously demonstrated in the history of preventive methods, it is certainly not the case that custom or law has always supported the fulfillment of that desire.

# 2
# Political and Philosophical Perspectives on Birth Control

## INTRODUCTION

As we have already seen, the distinction between procreational and other functions of sexual interaction seems always to have been with us. Although many ancient civilizations openly accepted this distinction and legally protected various forms of birth and population control, as we approach the modern world — particularly in the West, with its deep Judeo-Christian roots — sexual interaction for purposes other than procreation falls into disrepute. Although some of the early laws and customs barring practices such as extraspousal intercourse and prostitution developed for reasons pertaining to tribal or societal preservation, modern societies have often forgotten those origins, and today many people are morally concerned about the ready availability of contraception and about the abortifacient nature of some existing and developing birth control technologies.

Despite the advances in contraceptive science made in the nineteenth and early twentieth centuries, social resistance to the development of effective, widely available contraception and to nonreproductive sexual interaction was strong. Initially condemned as obscene, both were dubbed "social evils" in the Victorian Age, and contraception became associated with promiscuity and the sacrifice of traditional family values. These attitudes persist in large segments of contemporary society. Many people today want not only contraceptives but also reproductive information withheld from potentially sexually active teenagers. Indeed, in the past several years in the United States we have seen a steady shift away from the short-lived "sexual revolution" of the late 1960s and early 1970s to a renewed conservatism regarding sexual interaction and to a more and more strident opposition to sex education in America's public schools. In 1986, Surgeon General C. Everett Koop claimed that sex education is crucial for protecting minors from deadly sexually transmitted diseases such as AIDS (Acquired Immune Deficiency Syndrome). But it remains to be seen whether the fear of so deadly a disease will be sufficient to overcome the fear of formally explaining to minors how to have intercourse while minimizing the probability of pregnancy or disease transmission. One underlying fear is that providing information about sexual interaction and reproduction (to say nothing of making contraceptives readily available to minors) will lead to increased sexual activity among adolescents and increased multipartnered sexual activity. But as one looks at the rising world population (now at five billion and doubling every three to four decades, with the doubling time steadily decreasing[1] and at the numbers of reported abortions,[2] teenage pregnancies,[3] and new cases of AIDS in the United States alone,[4] one cannot help

---

[1]On 11 July 1987, a Yugoslavian baby boy, Matez Gaspar, was declared the five billionth person on earth by U.N. Secretary General Javier Perez de Cuella. Zagret, Yugoslavia was chosen as the place to mark the event because 129 countries participating in the 14th World University Games were represented there at the time (*Lexington Herald Leader*, 12 July 1987).

[2]Known legal abortions in the United States stood at 1,588,500 in 1985 (Henshaw 1987b).

[3]The rate of pregnancy in American young women between the ages of fifteen and nineteen was 96 per 1,000 in 1985, double the rate in Canada, England, and France (Hartmann 1987).

[4]On 12 June 1986, the U.S. Public Health Service reported that 21,517 cases of AIDS had been reported in the United States, involving 11,713 deaths. It also projected that a cumulative total of 270,000 cases of AIDS will have been diagnosed by 1991; and of these, some 179,000 persons will have died (Hoffman 1986). In December 1987, the U.S. Centers for Disease Control (CDC) estimated that 945,000 to 1.4 million Americans were infected by the human immunodeficiency virus (U.S. Centers for Disease Control 1987). In November 1988, the CDC reported that 78,312 cases of AIDS had been reported in the United States (U.S. Centers for Disease Control 1988b). 1988 estimates for the United States from the Public Health Service project a cumulative total of 365,000 diagnosed and reported cases of AIDS by the end of 1992, with 80,000 new cases anticipated during 1992, AIDS-caused deaths during 1992 projected to reach 66,000, and the cumulative number of AIDS-caused deaths expected to total 263,000 by the end of 1992 (U.S. Centers for Disease Control, 1988a). By August 1987, the known dead were 22,548 (Goldman 1987); by November 1988 the known dead were 44,071 (U.S. Centers for Disease Control 1988b).

but wonder how we could do worse. Still, the societal fear of widely available, effective contraception is an old one—as old, perhaps, as the opposing desire of individuals to control their reproductive capacities. And it is this fear, rather than the desire of individuals to control their fertility, which has tended to be reflected in public customs, religious mandates, and secular laws.

The early rabbis attempted to place strict limits on acceptable contraception, and the view that sexual interaction was acceptable only because of its link to procreation passed over to Christian interpretations of the Judeo-Christian scriptures. The *Summa Theologica* of St. Thomas Aquinas (1225–1274) systematized Roman Catholic teachings, and it associated sex for purposes other than procreation with sin—an association which also occurs in Protestant traditions. Indeed, after the Reformation, not only abortion (which was often undertaken to conceal fornication) but adultery and even the use of contraceptives were, for a time, capital crimes in Britain. Religious attitudes in the West dominated secular law throughout the nineteenth century and as recently as the summer of 1986, the u.s. Supreme Court ruled that statutes making sodomy (oral and anal sex, neither of which, obviously, can result in procreation) a crime, punishable by a prison term, are permitted under the American Constitution (*Bowers v Hardwick* 1986). As of 1986, twenty-three American states and the District of Columbia still had statutes making sodomy (in some cases only homosexual sodomy) punishable by fine (in Texas) or imprisonment, with terms ranging from thirty days in Arizona to a five-year minimum in Idaho and as much as twenty years in Georgia and Rhode Island (McDaniel, Raine, and Carroll 1986). The common classification of sodomy as a "crime against nature" reflects the persistent view that coitus which precludes reproduction is evil—sufficiently evil to justify a legal proscription against it.


THE BRITISH AND AMERICAN BIRTH CONTROL MOVEMENTS

As birth control techniques were becoming progressively more effective in the nineteenth century, movements to bring contraceptive knowledge to the public began in earnest. In Britain, Francis Place's "diabolical handbills" were among the first large-scale attempts to provide contraceptive information to the working poor (see Chapter 1; Himes 1936). Inspired by the work of Thomas Malthus

(1766–1854), who argued that unrestricted population growth has devastating effects on societies, reformers such as Place defied the public attitude of nineteenth-century society toward contraception.

Even Malthus was opposed to contraception and advocated instead "moral restraint" on the part of the poor — that is, delaying marriage until the would-be parents were in an economic position to adequately support and properly educate their children. Departing from Malthus, Place stands out as the first to base arguments for widespread contraceptive practice on a social theory and to identify measures that, according to the theory, would be both necessary and sufficient to eliminate poverty and other social problems. He argued that decreasing the number of workers would increase salaries, that early marriages would decrease the incidence of sexually transmitted diseases as well as the demand for prostitution, and that such marriages would be more congenial (since the young are better able to adapt to partners). Child labor was a serious concern to many in nineteenth-century Britain, and Place, like some others, thought that large families contributed to its existence and abuse. Widely practiced contraception, he believed, would do away with this social evil as well. As we have seen in Chapter 1, the primary method Place recommended was use of the vaginal sponge (e.g., Himes 1936; Green 1971).

Place was followed in Britain by Richard Carlile (1790–1843), who published the first English book on the medical, social, and economic aspects of contraception (Carlile 1826). Although Carlile spent nine years in prison for his efforts to secure freedom of the press, he was never prosecuted for his attempt to educate the masses on birth control methods. He was, on the other hand, subject to societal scorn, as were Bentham and Place. Ironically, it was the legal prosecution of several reformers which probably gave the British birth control movement its greatest boost.

We have already mentioned Charles Knowlton, an American physician who was moved by the plight of his poor patients to publish a tract on birth control (see Chapter 1). Knowlton was slightly preceded in America by Robert Dale Owen, a textile industrialist, who published the first American book on birth control (Owen 1831). Like so many nineteenth-century authors, Owen shared the utopian orientation and the optimistic, evolutionary view of human progress that was part of the heritage of the French Revolution:

In the silent, but resistless progress of human improvement, . . . change is fortunately inevitable. We are gradually emerging from the night of blind prejudice and of brutal force; and, day by day, rational liberty and cultivated refinement, win an accession of power. Violence yields to benevolence, compulsion to kindness, the letter of the law to the spirit of justice: and, day by day, men and women become more will-ing, and better prepared to entrust the most sacred duties (social as well as political) more to good feeling and less to idle form — more to moral and less to legal keeping. . . . It is no question whether such reform will come: no human power can arrest its progress. (Owen 1831).

Among the changes Owen thought to be inevitable were the ultimate social acceptance of birth control and the eventual univer-sal refusal of women to have intercourse with men "devoid of honor" — men unwilling to use condoms or practice coitus inter-ruptus (the method Owen most emphasized) to prevent concep-tion. Owen was aware that one reason (which persists today) that some men oppose the dissemination of contraceptive knowledge and the availability of contraceptive aids is that, with such knowl-edge and aids, women are free to commit adultery and fornication without the fear of pregnancy accompanying unprotected intercourse and hence without fear of their husbands or fathers or brothers find-ing out. Owen attacked this motive for opposing contraception, pointing out that chastity based on fear has little to do with virtue and that such reasoning profoundly degrades the women to whom such men are purportedly devoted.

Although Knowlton and Owen disagreed importantly on what methods were to be recommended (Knowlton, like Place before him, believed that contraception should be controlled by the woman), both were widely read in England and America. It was Knowlton, however, who ran into trouble with the law.

Knowlton was out of step with the nineteenth-century medical profession, which condemned elective birth control by either abor-tion or contraception (e.g., Field 1983; Luker 1984). The profession's stance was clearly articulated in an 1869 *Lancet* editorial: "A woman on whom her husband practises what is euphemistically called 'pre-ventive copulation' is necessarily brought into the condition of mind of a prostitute. . . . As regards the male, the practice, in its actual character and in its remote effects, is in no way distinguishable from masturbation." (See Glass 1940; Fryer 1965; Wood and Suitters 1970; Green 1971; Field 1983.)

Knowlton was the first of the modern supporters of birth control to be incarcerated for disseminating contraceptive information. He spent three months at hard labor for his efforts. In England, the most famous arrests and trials were those of the late 1870s, involving Annie Besant and Charles Bradlaugh in 1877 and Edward Truelove in 1878.

The British prosecutions were brought under the common law on obscenity. Besant and Bradlaugh were prosecuted for republishing Knowlton's *Fruits of Philosophy*, Truelove for distributing Owen's *Moral Physiology* and publishing J. H. Palmer's *Individual, Family and National Poverty* (1875). Truelove was convicted, and sentenced to four months in prison and a fifty-pound fine. His conviction and sentence generated considerable public outrage. Things, however, went better for Besant and Bradlaugh, who conducted their own militant defense. After initially receiving an ambiguous judgment, they appealed and emerged victorious when it could not be shown by the prosecution that Knowlton's book was obscene. The case not only established a legal right in Britain to publish and distribute contraceptive information, but in combination with the Truelove case it fired tremendous public interest. The number of tracts on contraception skyrocketed, and among them was a new book by Annie Besant that was issued to replace Knowlton's somewhat outdated *Fruits of Philosophy* (Besant 1879). What Himes (1936) has called "the democratization" of contraceptive knowledge was finally fully under way in Britain. Things were, however, quite different in America.

After Knowlton's arrest, there were several decades of quiet dissemination of contraceptive literature, much of it through the American post. In 1873, however, Anthony Comstock, leader of the New York Society for the Suppression of Vice, managed to get passed a federal law prohibiting the sending of contraceptive information through the mails. Comstock also helped enforce the law by astonishingly gaining permission to open suspicious mail and by writing to shopkeepers and physicians and getting them to break the law by forwarding him information, and then sending (or often bringing) the police to arrest the criminals he'd uncovered.

Meanwhile, back in England, the success of the Bradlaugh-Besant defense was followed by the establishment of the misnamed

Malthusian League in 1878 (misnamed because Malthus, as we
seen, was opposed to aided contraception). As its name sugg
the league proposed controlling reproduction for Malthusian or
nomic reasons. It was the league which first organized international
communication regarding birth control by setting up a meeting of
its medical division and the International Medical Association, which
was convening in London in 1881. A second, larger neo-Malthusian
conference met in Paris in 1900. By World War I, the Malthusian
League had member organizations in France, Holland, Germany,
Spain, Sweden, Belgium, Switzerland, Bohemia, Portugal, Brazil,
Cuba, and North Africa (Field 1983). The movement to limit populations had become international.

In the early twentieth century, however, the population control
movement also began to change direction. As Western populations
began to decline, particularly during and following World War I,
the economic arguments and Malthusian fear of overpopulation
began to lose what force they had had. In 1921, Marie Stopes founded
the Society for Constructive Birth Control in England, taking the
term "birth control" from Margaret Sanger, who had chosen it for
the name of her own new society, the National Birth Control League,
founded in 1914 (Sanger 1938). The groups' names reflected a shift in
rationale for pursuing readily available birth control, namely, away
from Malthusianism or *population* control to *birth* or *reproductive* control, with the emphasis on health, family life, and women's reproductive freedom.

Today, this difference in rationale for making birth control technologies readily available is reflected in talk about population control programs on the one hand and talk about family planning programs on the other. The difference is more than semantic, since a
moral justification for a national population control program rests
on the moral principle of utility, which holds that morally correct
choices are those which will most likely produce the greatest good
for the greatest number. On the other hand, the direct moral justification for national family planning programs rests on the moral
principle of autonomy, which holds that morally correct choices (in
the relevant cases) are those that most fully respect the autonomy,
freedom, or self-direction of individuals. Fully respecting autonomous choice may not be compatible with attempting to bring about
the greatest good for the greatest number, although it may be.
Attempts to limit population growth have sometimes included

extremely coercive practices, as we shall see. It has become clear to many people, however, that creating the social conditions which maximize individual choice generally and reproductive choice in particular tends to result in decreased birthrates. This is especially true of social conditions influencing the lives and viable options of women (e.g., whether women have ready access to education and to meaningful work outside the home).

The historical shift to a concern with individual choice in reproduction is clearly reflected in an inscription appearing on the wall of Britain's first birth control clinic, opened by Stopes and her husband, H. V. Roe, on March 17, 1921:

> . . . to show by actual example what might be done for mothers and their children . . . and what should be done all over the world when once the idea takes root . . . that motherhood should be voluntary and guided by the best scientific knowledge available (Wood and Suitters 1970).

The new motivation for widely available birth control is made exquisitely clear by a story Margaret Sanger tells in her account of why she left nursing for political battle. Sanger was working as an obstetrical nurse on the impoverished lower East Side of Manhattan. It was 1912, and people were adverse to going to hospitals except for the greatest emergencies. Sanger was called to a poor, small Grand Street tenement flat by a young man, Jake Sachs, whose twenty-eight-year-old wife was unconscious from the effects of a self-induced abortion. Sanger and a physician attended Sadie Sachs constantly for two weeks, finally overcoming the septicemia (a widespread, systemic infection which is caused by pathogenic bacteria and commonly follows abortions not performed under antiseptic conditions). After another week, Sanger was ready to leave. Mrs. Sachs was desperately afraid of another pregnancy and asked the physician what she could do to prevent it. He laughed (Sanger says not unkindly) and said, "Tell Jake to sleep on the roof." The physician left, and Mrs. Sachs turned to Sanger. "Please," she begged, "tell me the secret and I'll never breathe it to a soul." But Sanger had no more answer to offer than had the physician. Mrs. Sachs fell asleep, and Sanger quietly left. Three months later, Jake Sachs called once more. His wife was again ill from a self-induced abortion. Sanger reluctantly returned to the dingy apartment. Mrs. Sachs was in a coma. She died within ten minutes of Sanger's arrival. Her death had a profound effect on Sanger.

I folded her still hands across her breast, remembering how they had pleaded with me, begging so humbly for the knowledge which was her right. I drew a sheet over her pallid face. Jake was sobbing, running his hands through his hair and pulling it out like an insane person. Over and over again he wailed, "My God! My God! My God!" I left him pacing desperately back and forth, and for hours I myself walked and walked and walked through the hushed streets. When I finally arrived home . . . I looked out my window and down upon the dimly lighted city. Its pains and griefs crowded in upon me, a moving picture rolled before my eyes with photographic clearness: women writhing in travail to bring forth little babies; the babies themselves naked and hungry, wrapped in newspapers to keep them from the cold; six-year old children with pinched, pale wrinkled faces, old in concentrated wretchedness, pushed into gray and fetid cellars, crouching on stone floors, their small scrawny hands scuttling through rags, making lamp shades, artificial flowers; white coffins, black coffins, coffins, coffins interminably passing in never-ending succession. . . . I went to bed knowing that no matter what it might cost, I was finished with palliatives and superficial cures; I was resolved to seek out the root of evil, to do something to change the destiny of mothers whose miseries were as vast as the sky (Sanger 1938).

With the death of Sadie Sachs, Margaret Sanger left nursing to begin a political struggle to make contraception readily available in America. Her struggle would last a quarter of a century.

As Sanger began her work, she knew nothing about Malthus. And although she fell into inconsistency by eventually arguing on eugenic grounds that birth control should be readily available, her initial commitment was to making genuine reproductive choice a reality for all women.

I was not looking for theories. What I desired was merely a simple method of contraception for the poor. . . . I knew something must be done to rescue those women who were voiceless; someone had to express with white hot intensity the conviction that they must be empowered to decide for themselves when they should fulfill the supreme function of motherhood (Sanger 1938).

This motive for pursuing readily available contraception became the cornerstone of the birth control movement in the United States, which culminated in the Supreme Court's judgment that a woman has a right to decide if she will continue a pregnancy — a right which is compelling through the second trimester of pregnancy (*Roe v. Wade* 1973; see Chapters 7 and 9).

Sanger ultimately decided that clinics which would give women individual instruction in contraception (on the model of the Dutch clinics) were the key. But the Comstock Law had spawned a number of other laws, and giving contraceptive advice except "for the cure and prevention of disease" was illegal in most jurisdictions. Short of repeal of all such laws, what Sanger needed in order to open the way to the proliferation of the kinds of clinics she envisioned was a broad interpretation of "for the cure and prevention of disease." She tested the laws, first by opening a lay-run "clinic," since she was unable to find physicians who would assist her. The first American birth control clinic of this sort was opened in the Brownsville section of Brooklyn in 1916. It functioned for just nine days before it was raided by the vice squad and Sanger and her co-workers were arrested. Among them was Sanger's sister, Ethel Byrne, who was sentenced to thirty days in the workhouse on Blackwell's Island in the East River. Byrne responded by going on a hunger strike. She has the dubious distinction of being the first American woman to be force-fed in prison.

Sanger finally succeeded in winning several physicians to her cause, and she opened other clinics — this time real ones, where more than just general contraceptive information could be given. It was a raid in 1929 which finally gave Sanger her first substantial legal victory, when a New York magistrate ruled that the clinic physician had acted in good faith and had attempted to prevent conception for the sake of the "health and physical welfare" of patients. But it was not until 1936, after years of working for reform on the federal level, that Sanger and her associates succeeded in taking the teeth out of the Comstock Law when an appellate court ruled that contraceptives could be advertised and sent through the mails. In 1937, the American Medical Association was able to inform its membership that physicians now had the legal right to give contraceptives routinely and that contraception was now to be taught in American medical schools.

Perhaps more intriguing than the American birth control movement's struggle against the Comstock Law and the various state statutes that it helped spawn is the fact that Comstock's legal legacy actually lasted nearly a hundred years. Although a series of judicial decisions instigated by Sanger and her associates had taken much of the clout out of the Comstock Law by the late 1930s, the law itself was not formally repealed until 1971. And it was only in 1965 that the Supreme Court made it clear that states could not make it illegal for married couples to obtain and use contraceptives and only in 1972 that the Court ensured that unmarried persons would be at legal liberty to obtain and use contraceptives (*Griswold v. Connecticut* 1965; *Eisenstadt v. Baird* 1972). While it might seem natural to most people in the late twentieth-century Western world to assume that contraceptive choice should belong to individuals, it needs to be pointed out that this is not, even now, the universal position and it needs to be asked why governments might be so interested in controlling such choices.

## THE POLITICS OF BIRTH CONTROL

*Religion and Politics*   Religious influences on state attempts to control contraception and sexual practices more generally can never be underestimated. We have already suggested that the Judeo-Christian tradition, which associates nonreproductive sexual interaction with moral evil, has been highly influential in shaping public policy on the availability of contraceptive information and contraceptive aids. That influence is still in evidence today in laws against sodomy as well as in laws proscribing prostitution, fornication, and even cohabitation of unmarried couples. It is not surprising that two of the groups most helpful to Anthony Comstock and his Society for the Suppression of Vice were the Women's Christian Temperance Union and the New York Young Men's Christian Association. Wedded to the theological influences on state regulation is a philosophical position on the proper tasks of government which holds that one of the state's responsibilities is to protect the morals of its citizens — a view known as *legal moralism* (see, e.g., Devlin 1959; Hart 1963; Feinberg 1985b, 1988). This position, combined with the widely shared moral content of the Judeo-Christian tradition, goes a long way toward explaining governmental attempts to suppress contraception (and various forms of sexual interaction) in the West.

Not only was contraception thought to encourage amateur prostitution and promiscuity, but the use of contraception implied a lack of control — a vice not to be encouraged in Christian countries. Turn-of-the-century English Anglicans, for example, worried that contraception would "eat away the heart and drain away the life-blood of" their country and lead to "what may be called free love . . . and other evils of that sort" (Fryer 1965). The term "free love" itself reveals the traditional religious view that coitus without the "purchase price" of potential pregnancy is sinful, a view which is rooted in the belief that the natural world reflects the will of God, who has given to all things a proper function or purpose, and that intentional frustration of such purposes is a violation of God's will. In this way, "natural law" and divine law become conjoined, and although the United States is purportedly a secular nation committed to the separation of church and state, a residuum of religious taboo is undeniably (and unjustly) responsible for its laws against sodomy (as well as other forms of nonreproductive sexual interaction between adults) and for much of the American reaction to the liberalization of abortion and the ready availability of contraceptive aids. But religious tradition is not the only explanation for government attempts to control sexual behavior.

*Population and Politics*  Despite the worries of Malthusians and neo-Malthusians, there is a tradition which associates increases in population with increases in social good. Included in this tradition is Adam Smith, who held that increasing population is both the cause and effect of increasing public prosperity (Smith 1776). And even though he could not be farther from Smith in political economy, Friedrich Engels called the Malthusian doctrine a "repulsive blasphemy against man and nature . . . children are like trees, returning abundantly the expenditure laid out on them." Large families, said Engels, are gifts to the community (Meek 1955). Currently, this view is supported by theorists who point out that, in general, the standard of living has increased alongside steady increments in world population and that such population increases are accompanied by less severe shortages, lower costs for goods, and better ways of avoiding shortages. Adding more people presents problems, but it also adds to the pool of problem solvers. People are the ultimate resource (see, e.g., Simon 1981; Clark 1967; Boserup 1970; North and Thomas 1973). A position like this can encourage governments to adopt pronatalist policies (e.g., disallowing contraception and elective abortion, precluding women from obtaining meaningful work outside the family, etc.) and to reject individual inclinations to severely limit family size.

The argument from increased prosperity is not the only secular argument that has been given for pronatalist public policies. There are also arguments from societal preservation and political dominance. As recently as 1920, the French legislative assembly passed an act which gave France the most oppressive laws in Europe regarding abortion and the diffusion of contraceptive information. The assembly's move was precipitated by the loss of French lives during World War I and the fear of Germany's population superiority (McLaren 1983).

Germany was aware of its population superiority. Hermann Goering (founder of the Gestapo) made it clear that according to Nazi leadership, the territory occupied by sixty-six million Germans was already too little; it was certainly not sufficient for ninety million, which was the intended population size (Sanger 1938). Benito Mussolini, who held that the fate of any nation is tied to its demographic powers (Organski and Organski 1961), contended that if Italy were to amount to anything, it would need to enter the second half of this century with at least sixty million citizens (Sanger 1938). Depopulated nations are subject to control by other nations, and pronatalist public policies are often linked to concerns about political survival and darker interests in expansion and political dominance. Today, for example, as the relatively tiny nation of Israel fights for political survival, marriage and procreation are continually encouraged by the government; likewise as the war between Iran and Iraq drags on, both countries are stridently pronatalist (e.g., Women's Global Network on Reproductive Rights 1987a).

Readily available contraception is also often held to encourage sexual excess, to lead to the decline of the family, and to contribute to the growth of materialism and increase the greed, "softness," and self-indulgence that are often held to accompany lives of luxury. The secular moralists of nineteenth-century France provide a good example of the displacement of religious motivations for condemning contraception by utilitarian appeals to the public interest (see, e.g., McLaren 1983). Contraception (as well as readily available abortion) has been held to foster decadence and selfishness, since it permits people to avoid the expenses connected with raising children and allows them to become preoccupied with fulfilling their own self-serving interests. A society of people pursuing luxury is feared to be weak and to invite domination. As recently as 1949, the Royal Commission on Population asserted such a connection between birth control and war:

> There is much to be said for the view that a failure of a society to reproduce itself indicates something wrong in its attitude to life which is likely to involve other forms of decadence. The cult of childlessness and the vogue of the one-child family were symptoms of something

profoundly unsatisfactory in the *zeitgeist* of the inter-war period, which it may not be fanciful to connect with the sophistications and complacencies which contributed to the catastrophe of the second world war.

Governments adopt pronatalist policies, then, not only to avoid what are perceived to be dangerous decreases in populations, but also to discourage what are feared to be characteristics and life styles that make citizens morally and physically weak. Indeed, we have already seen in Chapter 1 that coitus interruptus was identified with masturbation and that both were held by eighteenth- and nineteenth-century physicians to lead to physical and mental deterioration as well as lack of control. Thus, not only contraception but sexual interaction more generally becomes an object of state interest because of its perceived ties to the public interest.

These purported ties are not limited to the adoption of pronatalist policies and practices, however, and it is sometimes the case that governments adopt rigorous antinatalist policies and practices or a combination of pronatalist and antinatalist policies and practices. Such combinations of policies and practices are often linked to concerns about maintaining racial dominance within a society and the elimination of the "unfit." In the early part of this century, for example, a eugenics movement sprang up in the United States. By 1932, twenty-seven states had laws allowing involuntary sterilization of the feeble-minded, insane, criminal, and physically defective (see Chapter 1). Sadly, even Margaret Sanger moved away from her initial emphasis on reproductive choice to join the eugenicists. As early as 1919, she claimed that "more children from the fit, less from the unfit" is the "chief issue of birth control" (Sanger 1919). In 1922, she warned that uncontrolled reproduction of the illiterate and "degenerate" threatened "our way of life" (Sanger 1922). And in 1932, she called for sterilization or segregation by sex of those whose offspring would be unfit — in her words, "the whole dysgenic population" (Sanger 1932). Sanger never seemed to realize that it is logically inconsistent to advocate reproductive choice *and* eugenics policies.

Sanger's slogan "more children from the fit, less from the unfit" mentions both of the strategies advocated by those concerned to ensure the primacy of a certain group in a society. Antinatalist pressures are put on the group to be held back (or done away with), while pronatalist pressures are put on the group to be nurtured (or expanded). Nazi Germany provides a stunning example of this kind of reproductive policy. There, sterilization laws were adopted to help preclude reproduction by "inferiors," while strident pronatalist, antifeminist policies and a propaganda campaign were adopted to push women of the desired heritage out of public life and the work force and back to the home to reproduce (e.g., Field 1983).

Among the most striking examples of antinatalist policies and practices are those in contemporary China, where, since 1979, families have been instructed to refrain from producing more than a single child without special permission. China's concern is with overpopulation, and despite the view that people are the ultimate resource, the concern is completely reasonable. Its population has been growing at alarming rates, and the government has decided that the only way of avoiding a crushing famine in the future is to radically decrease its birthrate. But just as severe pronatalist policies put individuals in conflict with society by attempting to keep birth control out of individual hands, severe antinatalist policies like those in China also put individuals in conflict with society. Many Chinese couples desire to have more than one child, and the government must keep a constant watch on individuals to ensure that the desire to procreate is kept in check. The result is a morally troubling set of highly coercive methods, including the utilization of "granny police," whose tasks include ensuring that fertile women maintain contraceptive use, persuading women who are pregnant without permission to procure abortions, and persuading women who have had a child to agree to sterilization following childbirth or an abortion. The methods of persuasion include making repeated visits to a woman's home until she is worn down and submits.

Intrauterine devices (IUDs) are widely used in China, accounting for as much as 85 percent of all contraceptive use. A modified stainless steel Ota ring is the most common IUD. Made without a tail (see Chapters 1 and 6), it cannot be removed by the woman herself, and it is illegal for medical personnel to remove the devices at a woman's request without authorization from the proper birth control official. Medical personnel who do remove IUDs without permission are subject to severe punishment. For a woman using an IUD, the periodic medical checkup consists of an X-ray to ensure that the device has not been removed and is in a functional position. Given the risks associated with IUDs (see Chapters 1 and 6), government pressure on women to accept them on such a wide scale raises serious worries about informed consent to assuming their risks (see Chapter 9).

Sterilization is second only to the use of IUDs. Despite China's egalitarian political philosophy, female sterilization is two and a half times as frequent as male sterilization. Several varieties of hormonal contractives are also in use, and they are commonly distributed by nonmedical birth control officials, which is also worrisome, given the potential side effects of many preparations (see Chapter 5). Condoms are used, but infrequently. Given that both hormonal contraceptives and condoms must be resupplied constantly, it is not surprising that the government has strenuously encouraged sterilization and the use of IUDs.

There are some exceptions to the one-child family rule in China. If a first child has died or has a serious handicap (provided the handicap is not the result of a genetic defect), then a couple may gain permission to have a second child. Couples in second marriages can apply for permission to have a child of their own. And where a family name is about to die out and a couple has not had a son, they may be given permission to try to have a son. The desire to produce sons remains strong in China (see Chapter 1), and it raises serious concerns about infanticide of female offspring.[5] Since couples still depend on being taken care of by their children in their later years, there is considerable motivation to attempt to have more children secretly. As might be guessed, the one-child policy has enjoyed more success in urban areas, where women can be more easily monitored, than in rural areas (see, e.g., Croll, Darin, and Kane 1985).

China is not alone in its worries about population increases. Although international birthrates have fallen in recent years, death rates have declined more, leading to substantial net increases in world population. Unless birthrates subside, the world population, which is growing by eighty million annually, may well double to ten billion in as little as forty years (Population Institute 1987). Current population increases tend to be concentrated in precisely those nations where most citizens lead lives of unacceptably low quality. Limiting population growth in an underdeveloped country seems a logical way to increase per capita income and availability of food and

---

[5] For a discussion of the implications of using sex selection technologies and the general preference for sons over daughters, see Warren (1985).

essential services. To most of us, providing famine relief and reducing the death rate in an underdeveloped nation are noble and humane actions. However, aid in the form of population control is sometimes interpreted by recipient nations as attempts by wealthy nations to suppress development of poorer ones by a form of "legalized genocide." Those who have taken the Malthusian argument to heart and who have worked to reduce population growth in developing nations are genuinely puzzled by such a response.

But developed nations need to take such reactions seriously, and they need to rethink the whole question of the sources of the destitution that controlling population growth is assumed to diminish. Serious questions have been raised about the causal connection held to obtain invariably between large populations and low quality of life and also about the effectiveness of often coercive population control policies that have been adopted in a number of developing nations, more often than not with the encouragement and aid of the United States. For example, it has been persuasively argued that most frequently the destitution held to be associated with uncontrolled population growth is in fact a function of the distribution of power and wealth within societies (see Lappe and Collins 1977; Perelman 1977; George 1977; Simon 1981; Petchesky 1984; Hartmann 1987). As Hartmann (1987) points out, the Sahelian famine in the late 1960s and early 1970s, which resulted in hundreds of thousands of deaths and massive migrations southward, serves as an example. The famine was not a result of inadequate resources in the region, since nearly all the affected countries had enough food to feed their people and, astoundingly, agricultural exports from the region actually increased during the famine years (Sen 1981). The problem of poverty is too often not the result of absolute scarcity but of the distribution of resources and services in a society. (Consider the phenomena of poverty and homelessness in the United States today.) The real key to development and prosperity lies not in simply attempting to control population growth but in changing the social and economic conditions which breed destitution for segments of a society. The focus on controlling numbers of births leads to overlooking questions about the social and economic conditions under which people tend to produce families too large for the resources to which they have access. Attempting to find a quick, technological "fix" by pouring millions of contraceptive aids into so-called overpopulated and underdeveloped nations is too simplistic a solution. As long as parents will need to rely on their children for support in their later years and as long as women are in subservient social positions (which is the case in virtually all of these societies), nations will indirectly encourage continued reproduction while directly trying to slow or halt it. Warwick (1982) points out several cases where population control programs failed miserably because planners ignored the sociocultural and economic context into which the programs were introduced. The examples make clear that it simply cannot be assumed, even in the poorest segments of these societies, that large numbers of children are less economically desirable than smaller numbers. Of the study he and his associates conducted in Egypt, Kenya, the Philippines, Mexico, Lebanon, the Dominican Republic, Haiti, and India, Warwick says,

> This research confirms previous evidence that the value of children to their parents depends heavily on the parents' circumstances. In situations in which children make direct contributions to the household economy, are the main source of old age security, are crucial to establishing a parent's sexual identity, or have deep religious meaning, parents are likely to be ambivalent about or even hostile to birth control, if they have thought about it at all. In situations where parents receive few economic benefits from another child, an employer or the state provides adequate social security, women are employed outside the home, and the traditional hold of religion has weakened, the premium on large families is much lower. (Warwick 1982; see also Hartmann 1987).

Developed nations need to realize more clearly, too, that many of the techniques used to limit population growth in developing nations (including widespread implantation of IUDs, widespread sterilization, widespread dissemination of various chemical compounds without careful consideration of individual and family medical histories and without continuing access to proper medical follow-up or appropriate safety provisions, and widespread abortion) are deeply morally troubling. Further, the excessive emphasis on population control in developing nations has often led, as in the case of China, to methods for finding contraceptive "acceptors" that work against seeking genuinely informed consent; this raises serious concerns about whether many (perhaps most) people in developing nations to whom contraceptive techniques are being applied are given sufficient information to adequately understand the mode of action and potential side effects and long-term health hazards of many birth control measures. And even if adequate information is given, the coercive nature of many antinatalist practices raises additional worries about voluntariness in accepting birth control (see Chapter 9). The distinction between population control and facilitating reproductive choice is conceptually and morally an important one, and reproductive choice is often precluded when population control is high on a government's agenda. What needs to be realized is that creating the social and economic conditions which make genuine reproductive choice possible is the most effective way of avoiding problems of "overpopulation."

National prosperity, various concerns about national protection, and internal concerns about group primacy, then, can lead and have led governments to try to force their citizens to reproduce or refrain from reproducing. But there are still other explanations for governmental attempts to control contraception, abortion, and sexual interaction. Not the least among these explanations are those having to do with the position of women in a society.

*The Philosophy of Woman and the Politics of Motherhood* At various points in history, the dominant position in the medical profession has been one of opposition to both readily available contraception and elective abortion. Such opposition played an important part in the profession's gaining a licensed monopoly on providing medical care and in its rise in social authority in both America and Europe (see, e.g., Mohr 1978; McLaren 1983; Luker 1984). But it has also sometimes been the case that segments of the profession have opposed readily available contraception while supporting abortion. Sanger, for example, was surprised to find that the German medical establishment was not supportive of her commitment to finding a universally and easily usable contraceptive for women. But the lack of support was clearly explained by an unnamed German gynecologist in 1918: "We will never give control of our numbers to the women themselves. What, let them control the future of the human race? With abortion, it is in our hands; we make the decisions and they must come to us" (Sanger 1938).

Traditionally, such decisions have not been afforded to women. And they have not been afforded to women in no small part because of a persistent view of human nature which stretches back to Aristotle and beyond and according to which women, in nature and value, are very different from men. Luker (1984) has forcefully argued that this traditional view is intimately linked to the intractability of the contemporary abortion debate and the continuing opposition of many people to readily available birth control aids. According to the view, the purported intrinsic differences of men and women make men and women naturally suited to different roles. Furthermore, these roles require different virtues or excellences for their fulfillment. Women, it is held, are suited by nature to create and nourish a home and to bear and rear children. As excellent "specimens of their natural kind," women must foster in themselves the virtues or excellences which make them fit to do their work well. A woman's value, then, lies in doing well that which she is held to be naturally suited to do — to act as a wife and mother. But the ready availability of contraceptive aids and abortion leaves women free to avoid their natural roles. When a society protects reproductive choice by accepting birth control in either or both of these forms, those who subscribe to the traditional view of woman are disturbed to find it being rejected. The stakes are high for both men and women, but they are particularly high for women who consider their value to lie in what they take to be their "natural" roles as wife and mother. When society accepts widely practiced birth control, the very lives of these women are devalued. Legal restrictions on the availability of contraceptive aids and abortion shore up the social recognition of the value of their lives. Thus, despite the heavy burdens women have borne under coercive pronatalist policies, such policies make women's place and value in the social order unambiguous, and many women have supported and continue to support such policies.

On the other hand, more and more women have come to reject the traditional view of woman. Seeing men and women as essentially the same and hence equal, women have increasingly come to view being limited to family roles as a barrier to the full equality with men to which nature entitles them, including an equal freedom to engage in intercourse without fear of pregnancy. Women with this understanding of the nature of woman see themselves and their lives as valuable independent of considerations having to do with family roles. Pronatalist public policies devalue *their* lives by relegating them back to a secondary status, and reducing them to their procreative capacity (Petchesky 1984). In attempting to prevent women from escaping childbearing, pronatalist policies attempt to force women to be what Corea (1985) has called "mother machines."[6]

Luker's suggestion that a conflict between these radically different world views underpins the contemporary abortion debate and explains its recalcitrance is eminently plausible. Such conflicts frequently get played out in the political arena as proponents of both positions seek to use the massive powers of the state to affirm their world views and protect the social recognition of the value of their lives. Thus, the dominant view in a society on the nature and value of women also influences the politics of contraception.

.    .    .    .    .    .

Religion, legal moralism, social prosperity, political and societal survival, political domination, racism and group primacy, elimination of perceived undesirables, and a society's view of woman, then, all figure in the complex question of why governments attempt to control sexual activity in general and birth control practices in particular. We shall return to some of these issues in the chapters to come.

As we have already mentioned, one of the most controversial features of some existing and developing birth control technologies is that they function as abortifacients rather than as contraceptives in the proper sense (see Chapters 5 and 6). Imbedded in the world views we have just been discussing are different positions on the moral status of the human conceptus. In discussing abortifacient technologies, we shall therefore need to take up the moral controversy surrounding abortion, including the question of prenatal

---

[6] Corea's focus, however, is not on coercive pronatalist policies, which attempt to limit access to contraception and abortion. Rather, she offers a provocative analysis of how new reproduction-enhancing technologies, as well as widely used contraceptives like the pill and the IUD, perpetuate the treatment of women as mere material. Many feminists have become increasingly condemning of reproduction-enhancing technologies, such as in vitro fertilization, embryo transfer, and surrogate motherhood, arguing that these technologies manipulate and exploit women and that they constitute a powerful new means by which men can control women's reproductive capacities. See, e.g., Overall (1987), Stanworth (1987), Spallone and Steinberg (1987), and the bibliographies in these books.

human rights. We shall focus on this question in Chapter 7 and, at least in part, in Chapter 9. First, however, we need to give a basic account of human reproduction in order to provide the necessary background for a precise understanding of the birth control technologies we shall discuss in succeeding chapters. We turn now to that account.

# 3

# An Overview of Human
# Reproductive Anatomy

## INTRODUCTION

The reproductive anatomy of human adults is among the most striking known examples of sexual dimorphism. However, as with other
less obvious examples of sexual dimorphism, it is a fascinating par-
adox that such phenotypically diverse and functionally complemen-
tary structures actually arise from identical dual duct systems and
common embryological analogues.

Sex determination involves a gradual sequence of events which
is complex yet logical. The progression to sexual dichotomy begins
early in prenatal development with the differentiation of the gonads
(sex glands) into either testes or ovaries, and it continues throughout gestation as changes (initially local and subsequently systemic)
are elicited by gonadal hormone production (in males) or lack thereof
(in females), as we shall see in more detail shortly. Testicular and
ovarian hormones continue this process of differentiation during
pubertal and adult life in such a way that eventually the embryo,
which intially had the potential of developing into a male or female,
becomes an adult that displays some degree of sexual dimorphism
in virtually every tissue and organ of the body. That is, fundamentally every human being is physiologically androgynous.

## SEX DETERMINATION AND DIFFERENTIATION

Both the similarities and the differences between female and male
functional reproductive anatomies may be best appreciated by first
briefly considering their common origin and the subsequent events
which (usually) modify the reproductive tract to conform to the
genetic sex of the individual.

Although genetic sex is determined at the moment of union
between an X-chromosome-bearing ovum and either an X- or a

Y-chromosome-bearing sperm cell, in reality this only establishes the potential sexual development of an individual. Indeed, even determining the sex of a person is a far more complex task than is commonly thought. In addition to genetic constitution, sexual categorization may also be determined on the basis of types of gonads, internal and external reproductive structures, hypothalamic differentiation, secondary sex characteristics, behavioral sex, and psychosexual orientation. Classification by sex based on one or more of these traits may well be in conflict with classifications based on other traits. The sexual identity of individuals, then, should not be viewed as falling into one of two completely discrete categories. Rather, an individual's true sexual identity (both physiologically and psychosocially) lies at some point along a continuum between the two traditionally idealized absolutes of male and female.

All reproductive tract structures initially exist in a sexually undefined form. In regard to all aspects of sexual differentiation, some product(s) must be *actively* imposed to initiate and maintain male development. Conversely, only the *absence* of some male inducer(s) is necessary for female-type development. In other words, the inherent direction of the development of all offspring is toward femaleness. Only active intervention of an appropriate male inducer will alter the inherent pattern and cause the development of a male.

It is well established that it is not the presence of a Y chromosome per se that causes indifferent gonads to differentiate as testes but rather the presence of a product of the Y chromosome, H-Y antigen (Wachtel 1977, 1979; Ohno et al. 1979; Wachtel and Ohno 1979). Normally, testicular differentiation under the influence of H-Y antigen occurs by the seventh week of gestation (Jaffe 1986). Jost (1970) first postulated that a gonad would passively become an ovary unless an inducer substance intervened to cause testicular organization. In humans, ovarian differentiation does not begin until approximately weeks 13 to 16 of gestation (Jaffe 1986). The role of H-Y antigen is crucial then, since hormonal secretions by the testes are ultimately directly or indirectly responsible for (1) determining whether the Wolffian (male) internal duct system develops or the Mullerian (female) internal duct system persists, (2) controlling whether the common "ball of clay" from which the external genitalia will be formed is molded in the male or female direction, and (3) determining the ability of the so-called higher centers (especially the hypothalamus and pituitary) to respond to endocrine signals and elicit either characteristically male or female patterns of gonad-otropic hormone release, which influences the form of sexual behavior displayed in the adult (Edwards 1980). Thus, again, absent active intervention on the system by the appropriate male inducer, an off-spring will become, or more accurately, will remain female. This is partly why determining sex is not always straightforward. For example, an individual may be genetically male (i.e., possess an X and a Y chromosome), yet if the production, release, or activity of H-Y antigen does not occur normally, the individual will develop phenotypically (i.e., regarding appearance), psychologically, and culturally into what we recognize as a female. Likewise, if the hormone testosterone produced by the testes is not "recognized" at the cellular level and does not cause active differentiation of male characteristics, female traits will passively develop.[1]

FUNCTIONAL FEMALE REPRODUCTIVE ANATOMY

*Ovaries* The human ovaries (female gonads) are paired, almond-shaped organs, measuring approximately 4 cm in length, 2 cm in width, and 1 cm in thickness, and weighing approximately 7 g each

---

[1] This condition is known as *testicular feminization syndrome*, and it can pose some ethical problems for the physician. The condition, for example, may be first suspected during a gynecological examination of a teenage girl complaining of primary amenorrhea (never having had a menstrual period). Further examination and testing may well reveal cryptorchid (internal and undescended) testes and a blind–ending vagina. Because of the very real danger that the cryptorchid testes will develop malignant tumors, it is usually recommended that they be removed. In essence, this places the physician in a difficult position, since a full and candid explanation of the condition would involve telling this woman that her failure to menstruate is a result of her being genetically male. The difficulty can be minimized and the woman's right to be given information adequate to provide a genuine understanding of her condition can be respected, however, by helping her understand the distinctions among various modes of sexual classification and by helping her realize that such classifications are made for various purposes and that, for the purposes of psychological and cultural sexual classification, an individual with this condition (i.e., someone whose hormonal development has not been influenced by a male inducer, whose appearance is female, who has been raised as a female, and whose psychological and social identity is female) is unequivocally female.

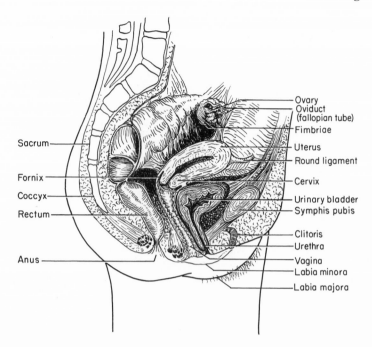

**Figure 1** Female reproductive tract seen in sagittal section.

during the reproductive years (Woodburne 1965; Bloom and Fawcett 1966; Mossman and Duke 1973). Figures 1 and 2 depict the anatomical relationship between the ovaries and other reproductive tract structures. The ovaries lie against the true pelvis, lateral to the uterus, and are suspended from a backward extension of the broad ligament (the general supporting structure of the female reproductive tract) by the mesovarium. The upper lateral, superior, and medial ovarian borders are largely covered by the oviducts (Fallopian tubes).

Each ovary is composed of a central medulla (a central portion made up of connective tissue and containing nerves, blood vessels, and lymphatic vessels) and a surrounding cortex (an outer portion which contains the immature germ cells enclosed in cellular complexes). Except at its point of attachment to the broad ligament (termed the *hilus*, which is also the point at which nerves and blood and lymph vessels enter the ovary), the outer surface of the ovary is covered by a single layer of cuboidal cells (this layer is often called the *germinal epithelium*, which is misleading because no germ cells are contained in this layer). Figure 3 illustrates ovarian anatomy and

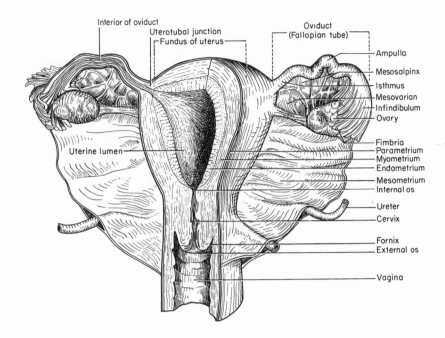

**Figure 2** Frontal view of internal female reproductive tract.

the progressive structures which appear on the surface during an ovarian cycle. Note that the various structures illustrated do not appear at different locations on the ovarian surface but rather occur successively at the particular site where the primordial follicle originated. In other words, at any particular site in the ovary, there may be a complete progression from a primordial follicle through the various stages of folliculogenesis (growth and development of the follicle), and the process may culminate in ovulation (release of the ovum from the ruptured, mature follicle) and formation of a corpus luteum. The corpus luteum, which derives its name from its visual appearance (yellow body) will subsequently regress, leaving a nonfunctional remnant, the corpus albicans (white body).

However, only a relatively few follicles ever complete maturation and ovulate. By far the most common fate is to undergo the normal process of follicular attrition or degeneration, appropriately termed *atresia*.

It is a little-known fact that women "lose eggs" throughout their lifetimes. At about the fifth month of gestation, female fetuses have

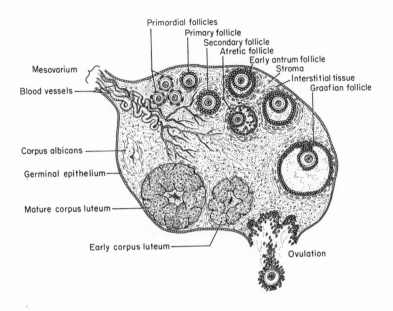

**Figure 3** Internal anatomy of the ovary and a composite diagram of ovarian structures.

a peak content of approximately 7 million germ cells in their ovaries. The germ cell population then declines precipitiously to about 1 million normal oocytes at birth. By seven years of age, this number has dropped to approximately 300,000. By sixteen to twenty-five years of age, the number has declined to approximately 159,000, and by twenty-six to thirty-five years of age, it is down to about 59,000 (Edwards 1980). The number of oocytes continues to decline until menopause. Of the 7 million oocytes that were initially present, only some 400 to 500 will ever undergo the full range of changes which culminate in ovulation. The remainder will undergo atresia (Holmes and Fox 1979; Baker 1982). Thus, a marked difference between female gametogenesis (oogenesis) and male gametogenesis (spermatogenesis) is that in the female there is a finite supply of germ cells which are decreasing in number from midfetal development, while in the male spermatogenesis does not begin until puberty and the number of germ cells which may be produced is virtually infinite, since the stem cells (spermatogonia) are continually being replaced throughout life by mitosis (cell division). It is because a woman's oocytes are aging as she ages and because an egg which has begun to degenerate may be released and fertilized that there are special worries about genetic defects in fetuses conceived by women during their later reproductive years (e.g., over forty years of age). As we mentioned in Chapter 1, it has been assumed in the scientific community that prevention of pregnancy will be most effectively directed toward preventing the 400–500 ovulated eggs from either being fertilized or, if fertilized, from continuing to develop. As we shall see, ovulation is most effectively prevented through interfering with the sequence of neuroendocrine events which are necessary for its occurrence.

*Oviducts (Fallopian Tubes)* The oviducts are bilateral tubes approximately 10 cm in length, suspended in the mesosalpinx, a peritoneal fold derived from the lateral layer of the broad ligament. Each oviduct can be subdivided into (1) the infundibulum, the most lateral portion consisting of a funnel-shaped opening surrounded by fingerlike fimbriae in a fringelike manner; (2) the ampulla, a relatively wide, flacid, tortuous, highly folded portion which is the longest oviductal section; and (3) the isthmus, a narrow, straight, muscular portion which connects directly to the uterus (Figures 1 and 2). Medially, the tube passes through the uterine wall as the intramural segment (Hafez 1978; Tortora and Evans 1986).

The epithelial (covering) lining of the oviduct is columnar and made up of (1) ciliated cells, which have slender, highly motile cilia (kinocilia) extending into the lumen, and (2) secretory cells. The percentage of ciliated cells (which are important for ovum transport) decreases gradually down the length of the ampulla so that in the isthmus there are only a few ciliated cells located deep between the tall secretory cells, which are important for secreting substances to nourish the fertilized egg. The histological (tissue-level) appearance of the epithelium, especially the height of the columnar cells, varies dramatically during the different phases of the menstrual cycle (Bloom and Fawcett 1966).

The oviduct has the role of transporting the ovulated ovum and the deposited spermatozoa in opposite directions (i.e., toward one another) in order to facilitate fertilization. Further, it maintains the fertilized egg within its confines during the initial developmental stages and then propels it into the uterus when the uterine environment is right for continued development. The unique features of (1) the epithelial lining described above; (2) the oviductal musculature, consisting of an inner circular layer and outer longitudinal layer of smooth muscle which increases in prominence from the infundibulum to the isthmus; and (3) the extensive neural control of differential oviductal segments all contribute to control of this multiple function. In the meantime, the changing milieu of ovarian steroid hormones provides the endocrinological background essential to control transport of gametes and conceptuses.

At ovulation, a mature ovum is released from the ovary and adheres to the ovarian surface until it is swept off by the ciliary action of the fingerlike infundibular fimbriae. The ovum is then moved along by the combined action of the cilia, which beat toward the uterus, and the wavelike contractions of the comparatively weak musculature of the ampulla. If the ovum is fertilized, this takes place in the upper one-third of the oviduct, above the ampullary-isthmic junction. The pattern and rate of sperm transport through the oviduct to the site of potential union with the ovum are controlled by several mechanisms, including wavelike circular contractions of the oviductal musculature, complex contractions of the oviductal mucosal folds and the mesosalpinx, fluid currents and countercurrents created by ciliary action, and possibly the opening and closing of the intramural portion. Oviductal contractions are independent of uterine contractions. The frequency and amplitude of oviductal contractions are controlled by ovarian hormones, neural transmitters, and various seminal plasma components (such as prostaglandins). Prevention or alteration of the normal pattern of either ovum or spermatozoa transport such that fertilization is interfered with is a second potential means of achieving contraception.

The fertilized egg will remain in the area of the ampullary-isthmic junction of the oviduct for three to four days before being transported into the uterus. During this time, the cleaving egg (or zygote in the stage of rapid cell division) is maintained in constant rotation to prevent adherence to the oviductal wall. The timing of the entry of the conceptus into the uterus is critical for its successful implantation and survival. Tubal motility and transport of the conceptus into the uterus is under hormonal control, which occurs through the combined action of ovarian steroid hormones and local neurotransmitters. Various methods for interfering with the normal movement of the conceptus through the oviduct into the uterus (including accelerating and delaying transport) have been examined as possibly providing a third means of birth prevention. We shall consider this approach in detail in Chapter 5, but notice that these methods of birth control do not prevent fertilization. Rather, they prevent continued development of the conceptus beyond initial cleavage divisions and are therefore considered by many to constitute a method of aborting pregnancies in their earliest stages.[2]

*Uterus*  The uterus, a thick-walled, muscular, hollow, pear-shaped organ occupies a central position in the pelvic cavity. The human uterus weighs approximately 60–80 g and is approximately 7.5 cm in length, 5 cm in width, and 3 cm in thickness. The long axis of the uterus is inclined superiorly and anteriorly so that it lies approximately 60° above the horizontal plane when a woman is standing. The uterus is freely mobile and its position varies considerably with distention of the bladder or rectum, with varying body posture, and during pregnancy (Jacobsen and Krieger 1977; Hafez 1978).

The uterus consists of three divisions: (1) a rounded fundus, which is the dome-shaped segment of the corpus which lies superior to the entrance points of the oviduct; (2) the corpus or main body; and (3) the cervix, which projects into the vagina (Figures 2 and 4).

The uterine wall consists of three concentric layers: (1) the perimetrium or serosa, which is the thin outer layer derived from the peritoneum; (2) the myometrium, the thick layer of smooth muscle fibers and collagenous tissue; and (3) the endometrium, the thick mucosal layer which changes dramatically in thickness (1–6 mm) and cellular type during the menstrual cycle in response to changes in the systemic concentration of steroid hormones secreted by the ovaries. The endometrium actually consists of two layers: (1) the stratum functionalis (or superficial layer), the layer closer to the uterine cavity, which is shed during menses, and (2) the stratum basalis (or basal layer), which is maintained and produces a new stratum

---

[2] At this very early stage, the product of conception is referred to as a *conceptus*, and it includes the cells which will only later differentiate into two cell masses — one comprising the cells which will become the placenta and one comprising the cells which will become the embryo. Because this differentiation into placenta and embryo has not yet occurred, some (including many physicians) hold that birth control intervention at this stage does not constitute abortion. Again, we shall take up discussion of this distinction in Chapter 5.

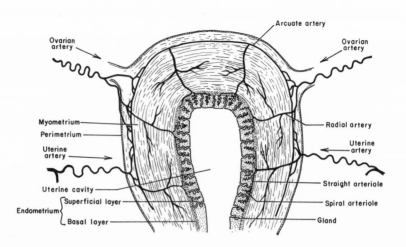

**Figure 4**  Blood supply and internal anatomy of the uterus.

functionalis following menses (Figure 4). The endometrium also contains numerous glands which produce various biochemical products essential for nourishment of the embryo (Jacobsen and Krieger 1977; Tortora and Evans 1986).

The major role of the uterus in reproduction is obvious, since it is the site of embryonic and fetal development for all of gestation except for the first three to four days, when the cleaving fertilized egg is still in the oviduct. Interference with implantation (i.e., interference not involving conceptus transport in the oviduct) is a fourth possible approach to birth control, and, as we shall see in detail in Chapter 6, this is the primary or a secondary mode of action of several methods of birth control. Insofar as these methods involve interference with implantation of the conceptus, they are also considered by many to be abortifacient rather than contraceptive methods of birth control (see Chapter 5).

In addition to serving as the site of embryonic and fetal development, the uterus and endometrial secretions play other roles in reproduction and thus offer other potential avenues of intervention. As sperm are transported through the uterus to the oviducts, they undergo a series of biochemical and physiological alterations as a result of exposure to endometrial secretions essential for fertilization. This process is termed *capacitation*. Interference with the process of sperm capacitation is a fifth possible means of birth control.

*Cervix*   The cervix, technically the lower part of the uterus, differs markedly (both structurally and functionally) from the uterine body and fundus. The cervix is a sphincterlike structure characterized by a thick wall and constricted lumen. The upper portion of the cervix contains smooth muscles condensed in a circular pattern to form the internal cervical os (sphincter). The cervical mucosa (or lining) consists of primary and secondary mucosal crypts which run in transverse, longitudinal, and oblique directions. The cervical mucosa is 2–3 cm thick and contains numerous large, branched, mucus-secreting glands (Tortora and Evans 1986).

The tightly constricted cervix and the cervical mucus form a barrier to infection between the vagina and the cervix and, throughout most of the cycle, represent a hindrance to the passage of sperm. However, during midcycle (around the time of ovulation), the external cervical os (formed where the cervix protrudes into the vagina) is dilated and filled with watery cervical mucus, which facilitates sperm transport. Due to its unique rheological (flow-controlling) properties, the cervical mucus plays a major role in sperm transport. Changes in this mucus can be detected by women, and these are changes relied on by those using the symptothermal method of birth control described in Chapter 1. Cervical crypts are considered "sperm reservoirs," since motile sperm are stored there following intercourse and then released to migrate toward the uterine lumen (Hafez 1978). These crypts are considered less hostile to sperm than either the vagina or the uterine body.

Since the secretion of cervical mucus is stimulated by estrogens and inhibited by progesterone, cyclical quantitative and qualitative variations in production occur during the menstrual cycle. As we shall see, this normal pattern is altered by administration of exogenous hormones, such as oral contraceptives.

*Vagina*   The vagina is a remarkably distensible fibromuscular canal, approximately 7–10 cm long in its anterior wall and 12–15 cm long in its posterior wall. The anterior wall is shorter because of the intrusion of the cervix. The vagina, rather like a balloon, may be thought of as a potential, rather than an actual, space. It can adjust in size to fit snugly around a finger or expand to allow the passage of a baby. Likewise, it can adjust equally well to penises of various sizes. The vaginal surface is corrugated by the presence of longitudinal ridges, which are especially prominent in the outer two-thirds of the vagina. These ridges (rugae) are functionally important during intercourse since they aid the various muscles associated with the vagina in gripping the penis to facilitate ejaculation. The outer one-third of the vagina contains nerve endings responsive to sexual stimulation (although the vagina is less sensitive than are the clitoris and the lips of the vulva), while the inner two-thirds of the vagina is practically devoid of nerve endings (Hafez 1978). This is why, contrary to popular belief, female orgasm is not achieved by deep thrusts into the vagina but rather by stimulation of the clitoris and the outer one-third of the vagina. Since the inner portion of the vagina and the cervix have few sensory nerve endings, the length of the penis and the depth of penetration are physiologically irrelevant to a woman's sexual satisfaction.

The secretions of the vagina have a low pH, which aids in retarding microbial growth. However, as we have already seen in Chapter 1, this low pH is also deleterious to sperm cells. For this reason, the buffering action of the higher pH of the semen (which is more alkaline) is very important to neutralize vaginal pH and aid sperm survival. Effective contraceptive vaginal spermicides take advantage of the rather delicate nature of the sperm cell to drastically reduce sperm survival.

FUNCTIONAL MALE REPRODUCTIVE ANATOMY

*Scrotum*   The scrotum is a loose sac of skin formed embryologically from an evagination of the abdominal wall. Internally, the scrotum is divided by a septum into two sacs, each of which contains a single testis. Unlike the rest of the abdominal area, the scrotum has little or no fatty insulation. It is sparsely covered with pubic hair and has an abundance of sweat glands and temperature receptors. These factors, plus a layer of muscle fibers (the tunica dartos, which is directly under the skin and which contracts and relaxes involuntarily in response to cold and heat respectively), function to maintain within the testes the optimum temperature for sperm production. Testicular thermoregulation is also aided by the complex convolutions of the arteries and veins located above the testes. This vascular network, called the *pampiniform plexus*, provides an effective countercurrent mechanism by which arterial blood entering the testes is cooled by venous blood leaving the testes. Intratesticular temperature needs to be $3°$ to $5°$ F cooler than body temperature

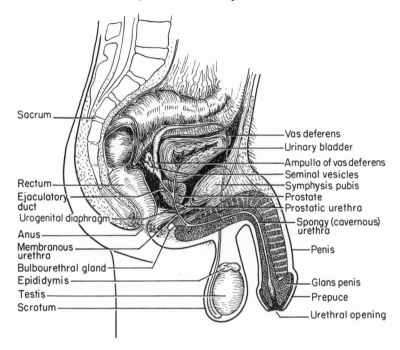

**Figure 5** Male reproductive tract seen in sagittal section.

for production of fertile human sperm. Wearing tight clothing, which forces the testes to remain close to the body cavity, may impede testicular cooling and thus may contribute to temporary subfertility. In addition to exposure to cold, sexual stimulation, fear, and physical exercise also cause the scrotum to tighten, wrinkle, and draw the testes up against the body.

*Testes* The testes (male gonads) are paired oval glands (Figure 5), measuring about 5 cm in length, 2.5 cm in diameter, and weighing 10–15 g (Tortora and Evans 1986). Although the testes are usually equal in size, in most men the left testis hangs lower in the scrotum than the right one. Interestingly, in left-handed men the reverse is usually true (Masters, Johnson, and Kolodny 1986).

The testes initially develop internally at the same anatomical site as do the ovaries. Under normal circumstances, the testes descend through the inguinal canal, a passage formed in the abdominal wall by the seventh month of gestation, and emerge into the scrotum shortly before birth. In approximately 10 percent of human males,

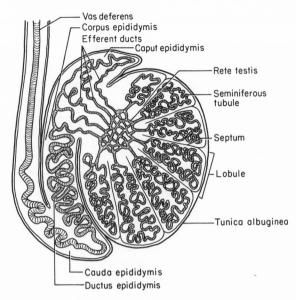

**Figure 6** Internal anatomy of the testes and epididymis showing the duct system.

the testes are undescended at birth, but by the end of the first year of life, testicular descent occurs in all but about 2–3 percent of male infants (Hafez 1978). Failure of testicular descent is termed *cryptorchidism* (from *kryptós* meaning hidden and *orchis* meaning testis), and if it is not surgically corrected, individuals with the condition are sterile as adults, because the lower testicular temperature required for spermatogenesis cannot be achieved. Cryptorchidism does not affect hormone production by the testes, so cryptorchid individuals have normal libido.

The testes are covered by a dense layer of white, fibrous tissue (the tunica albuginea) that extends inward, forming septa and dividing each testis into a series of some 250 internal compartments or lobules (Figure 6). Each lobule contains coiled seminiferous tubules, which, if stretched out, would be over a quarter mile in length. It is within the seminiferous tubules, which make up some 80 percent of the mass of the testis, that spermatozoa (male gametes) are produced by the process of spermatogenesis. The lining of the seminiferous tubules is composed of Sertoli (sustentacular) cells and the developing germ cells. Sertoli cells (named after the nineteenth-century Italian physiologist who first described them) provide support and

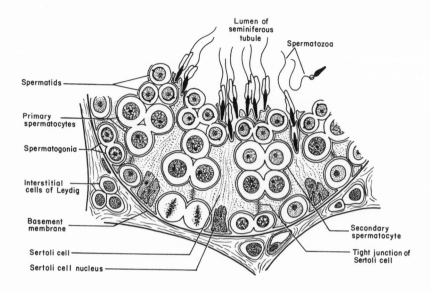

**Figure 7** Microscopic structure of a seminiferous tubule within the testes showing the progressive stages of spermatogenesis.

nourishment to the developing germ cells and perform numerous biochemical and endocrinological functions.

At birth, the seminiferous tubules are not fully developed, but with the onset of puberty and its concomitant hormonal changes, spermatogenic cells at various stages of development appear. A cross section through a seminiferous tubule reveals that it is packed with sperm cells at various stages of development (Figure 7). The most immature cells, the spermatogonia (which have been present since early embryonic development), are located against the outer boundary of the tubule, the basement membrane. Whereas a finite number of female germ cells (oogonia) are established prenatally, spermatogonia continually produce new germ cells by mitotic divisions. The production begins at puberty and continues throughout the reproductive life (which in most cases is the biological life) of the man. Spermatogonia that migrate away from the tubule lining enlarge to become primary spermatocytes. It is in these cells that meiosis (reduction division) first takes place; each primary spermatocyte produces two secondary spermatocytes, which in turn divide to produce two additional cells termed *spermatids*. Thus, one primary spermatocyte gives rise to four spermatids. Spermatids then undergo a complex morphological (structural) and biochemical transformation to become functional male gametes, now appropriately call *spermatozoa* (singular, *spermatozoon*). Spermatozoa, like the spermatids from which they arose, are haploid (i.e., have one sex chromosome). Approximately 50 percent of the spermatozoa carry the X chromosome and 50 percent carry the Y chromosome. In simple terms, the chromosomal sex of an offspring is determined by whether the spermatozoon which ultimately fertilizes the X-chromosome-bearing ovum is itself X-bearing (resulting in an XX genetic female) or Y-bearing (resulting in an XY genetic male).

In men, it takes approximately seventy-two days for a spermatogonium to become a mature spermatozoon. The various cell types within any cross section of the seminiferous epithelium form well-defined cellular associations that undergo cyclic changes. Six stages have been identified in man (Clermont 1963). Stages of the cycle of the seminiferous epithelium change not only with time but also along the length of the tubular loop. Thus, spermatogenesis is a continuous process and all stages of developing germ cells are present at all times. Over a lifetime, a man produces an astounding number of sperm, perhaps as many as twelve trillion (Jensen 1982). Sperm production is affected by several factors, including general health, age, frequency of ejaculation, season of the year, temperature, photoperiod, nutrition, stress, exposure to toxic substances, and individual variation.

In addition to gamete production, the other major function of the testes is production of androgens (19-carbon steroid hormones), which occurs in the interstitial cells of Leydig (Figure 8). Testosterone is, in regard to biological activity, by far the most important of the androgens produced by the Leydig cells. Androgens were so named because of their stimulatory effect on male secondary sex characteristics.

To digress for a moment, while testosterone is commonly referred to, both in numerous publications and general conversation, as the "male hormone: and estrogens and progesterone as "female hormones," such language is seriously misleading. Hormones are not male or female. A common pathway leads to the production of all steroid hormones in both sexes (Figure 8). Indeed, a small quantity of the testosterone produced by the interstitial cells of Leydig in men is subsequently converted by the Sertoli cells into estrogen. Testosterone is produced in men only through the con-

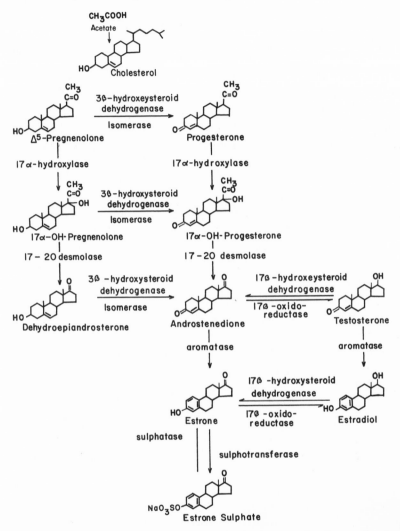

**Figure 8** Biochemical pathway utilized by both sexes for the production of steroid hormones.

version of the $C_{21}$ steroid progesterone (or pregnenolone, another $C_{21}$ steroid). Similarly, in order to produce estrogens ($C_{18}$ steroids), females must first produce precursor androgens ($C_{19}$ steroids). Therefore, while it is appropriate to say that testosterone and estrogens are key regulators of male and female reproductive functions respectively, it is not appropriate to designate testosterone as a "male hormone" and estrogens as "female hormones," thereby implying that they are specific to that gender. This reaffirms an observation made earlier — that even physiological sexual differentiation is not absolute in any individual human being.

To return to our discussion of testicular function: testosterone secretion by the Leydig cells is stimulated by the gonadotropic hormone LH (luteinizing hormone), which is produced and released by the anterior pituitary in response to the release of its controlling hormone, gonadotropin releasing hormone (Gn-RH) from the hypothalamus. As we shall see in the following chapter, reproductive function in both sexes is the result of a very delicate interplay among the hypothalamus, anterior pituitary, and gonads. However, as we shall also see, in men this relationship is not subject to cyclical variation and is much more straightforward than in women. The interaction between LH and testosterone is basically a simple institution or removal of negative feedback. LH stimulates the production of testosterone, but once the circulating concentration of testosterone in the blood reaches a certain level, it inhibits further Gn-RH release by the hypothalamus and hence further release of LH from the anterior pituitary. Absent LH to maintain production, testosterone production decreases. As testosterone concentration in the blood falls, the inhibition on the release of Gn-RH is removed, stimulating renewed release of LH. As blood levels of LH increase, the testes are once again stimulated to produce more testosterone. In a mature male, this episodic pattern is repeated continuously.

The androgenic hormones, principally testosterone, cause changes in most tissues of the body. As we have already mentioned, the influence of testosterone begins early in embryonic development, for it actively triggers the development of male internal genitalia (i.e., the duct system and accessory sex glands). Another androgen, dihydrotestosterone (DHT), produced from testosterone by the enzyme 5α-reductase, is responsible for the development of male external genitalia (i.e., the penis and scrotum). Absence of 5α-reductase (and hence DHT) produces an individual who is genetically male (XY) and has internal (or inguinal) testes, internal male ducts and accessory glands, and normal testosterone production but has genitalia that are highly undermasculinized.[3]

---

[3] Imperato-McGinley et al. (1974) first reported this 5α-reductase deficiency syndrome, which had affected several families in an isolated community in the Dominican Republic. At birth, individuals with the

In addition to its roles in the development, growth, and maintenance of male sex organs and secondary sex characteristics, testosterone is also essential for spermatogenesis. Follicle-stimulating hormone (FSH), a second gonadotropin produced and secreted by the anterior pituitary in response to Gn-RH, is also involved in spermatogenesis, probably through its effects on the activity of Sertoli cells.

*Duct System*   Once the sperm mature, they are released into the lumen of the seminiferous tubules (a process called *spermiation*) and enter into a series of collecting ducts in the center of the testis (the rete testis). Sperm are next transported out of the testis through a series of coiled efferent (away from) ducts that empty into a single highly coiled tube, the epididymis (Figures 5 and 6).

The epididymis (which means on the testes) measures 6 m in length (if stretched out) and 1 mm in diameter (Tortora and Evans 1986). It consists of three distinct anatomical regions, the caput (head), corpus (body), and cauda (tail). Transport of sperm through the epididymis takes about three weeks. During transport, sperm undergo various maturational changes which are required to attain fertilizing capacity. Sperm storage is primarily in the cauda epididymis, and sperm are capable of surviving there for several weeks. The epididymis is also the site of reabsorption of testicular fluid, aged sperm, and products of sperm breakdown.

The terminal portion of the cauda epididymis becomes thicker and less coiled. At this point it is referred to as the *vas deferens*

---

syndrome are often classified as females, since the visual appearance of the external genitalia is likely to be the only criterion used for gender determination. Naturally, the parents rear these children as females, bringing, no doubt, some degree of sexual stereotyping to the process. At puberty an interesting phenomenon occurs, referred to by the townspeople as *quevedoces* (meaning penis at twelve). Virtually overnight, the voices of affected individuals deepen and the individuals develop a typical male phenotype, with a substantial increase in muscle mass. The phallus, previously appearing as a slightly enlarged clitoris, enlarges to become a functional penis. Labial masses enlarge into a scrotum and testes descend from the inguinal canal. These changes are apparently due to the marked increase in testosterone occurring at puberty, which overcomes the continuing deficiency of DHT.

These individuals are subsequently treated as males, and postpubertal psychosexual orientation in most of them has been reported to be male despite their initial rearing as female (Imperato-McGinley et al. 1974).

(Figures 5 and 6). The vas deferens, about 45 cm long (Tortora and Evans 1986), ascends along the posterior border of the testis, penetrates the inguinal canal, and enters the abdomen, where it loops over the top and runs down the posterior surface of the bladder. This circuitous route is necessitated by the original journey of the testes during testicular descent. A vasectomy is a simple procedure in which portions of each vas deferens are removed and the ends of the remaining portions of the duct are occluded following excision. Basically, a vasectomy prevents the spermatozoa from getting from the site of production and storage to the site of ejaculation. Vasectomy procedures will be discussed in greater detail in Chapter 10.

Each vas deferens joins its ejaculatory duct prior to the urinary bladder. Each duct is about 2 cm long (Tortora and Evans 1986). Both ejaculatory ducts eject spermatozoa into the prostatic urethra. The urethra is the terminal duct of the system and serves as a common passage for both spermatozoa and urine. The urethra continues through the prostate gland, urogenital diaphragm, and the penis (Figures 5 and 9).

*Accessory Sex Glands*   The accessory sex glands secrete the liquid portion of the semen, properly call *seminal plasma*. Thus, ejaculated semen consists of two primary components: spermatozoa, produced in the testes and transported by the duct system, and seminal plasma, produced by the accessory sex glands. Of the 3 to 6 ml volume of a normal ejaculate, at least 95 percent is seminal plasma and 5 percent or less is sperm. In a vasectomized male, the production and ejaculation of seminal plasma is unaffected; thus the volume of the ejaculate is not noticeably reduced.

The seminal vesicles produce 60 to 70 percent of the seminal plasma. They are paired, convoluted, pouchlike structures, about 5 cm in length (Tortora and Evans 1986), and they lie posterior to and at the base of the urinary bladder and in front of the rectum (Figures 5 and 9). They secrete an alkaline, viscous fluid, rich in the sugar fructose. Fructose is the primary source of energy for motile sperm.

The prostate is a single, doughnut-shaped gland about the size of a chestnut. It is inferior to (below) the urinary bladder and surrounds the upper portion of the urethra (Figures 5 and 9). The prostate secretes an alkaline fluid which, as we have seen, is important for lowering the pH of the vagina. Approximately 30 percent of

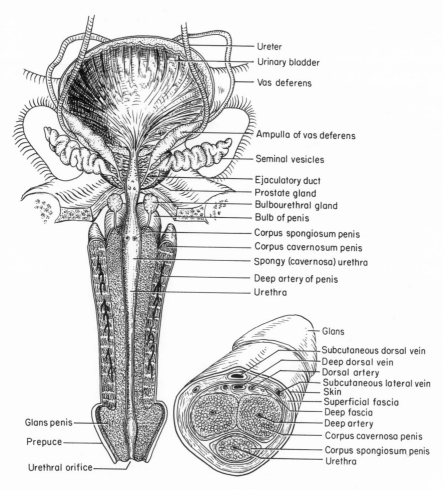

**Figure 9** (a) Sagittal view of internal anatomy of the penis and accessory sex glands. (b) Cross-sectional view of internal anatomy of the penis.

seminal fluid volume is of prostatic origin. The prostate also produces a clotting enzyme that acts on a substance produced in the seminal vesicles. This is what causes ejaculated semen to rapidly coagulate. Clotted semen liquifies in a few minutes when acted on by another enzyme produced by the prostate.

The bulbourethral glands, also referred to as *Cowper's glands*, are small, paired glands about the size and shape of peas and are located on either side of the urethra and beneath the prostate (Figures 5 and 9). They secrete only a few drops of alkaline fluid, which often appear at the tip of the penis during sexual arousal but before ejaculation. This fluid helps to neutralize acidic pH and provides some lubrication for sexual intercourse.

Semen has a pH range of 7.2 to 7.8 (which is slightly alkaline). It functions to provide spermatozoa with a transport medium and nutrients for energy metabolism. It not only buffers the acidic environment of the female reproductive tract but also neutralizes the acidity from urine in the male urethera. Semen also contains enzymes which can activate products of female reproductive tract secretions, thus making them available for sperm energy metabolism. Finally, semen contains prostaglandin hormones (especially prostaglandin $F_{2\alpha}$), which stimulate contractions of the female reproductive tract to aid sperm transport.

*Penis*   Internally, the penis consists of three parallel cylinders of spongy tissue bound together by fibrous tissue (Figure 9b). Each of the two dorsally located masses is called a *corpus cavernosum penis*. The smaller ventral mass, called the *corpus spongiosum penis*, contains the spongy urethra. All three masses consist of irregular, spongelike tissue filled with small blood vessels. With sexual stimulation, the arteries supplying the penis dilate and large quantities of blood enter the venous sinuses. Expansion of these spaces is aided by the constriction of the veins draining the penis; thus, most entering blood is retained and the penis becomes erect. In simple hydraulic terms, erection is a response to increased fluid pressure. The time required for erection is highly variable and dependent upon a vast number of factors, but it may occur as little as 3 to 5 seconds after the start of stimulation (Smith 1985).

Contrary to some common misconceptions and despite the slang reference to erections as "boners," there is no bone in the human penis. However, many animals (e.g., dogs, cats, bears, squirrels, opossums, whales, and numerous others) do have a penis bone, properly called an *os penis* or *baculum*. It may be composed of bone, cartilage, or a combination of both. The shape and position of the baculum within the penis tends to be species-specific. When present, it does aid in the attainment and maintenance of rigidity.

In addition to its extensive blood supply, the penis also has many nerves, which make it highly sensitive to touch, pressure, and temperature and contribute to rapid response to pleasurable stimuli. The glans penis (tip or head of the penis) has a higher concentration of sensory nerve endings than the shaft (body) of the penis, and it is thus particularly sensitive to physical stimulation. Two other areas particularly sensitive to touch are the coronal ridge (the rim of tissue that separates the glans from the shaft of the penis) and the small triangular region on the underside of the penis where the frenulum (a thin strip of skin) attaches to the glans.

Covering the glans is the loosely fitting skin called the *foreskin* or *prepuce*. *Circumcision* literally means cutting around and refers to the common practice of excising the foreskin from male infants.

Concern about penile size is perhaps one of the most unfounded obsessions. To quote Zilbergeld (1978), "in fantasyland [penises] come in only three sizes — large, gigantic, and so big you can barely get them through the doorway," a way of thinking reflected in advertisements for condoms. In reality, the average length of the flaccid penis of an adult male is approximately 9.5 cm, and the average length at erection is 16 cm, with a diameter at the base of 4 cm (Smith 1985; Masters, Johnson, and Kolodny 1986). There is relatively little difference in penile size among men, as compared to large differences in height and weight. Also, despite the recalcitrance of popular myths, there are no valid indicators (e.g., size of hands, feet, fingers) of penis size. As we have already seen, since the inner two-thirds of the vagina is relatively devoid of sensory nerves and since the vagina can accommodate its size equally well to an erect penis of relatively small or relatively large circumference, common concerns about penis size and its relation to giving sexual satisfaction have no physical foundation. It should be noted, however, that since human sexual behavior in general and human sexual gratification in particular are largely a function of psychology, if a woman, for example, genuinely believes that a "small" penis is likely to be associated with an inadequate sexual experience and also perceives her partner's penis as small, then the prophecy is likely to be self-fulfilling.

. . . . . .

We have presented above the primary physiological structures and functions involved in human reproduction. We turn next to an overview of the basic physiology and endocrinology of reproduction.

# 4

# An Overview of Human Reproductive Physiology and Endocrinology

## INTRODUCTION

Human reproduction is regulated by hormones and governed by the central nervous system. Most people today, even those with little or no knowledge of the biological sciences, are at least vaguely aware that mysterious chemicals called *hormones* are involved in reproduction and that the brain plays a major role in sexual response. However, our understanding of the role of hormones and of the brain is of fairly recent vintage. Indeed, the very term *hormone* (from the Greek *hormon*, meaning exciting or setting in motion) was first introduced into biology and medicine in 1904 by Bayliss and Starling, who the following year defined a hormone as "a substance produced in one part of the body and carried by the blood or lymph to some other part, the activity of which is thereby modified." The word *endocrine* (from the Greek *endon*, meaning within, and *krinein*, meaning to separate) first came into use in 1905, shortly after Bayliss and Starling designated the first so-called hormone *secretin* (which is produced by the upper gastrointestinal tract and stimulates the secretion of pancreatic juice to aid digestion). Pende employed the word *endocrinology* in 1909, and in 1913 Levi wrote a paper entitled "Glandes a secretion interne et morphologie" (see Rolleston 1936), which further described the concept of an endocrine system. Although as early as 1856 Claude Bernard referred to the constancy of the "milieu interieur," the concept that there was a coordinated relationship among endocrine glands controlled by "higher centers" functioning to maintain physiological homeostasis (equilibrium) is generally attributed to Cannon (1932). Thus, endocrinology is truly a science of this century.

## BASIC REPRODUCTIVE ENDOCRINOLOGY

The specific mechanisms governing the complex processes of reproduction have, until fairly recently, remained almost a total mystery. Certainly not until the discovery by Green and Harris in 1947 that the hypothalamus controls the activity of the anterior pituitary (previously thought to be an autonomous "master gland") have we had the necessary ingredients to formulate our current theory of reproductive control. Even to this day, many important aspects of this regulation are not fully understood, and the almost continual emergence of new information requires that the theory be constantly revised.

In simple terms, all reproductive processes are regulated by the hormonal secretions of three separate structures, each of which produces unique products. The members of this triad are (1) the hypothalamus, which secretes releasing and inhibiting hormones; (2) the anterior pituitary, which secretes gonadotropic (gonad-stimulating) hormones; and (3) the gonads (ovaries or testes), which secrete sex steroid hormones. Information from a variety of external cues (e.g., visual, olfactory, auditory, tactile) is channeled through the central nervous system and ultimately to the brain, where it converges on the hypothalamus. The information is then processed, integrated, amplified, and transduced to a hormonal signal (comprised of hypothalamic releasing or inhibiting hormones), which is transmitted to the anterior pituitary. In turn, the anterior pituitary responds by producing and secreting the gonadotropic hormones into the blood stream to be carried to the gonads. The gonads may then respond to this signal in a number of ways, for example, by secreting sex steroid hormones which may affect other portions of the reproductive tract as well as feed back to the hypothalamus and pituitary gland to modify their functions. While it is beyond the scope of this book to describe the specifics, it needs to be pointed out that there is a *very* complex positive and negative feedback system in operation which integrates these three structures to maintain physiological homeostasis. While there are some modifications of the basic system just outlined which are specific to each sex, it should be emphasized that there are far more similarities than differences between the sexes in regard to control of reproductive function (see Adler 1981).

The appearance of the hypothalamus belies its importance. The hypothalamus is an inconspicuous part of the brain, visible on the undersurface merely as an oval band of grey matter suspending the pituitary gland. Though it only weighs about 5 g (which is just 1/300th of total brain weight), this tiny structure controls pituitary functions governing sexual cycles, pregnancy, lactation, growth, and stress as well as temperature, water balance, sleep, and various emotional reactions (Cross 1972). The clue to the remarkable diversity of actions of the hypothalamus lies in the nature of its functional connections. Unlike any other brain region, it not only receives sensory input from almost every other part of the central nervous system, including the cerebral cortex, basal ganglia, thalamus, midbrain, and hindbrain, but also sends nerve impulses to several endocrine glands and to motor pathways governing the activity of skeletal muscles, the heart, exocrine glands, the smooth muscle of blood vessels, and many viscera. These various capabilities, which are unique to it, are made possible by neurosecretory neurons in the hypothalamus that allow it to receive messages from the nervous system (via electrical transmission) and convert those messages into endocrine responses (i.e., the release of hormones). The hypothalamus might perhaps best be understood as an enormously complex "switchboard" connecting the brain above to the endocrine system below.

Regarding reproduction, the relationship between the hypothalamus and the pituitary (or hypophysis) is crucial. The pituitary (from the Latin *pituita*, meaning phlegm) received its name as a result of the Galenic view that the gland excreted mucus from the brain and discharged it into the nasopharynx, a theory that was disproved in the seventeenth century. The term *hypophysis* (from the Greek *hypophyein*, meaning undergrowth) describes the location of the gland below the brain (Greep 1974). The pituitary gland consists of two major subdivisions or lobes, the anterior lobe (or adenohypophysis) and the posterior lobe (or neurohypophysis). The posterior lobe (which stores and secretes the hormones oxytocin and vasopressin, both of which are actually produced in the hypothalamus) is made up of neural tissue and is directly connected to the brain. The anterior pituitary synthesizes and secretes the gonadotropins luteinizing hormone (LH) and follicle-stimulating hormone (FSH) as well as prolactin, somatotropin, adrenocorticotropin, and thyroid-stimulating hormone. However, unlike the posterior lobe, the anterior lobe contains no nerve fibers and terminals and so is not in direct neuronal contact with the hypothalamus. Rather, there is a special vascular connection between the two, the hypothalamo-hypophyseal portal system.

A portal system, by definition, begins and ends in capillaries without entering the systemic circulation. Thus, the hypothalamo-hypophyseal portal system allows the small polypeptide releasing and inhibiting hormones produced in the hypothalamus to travel directly to the anterior pituitary located below (these hormones are composed of only a few amino acids and hence are very small). Since the hormones are not diluted in the blood stream, this permits an extremely rapid and powerful response to be elicited by a minute amount of hypothalamic hormones.

The existence of the hypothalamo-hypophyseal portal system was not recognized until the 1930s (see Greep 1974). At first, it was thought that blood flowed up the stalk from the pituitary to the hypothalamus. However, thanks mainly to the anatomical studies of Popa and Fielding (1930, 1933) and Wislocki and King (1936) and the later, more physiological studies of Green and Harris (1947) and Harris (1948), it was eventually established that blood flows down the stalk, thereby providing a route for information transfer from the brain to the anterior pituitary. In addition, we have recently come to realize that a small proportion of blood may actually flow in a retrograde manner up the pituitary stalk, thus providing a vascular link from the anterior pituitary back to the hypothalamus and allowing so-called short-loop negative feedback.

Although the existence of hypothalamic releasing factors was suggested in the 1940s, it was not until the 1970s that the first ones were characterized structurally and synthesized chemically. The leading scientists in this endeavor were Roger Guillemin (see Guillemin 1978) and Andrew Schally (see Schally 1978), whose competitive efforts to be the first to characterize the hypothalamic hormones eventually led (somewhat ironically, in view of their spirited rivalry) to their being named as co–Nobel laureates (see Wade 1981). In June 1971, Schally's laboratory was the first to announce the primary structure of porcine luteinizing hormone releasing factor or LRF (same as Gn-RH) (Matsuo et al. 1971). Guillemin's group soon after reported the identical primary structure for bovine LRF (Burgus et al. 1972).

It was originally thought that a separate hypothalamic hormone existed for each anterior pituitary hormone. However, once the structures of the hormones were determined and pure preparations became available, it was found that there is considerable overlap. This is especially true in regard to the gonadotropins. The same hormone that stimulates the release of LH also induces the release of FSH; thus it is called *gonadotropin releasing hormone* (Gn-RH). Some researchers still hold the view that there are selective factors for the release of each gonadotropin. Most researchers agree that the same cells (gonadotrophs) within the anterior pituitary synthesize and secrete both LH and FSH; however, there are some who claim that some gonadotrophs produce only one hormone (Karsch 1984).

MALE AND FEMALE DIFFERENCES

It is well established that secretion of LH and FSH (which control the functions of the gonads) are governed by two functionally separate but superimposable regulatory systems — the tonic system and the cyclic (or surge) system. In both men and women, the tonic system produces ever-present basal levels of circulating gonadotropins, which stimulate both the endocrine (steroid hormone production) and exocrine (gamete production) functions of the gonads. In contrast, the cyclic system is responsible for acute and dramatic (perhaps as much as 100-fold) but transitory increases above basal secretion of gonadotropins; these increases are evident for short periods (generally twelve to twenty-four hours) in each menstrual cycle. However, these short-lived changes, which have the primary function of causing ovulation, are the triggers which are responsible for drastic changes in the type of steroid hormones produced during the cycle. Endocrine changes during the menstrual cycle will be considered in detail shortly.

The capability for surges of gonadotropin secretion is what makes cycling possible in women. Although the hypothalamus of *both* men and women begins with this potential, the presence of testicular steroids in men and the subsequent exposure of the hypothalamus to them during a critical period of prenatal development renders the so-called cyclic center of the hypothalamus in men inoperative and incapable of responding to feedback effects in a surge-like manner.

In Chapter 3, we pointed out that it is a mistake to think in terms of male and female hormones. This fascinating bit of irony should clearly show why: In actuality, it is not testosterone per se which renders the potential cyclic center of the male hypothalamus inoperable. Rather, after testosterone enters the cells of the potential cyclic center of the hypothalamus, it is converted by an enzyme called *aromatase* (the process is called *aromatization*) into the estrogen estradiol-17$\beta$. It is actually estradiol, a so-called female hormone, which changes the "wiring diagram" within this portion of the male hypothalamus and organizes the neural connections within it in such a manner that the ability for a cyclic response is lost. Why does estradiol not do the same thing in women? The answer is that while estradiol is present in both sexes (from a placental as well as a gonadal source), estradiol in both sexes is bound in the blood by the estrogen-specific serum protein $\alpha$-fetoprotein. Estradiol bound by $\alpha$-fetoprotein cannot leave the blood and gain access to the hypothalamus. Therefore, the cyclic center passively develops in the female because there is nothing to interfere with its development. Testosterone, normally present in high concentrations in male but not in female fetuses, is not bound by $\alpha$-fetoprotein. Thus, testosterone (misnamed as the "male hormone") is in this case serving as a precursor to estradiol (misnamed as a "female hormone"), which then causes a male-type brain to develop (see MacLusky and Naftolin 1981). In recent years, several interesting examples of sexual dimorphism in human brain anatomy have been reported (e.g., DeLacoste-Utamsing and Holloway 1982; de Vries et al. 1984; Swaab and Fliers 1985).

The existence of a tonic system in both sexes and a surge system only in women is in harmony with the concept that these two centers reside in different regions of the hypothalamus. This spatial separation can be clearly demonstrated in other species, such as the rat, and numerous researchers have shown that cyclic function can be destroyed by lesioning the portion of the hypothalamus (the suprachiasmatic nucleus) known to be associated with cyclical Gn-RH release. Although the system is much more complex in women, it is possible to eliminate the LH surge responsible for ovulation without interfering with tonic gonadotropin secretion and this is in fact the primary mode of action of oral contraceptives. In men, however, since there is only the tonic center upon which to work, it is exceedingly difficult to prevent gamete production without also adversely affecting testosterone production and obtaining the highly undesirable side effects of that action. As we saw in Chapter 1 and shall see in more detail in Chapter 10, this is one of the factors that has led scientists to concentrate their efforts on female rather than male contraception, and it is one main reason why a male version of the pill is not possible.

## THE MENSTRUAL CYCLE

### Historical Perspective

Since antiquity, menstruation has been viewed as the single factor most distinctly separating men and women. Historically, men have often viewed menstruation as a "weakness" or "sickness" of women and have associated the cyclical nature of the female reproductive processes with general instability and erratic behavior. This view of women as congenitally defective has played an important role in the oppression of women and in maintaining discriminatory views of appropriate roles for women in society.

Menstruation, which does tend to recur at roughly monthly intervals, derives its name from the Latin word for month. In popular folklore, the moon was seen as regulating the emotional tides of women as well as the tides of the sea. This is but one of the many myths, legends, and taboos that have surrounded menstruation and female reproductive functions more generally.

According to Gruhn (1987), the uterus and menses were recognized by the ancient Sumerians, whose birth goddess, Nintu, was shaped like a uterus, and by the Egyptians, whose hieroglyph, Ankh, depicted on images of the birth goddess, Taurt, resembled a uterus. Thus, in order to reduce the threat of destruction by the unseen forces that directed a woman's bleedings, some early cultures first made the uterus a goddess. Views of women as "hysterical," as well as the view that reproduction is the natural function of women, are linked to a belief that persisted until the fourteenth century, namely, that the human uterus is a multichambered organ that could wander about the body causing hysteria. The purported cause of this restlessness was articulated by Plato (c. 347–266 B.C.), who thought that if a woman goes too long without becoming pregnant, her womb becomes indignant and wanders throughout her body, interfering with respiration, creating extreme anxiety, and causing all sorts of diseases (see Plato's *Timaeus* 9lb–c).

Aristotle (382–322 B.C.) believed that the "seed" contained in the male ejaculate developed in the "soil" of the menstrual blood. Male seed provides form, motion, and soul for the offspring while female soil provides matter and body. Aristotle reached his conclusion because he held that the rational soul (which distinguishes the human being from the lower animals) is inoperative in women. Lacking sufficient "soul heat," women cannot "cook" their menstrual blood into semen and thus do not contribute anything of essential character to the offspring (see Aristotle's *On the Generation of Animals* 1: 17–23; see also Gruhn 1987). The same view can be found in Aeschylus, articulated by Apollo in the *Eumenides*:

> The mother is not the true parent of the child. . . . She is a nurse who tends the growth of young seed planted by its true parent, the male. So, if fate spares the child, she keeps it, as one might keep for some friend a growing plant. And of this truth, that father without mother may beget, we have present, as proof, the daughter of Olympian Zeus, one never nursed in the dark cradle of the womb (translated by Phillip Vallacott).

On this view, man alone is parent; woman is mere custodian and nurturer of his seed. She is, as it were, (and at most) a kind of flower pot (Whitbeck 1976, 1983). Making the uterus a goddess is one way of managing the threat of unseen, "dark" forces; reducing it to a mere nutritious container is another.

It was also believed that milk was formed from menstrual blood, since lactating women do not menstruate (Short 1984). It was not until 1908 that the occurrence of normal cyclic changes in the human endometrium (uterine lining) were clearly illustrated by Hitschman and Adler (see Gruhn 1987) and that the menstrual process began to be scientifically understood.

In various societies, menstrual blood has been said to be able to ward off evil, cure diseases, possess supernatural powers, extinguish fires, temper metals, attract lovers, and protect men from being wounded in battle. In the folklore of various cultures, menstrual blood was believed to have the same powers that are claimed by modern-day faith healers, that is, that it can curb assorted ailments, including leprosy, warts, birthmarks, goiter, hemorrhoids, epilepsy, worms, and headache (see Delaney, Lupton, and Toth 1976). The first napkin worn by a virgin was believed to be especially effective as a cure for the plague.

However, the most predominant sentiment about menstrual blood in most cultures has clearly been to regard it as being unclean and even poisonous. Much of this folklore is described in *The Curse: A Cultural History of Menstruation* by Janice Delaney, Mary Jane Lupton, and Emily Toth (1976). One of the most graphic descriptions of the purported effects of menstrual blood comes from the folklore of the New Guinea Mae Enga tribe, who believe that it could "sicken a man and cause persistent vomiting, kill his blood so that it turns black, corrupt his vital juices so that his skin darkens and hangs in folds as his flesh wastes, permanently dull his wits, and eventually lead to a slow decline and death." A Mae Enga tribesman was said to have divorced his wife because she slept on his blanket while menstruating. This apparently did not appease him, since he later killer her with an ax. The Tinne Indians of the Yukon territory believed that men must avoid all contact with menstruating women since a woman in this condition was a serious threat to a man's virility. Women were not employed in the opium industry during the nineteenth century because it was believed that a menstruating woman would turn the opium bitter (Delaney, Lupton, and Toth 1976).

Several religions have specific edicts which apply to menstruating women. Moslem women cannot pray in a mosque during menstruation. Some Buddhists also think it wrong for a menstruating woman to enter a temple. Hindu women are forbidden to prepare food for their husbands during menstruation. The Church of England still has a special service in their prayer book for "The Churching of Women," a ceremony to be performed after a woman has cleansed herself by having her first menstruation following the birth of a child (Short 1984).

In many primitive societies, menstruating women were excluded from the tribe and forced to occupy a small menstrual hut set some distance from the village. It is possible that women perpetuated this practice, since it was likely their only break from their usual chores of cooking, cleaning, planting, harvesting, and fulfilling the wishes of their husbands.

Perhaps the most prevalent taboos in various cultures have been those involving food and menstruation. Various primitive societies have held menstruating women responsible for crop failure, bad luck in hunting and fishing, the death of livestock, and the failure of food to be successfully preserved, of cider to ferment, of sugar to be refined, and of bacon to be cured (Delaney, Lupton, and Toth 1976).

Purported scientists have contributed to perpetuating these myths. As cited by Fluhmann (1939), Schick reported in 1920 that a bouquet of roses given to a servant girl during her period had faded by the next day. Schick coined the term *menotoxins* for purported noxious substances that were exuded through the skin of women during menstruation that had the ability to kill plants and prevent dough from rising and keep beer from fermenting. Macht also reported in 1924 that menstrual blood had the power to inhibit plant growth (Fluhmann 1939).

While most of the myths and taboos have faded, others concerning sexual intercourse during menstruation still exist. Many people cite *Leviticus* 15:19 as a biblical injunction against intercourse during menstruation: "And if a woman have issue, and her issue in her flesh be blood, she shall be apart seven days: and whosoever toucheth her shall be unclean until the even." Orthodox Jews are especially scrupulous about observing this taboo. Many people today still hold long-standing magical and just plain erroneous beliefs about the effects of intercourse during menses. Fears include that ill effects might befall both men and women. In the nineteenth century it was widely believed that a man could get gonorrhea from sexual contact with a menstruating woman. In the twentieth century, man's punishment is said to be urethritis (an inflammation of the urethra). For women, intercourse during menstruation has long been viewed as a dangerous practice because of the chance of it leading to hemorrhage, injury, or infection (Delaney, Lupton, and Toth 1976). For members of both sexes, it is often avoided for purely aesthetic reasons, since many consider it messy, sloppy, and visually unappealing. In actuality, there is no physiological reason to abstain from intercourse during menses. In fact, since intercourse during menses tends to alleviate menstrual cramps and hasten the elimination of the products of menstruation, it may instead have a beneficial effect. Additionally, as we have seen in Chapter 1 and shall see in more detail below, menses is the "safest" period during the menstrual cycle.

*Overview and Cycle Length*

The menstrual cycle is a repetitive expression of a complex series of physiological events resulting from the operation of the hypothalamic-pituitary-ovarian system. The central nervous system integrates the various intrinsic and extrinsic factors which regulate the synthesis and release of the hypothalamic hormones and, hence, the production and release of the gonadotropins by the anterior pituitary. Ovarian activity, including steroid hormone production, follicular development, and gamete maturation, is dependent on gonadotropin stimulation. Ovarian steroid hormones act on the oviducts, uterus, cervix, vagina, and breasts as well as feed back to regulate the functions of the hypothalamus and pituitary. Menstruation, the periodic physiological bleeding from the endometrium, is clearly the major outward manifestation of these underlying cyclic endocrine changes.

The onset of menstruation, properly called *menarche*, usually occurs between the ages of 11 and 14. In the United States, the mean age at menarche is 12.65 ± 1.17 years (Zacharias, Wurtman, and Schatzoff 1970). There has been a steady decrease in the mean age at menarche in North America and Europe over the past century. In the United States, the decrease has been approximately two to three months per decade in the last century, although the trend has now slowed or perhaps ceased. A complex interaction of numerous factors, including genetics, social and economic factors, nutrition, degree of physical activity, health, and season of birth, have been shown to affect age at menarche (Nicholson and Hanley 1953; Damon 1974; Zacharias, Rand, and Wurtman 1976; Wyshak and Frisch 1982).

At the other end of the reproductive life of women is menopause, the termination of menstrual cycles. The average age at menopause has been reported to be 51.4 years (Jaszmann 1976). However, the age range is quite large, with approximately 50 percent of all women reaching menopause between ages 45 and 50, about 25 percent before age 45, and 25 percent after age 50 (Jones, Cohen, and Wilson 1972).

Although the median menstrual cycle length for women during the active reproductive years corresponds to the lunar month of twenty-eight days, each woman's menstrual cycle has an individual pattern of length, variability, duration, and intensity. The range of normal cycle lengths is twenty-four to thirty-five days (Hafez 1978). Cycles can be considered normal if they are regular and the interval does not vary by more than five days. As we mentioned in Chapter 1, many factors can cause irregularities in cycle length, including rapid weight loss, serious emotional stress, abrupt changes in climate, illness, and aging. Irregularity of cycle length is common during the first five or six years following menarche and preceding menopause. Minimal variation in cycle length occurs in women in their midthirties (Hafez 1978). Pregnancy and lactation are the only two nonpathological, naturally occurring events which suspend menstrual cycles in premenopausal women; thus breast-feeding is now commonly recognized as an unassisted (though not totally reliable) way of spacing births.

In essence, the subject of this book, preventing birth, is an example of how human beings attempt to foil one aspect of "Mother Nature's game plan." Menstrual cycles occur only because pregnancies either have not occurred or have been interrupted. If we assume a forty-year reproductive lifetime for a woman, which is about average, and also assume that she has a menstrual cycle roughly every twenty-eight days during that interval, then she will have over five hundred opportunities to exercise her capacity to reproduce or, alternatively, five hundred time periods during which she must exercise special care to avoid pregnancy. Each menstruation may be viewed as a dual declaration that a woman is not pregnant and that a new opportunity or risk awaits.

## Stages and Endocrinology of the Menstrual Cycle

Although, as previously discussed, a menstrual cycle involves the rhythmic fluctuations of the hormones of the hypothalamus and anterior pituitary as well as the ovary, classification of the stages of the cycle is based on the events happening on the surface of the ovary (the ovarian cycle) or at the primary target tissue for the ovarian hormones, the endometrium (the endometrial cycle). Naturally, endometrial changes merely mirror the changing profile of steroid hormones produced by the ovary. Figure 10 provides a summary of the ovarian and endometrial events and the hormonal changes that occur during a typical menstrual cycle. The three stages of the menstrual cycle which we shall discuss in detail are (1) menstruation or menses, the actual discharge of bloody fluid; (2) the follicular or preovulatory phase (based on ovarian morphology) or proliferative phase (based on endometrial changes); and (3) the luteal or postovulatory phase (based on ovarian morphology) or secretory phase (based on endometrial changes).

*Menstrual Phase* Although the beginning of menses is commonly regarded as the onset of a new cycle, from a physiological stand-

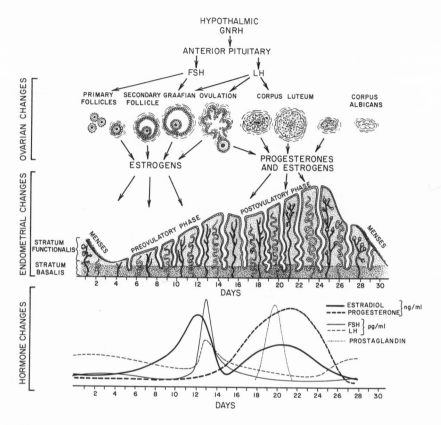

**Figure 10.** Ovarian, endometrial, and hormonal changes during a typical menstrual cycle.

point it actually represents the terminus of the previous cycle. However, since it is the only readily observable benchmark of cyclic change, it is the logical event to regard as the beginning of a new cycle.

The bleeding associated with menstruation is due to the actual sloughing off of the superficial layer of the endometrium (uterine lining), which exposes the blood vessels below and leads to bleeding. As we have seen in Chapter 3, the endometrium actually consists of two layers: a superficial one that contains glands and comprises some two-thirds of the endometrium and a thinner basal layer. The superficial layer, which is the layer that responds to steroids by increasing in cellular height during the proliferative phase and by producing the glandular secretions during the secretory phase, is almost completely lost during menstruation. The functional support of the superficial layer of the endometrium is dependent upon the hormone progesterone $(P_4)$, which is produced by the corpus luteum (CL) after ovulation. When the corpus luteum regresses and progesterone support for the endometrium is removed, the endometrium also regresses. As the endometrium shrinks due to lack of progestational support, it constricts the numerous spiral arterioles (blood vessels) which lie close to the surface and richly supply it with blood. In turn, these highly convoluted blood vessels also constrict, further reducing the blood flow to the tissue and causing it to, quite literally, die. As patches of the dead endometrial tissue are sloughed off, the blood vessels are exposed and they leak blood into the uterine cavity. Fortunately, only small patches of endometrium become detached at a time, so under normal conditions no major hemorrhage occurs. Menstrual blood does not clot because of the presence of fibrinolytic enzymes and the release of tissue heparin (a blood-thinning substance). Clots which may appear in some women during a heavy menstrual flow are a combination of red blood cells, cervical mucus, vaginal cells, and secretions. These clots form in the vagina, not in the uterus. Also aiding the elimination of sloughed endometrium and blood from the uterus is the local release of the hormone prostaglandin $F_{2\alpha}$ ($PGF_{2\alpha}$) concomitant with endometrial breakdown. This prostaglandin, which also triggers the regression of the corpus luteum, serves the two important uterine functions of causing constriction of the blood vessels to minimize blood loss and causing contractions of the myometrium (uterine muscle) to aid in expulsion of the products into the vagina. In essence, it is prostaglandin $F_{2\alpha}$ which causes menstrual cramps.

The duration of menstruation is somewhat variable; it ranges from three to seven days, with four to five days being the more typical length (Hallberg et al. 1966; Hafez 1978; Sloane 1980). Total volume of menstrual blood loss has been reported to range from 20 to 75 ml, with mean values of 30–50 ml more typical (Hallberg et al. 1966; Hafez 1978; Sloane 1980; Tortora and Evans 1986). Blood loss exceeding 80 ml is considered abnormal (Hallberg et al. 1966). Most blood loss occurs in the first few days of menses, with 78 percent during the first two days and 91 percent during the first three days (Jones and Wentz 1977). The length of the period does not appear to be an indicator of the degree of bleeding. Several forms of birth control can affect the volume of menstrual bleeding. For example, the use of oral contraceptives reduces blood loss by 50–70 percent (Ahmad 1979), while average blood loss has been reported to increase by 65 percent in nulliparous and 91 percent in parous women after one year of IUD use (Mishell 1977).

Although the period of menstruation is routinely considered separate from the follicular phase, folliculogenesis (growth of the follicle) actually begins early in the menstrual phase. Normally, 4 or 5 so-called primary follicles are "selected" each cycle to begin development from the total follicular pool of perhaps 100,000 or so follicles. By the end of menses, within each of these growing follicles an outer membrane around the ovum, called the *zona pellucida*, has developed. At this point, the follicle has also had a mitotic increase in the layers of follicular cells (more appropriately termed *granulosa cells*) which lie outside the zona pellucida and within the covering membrane of the follicle, called the *basement membrane*. This increase in follicular development is occurring at the same time that the corpus luteum from the previous cycle is continuing to regress and become a nonfunctional corpus albicans.

Not only does corpus luteum regression and progesterone withdrawal from the system cause the endometrium to regress and be sloughed off, triggering menses, but progesterone withdrawal also removes the negative feedback from the hypothalamus and anterior pituitary, facilitating a steady increase in gonadotropins. As tonic levels of FSH and LH increase, follicular growth results. As the follicle grows, it also begins to increase its estrogen (especially estradiol) production. In light of the increasing estradiol:progesterone ratio, responsiveness of the various target tissues (oviducts, uterus, vagina, breasts, etc.) also changes. By the end of menses (i.e., days 4–5 of the cycle), there are now four or five growing follicles and steadily increasing estrogen concentrations. New endometrial growth begins as soon as the old is sloughed off and eliminated.

*Follicular, Preovulatory, or Proliferative Phase*   Technically, this is the phase between the end of menstruation and ovulation. However, both follicular development and proliferation of new endometrial tissue have actually already begun. This phase is by far the most variable and it is the most responsible for the wide variation in cycle length among women. It may be as short as five days in a woman with a short cycle (e.g., twenty-four-day cycle) or as long as sixteen days in a woman with a long cycle (e.g., thirty-five-day cycle). In the idealized twenty-eight-day cycle, with ovulation on day 14 and a four-day period of menses, this phase lasts from day 5 through day 13.

As we have said, follicular development has already begun and has probably reached the secondary follicle stage by the end of menses. A cavity or antrum will now begin to form in the granulosa cells of each developing follicle. With the appearance of the antrum, the follicle is now called a *tertiary follicle*. This antrum begins to fill with follicular fluid, which is actually a transudate from the peripheral blood plasma modified by follicular metabolic activities and rich in steroids, glycoproteins, various enzymes, prostaglandins, ions, and salts. The follicle grows in size as the follicular fluid increases (much like a balloon being filled with water) and it begins to protrude above the surface of the ovary. The increasing estrogen production (primarily estradiol) by the granulosa cells facilitates this increase in follicular fluid and stimulates continued development of the follicle. Also occurring as the tertiary stage of folliculogenesis commences is a mitotic increase in the theca cell layer lying just outside the basement membrane of the follicle. Theca cells (which are analogous to interstitial cells of Leydig in the testes) produce androgens, primarily under the influence of LH. These androgens (the primary one is androstenedione) readily cross the basement membrane of the follicle and are aromatized (converted) to estrogens (mainly estradiol) by the granulosa cells (analogous to Sertoli cells in the testes). The activity of the granulosa cells is primarily controlled by FSH. This mode of describing follicular steroidogenesis is termed the *two-cell, two-gonadotropin model* and was first proposed by Fortune and Armstrong (1978). Again, theca cells and granulosa cells are the two types of cells and the two gonadotropins controlling their activity are LH and FSH respectively. Predominant products are androstenedione and estradiol respectively. Thus, as follicular growth continues toward ovulation, estrogen levels are steadily rising under the influence of tonic release of LH and FSH.

Occurring concomitant with folliculogenesis is the separate but related event of oogenesis (growth and maturation of the oocyte). Both folliculogenesis and oogenesis require gonadotropic support for completion. As the follicle approaches maturity, it is referred to as a *Graafian follicle*. Normally, only one follicle will complete maturation and ovulate, with the others undergoing the degenerative process atresia. Within the Graafian follicle, the oocyte and the specialized granulosa cells surrounding it have moved to the basal portion of the follicle opposite the site of stigma formation. The stigma is the thin, circumscribed area of follicular rupture. The oocyte, awakened from its hibernating state by the increase in gonadotropins, has completed its first meiotic division by the time of ovulation and is properly referred to as a *secondary oocyte*. It is not well understood why, in a particular cycle, a few follicles will suddenly arise from their years of slumber while others remain dormant. Nor is it understood why normally only one of these four or five follicles completes development and ovulates while the others become atretic.

Returning to the activity of the endometrium during its proliferative phase, repair in those areas of the endometrium that first sloughed off is underway even before menstrual flow ceases. The increasing concentrations of estradiol during this phase is the stimulus for reorganization and proliferation of endometrial cells. Cells in the basilar layer undergo mitosis and aid in the regeneration of a new superficial layer. Covering epithelium is regenerated first, and then the superficial layer grows until it becomes at least three times as thick as the basilar layer. Within approximately three days after the end of menstruation, the surface epithelium of the endometrium has been completely renewed and the torn vasculature and glandular elements have healed. The endometrial glands are characteristically narrow, tubular, and lined by cuboidal (cube-shaped) epithelium. As the preovulatory phase progresses, the epithelium becomes columnar (column shaped), distinct nuclei are present at the base of each cell, and conventional histological staining techniques indicate increasing capacity for secretion by the glandular epithelium. As ovulation approaches (i.e., at midcycle), the endometrial glands increase in size and become more convoluted. Increased vacuolation (the appearance of clear spaces) occurs at the base of the cells lining the glands, reflecting increased glycogen (stored carbohydrate) accumulation. Numerous enzyme systems which are critical to providing energy to the early embryo are also now present. The vasculature supplying the endometrium is becoming increasingly coiled. At the time of ovulation, the endometrium has increased in depth about threefold from its initial depth of 1 mm.

Ovulation is triggered by the rising estradiol concentration that, once requirements for threshold level and duration of exposure are met, causes a surge of LH release from the anterior pituitary. This surge (i.e., a virtually immediate six- to tenfold increase in LH) occurs approximately sixteen to eighteen hours before ovulation. Once the LH surge occurs, a complex series of events begins at the level of the mature Graafian follicle on the ovary and within the oocyte that ultimately results in the release of an ovum ready to be fertilized. This surge of LH release is absolutely necessary for ovulation; therefore, preventing its occurrence is a logical means of contraception and in fact is the primary mode of action of oral contraceptives.

*Luteal, Postovulatory, or Secretory Phase*   This is the phase between ovulation and the onset of the next menses. It is much more constant in duration among women than is the preovulatory phase, and it normally does not vary more than a day or so from the average duration of fourteen days. Thus, in an idealized twenty-eight-day menstrual cycle, it begins following ovulation on day 14 and lasts until the onset of menses on day 28.

Following ovulation, the structure of the follicle collapses and fills with blood and the blood coagulates (clots) to form a transitory structure called a *corpus hemorrhagicum* (bloody body). Since the basement membrane of the follicle previously separating the granulosa cells (inside) from the theca cells (outside) is ruptured at ovulation, these cells can now mix. Under the influence of LH, granulosa and theca cells combine and are transformed into functionally different cells, called *lutein cells*. Collectively, the lutein cells compose the structure now on the ovary at the previous site of follicular rupture, the corpus luteum. The lutein cells proliferate rapidly and quickly displace the transitory corpus hemorrhagicum. As corpus luteum formation occurs, progesterone levels rapidly increase. Therefore, following ovulation there is a drastic change in the estradiol: progesterone ratio, which now markedly favors progesterone. Some estradiol is produced by the corpus luteum, but its primary product is progesterone. The increased progesterone causes changes to occur in all other target tissues, including the tissues of the uterus.

Progesterone (which means favoring gestation) is responsible for preparing the endometrium to receive a fertilized egg and to sustain its development. In service of this end, progesterone stimulates filling of the endometrial glands with secretions rich in glycogen, lipids, and proteins to nourish the expected conceptus. This phase of the cycle is referred to as *secretory* because of the copious secretion of products by the endometrial glands. Compared with their appearance during the proliferative phase, endometrial glands are now more branched, more coiled, and deeper. The height of the endometrium has increased another twofold over its height at ovulation and now consists of three distinct layers: (1) the superficial compacted vascular-rich region, (2) a central spongy zone of the dilated and convoluted glands, and (3) a deep basal layer. These preparatory changes reach their apex about one week after ovulation, which is the anticipated time of arrival of a conceptus. Disruption of these endometrial changes is another and highly effective means of birth control, as we shall see in more detail in Chapter 6, when we discuss IUDs.

If fertilization does occur and a conceptus implants in the uterus, the corpus luteum continues to secrete progesterone, thereby sustaining endometrial activity and, hence, pregnancy. This occurs because a hormone called *human chorionic gonadotropin* (hCG) is produced by the developing conceptus as early as day 8 of pregnancy, or only one day after implantation (Jaffe 1978). This hormone is similar to LH and serves to maintain the corpus luteum during early pregnancy. Later, the placenta itself becomes capable of producing progesterone and various estrogens. Interfering with the action of hCG on corpus luteum maintenance is another way of interfering with a pregnancy. This approach to birth prevention will also be discussed in Chapter 6.

If fertilization does not occur (or if a conceptus dies or fails to produce hCG; see Chapter 6), the corpus luteum regresses (due, primarily, to the action of prostaglandin $F_{2\alpha}$) approximately two or three days preceding onset of the next menstruation. This is the period of "premenstrual tension" or "premenstrual syndrome" (PMS), which is held to affect a number of women. Concomitant with corpus luteum regression is a precipitous decline in progesterone. At this time there is an infiltration of polymorphonuclear leukocytes (a specific type of white blood cell) and degeneration of the connective tissue stroma of the superficial endometrium begins. The vasculature supplying the superficial layer becomes constricted and damaged in such a way that it will subsequently leak blood into the uterine lumen following endometrial sloughing. As soon as the blood breaks through the degenerating endometrial epithelium, the menstrual flow begins again and a menstrual cycle has come full circle.

PREMENSTRUAL SYNDROME

We have already seen that men have long feared that the impending onset of menstruation may cause women to become temporarily irrational while in the throes of their purportedly wildly raging hormones. This precept is still employed today to mask sexism and sexist discrimination. There are many men (and women) who feel that women should not occupy positions with crucial decision-making powers because of what they may do during periodic "hormonally deranged states." The belief that women experience such periodic lapses of control and reason has recently been supported by attempts to use premenstrual syndrome (PMS) to explain a great number of negative states and behaviors, ranging from grouch-iness to murder. For example, in 1980 and 1981, British courts reduced murder charges against two women to manslaughter charges because of a successful argument that PMS had lessened their responsibility for stabbing to death another woman in one case and running over a lover with a car in the other (Dalton 1980; Reid and Yen 1981; Allen 1984). PMS can now be grounds for a plea of temporary insanity in France (Yen 1986).

An English physician, Katharina Dalton, is probably the individual most responsible for popularizing PMS, which she has quaintly called "the curse of Eve" (Dalton 1964, 1970, 1971, 1976, 1977, 1980, 1984). Dalton claims that PMS is responsible for, among other things, increases in sick days of female workers, accidents, hospital admissions, psychiatric disorders, child abuse, misbehavior among school-girls, crimes of violence, alcoholism, and prostitution. Despite the absence of controlled studies to verify her approach, Dalton has been an enthusiastic advocate of administering large doses of exogenous progesterone to treat PMS (e.g., Dalton 1977, 1984). In expressing sympathy for men who enter marriage unaware of the purported perils of PMS, Dalton (1977) affirms the traditional stereotype with its traditional language: "Sudden mood changes, irrational behavior, and bursting into tears for no apparent reason are bewildering, while sudden aggression and violence are deeply disturbing when with little warning and no justification, his darling little love bird becomes an angry, argumentative, shouting, abusive bitch."

Although PMS, first called *premenstrual tension*, was described in the clinical literature in 1931 by American gynecologist Robert Frank, there is still considerable confusion as to the cause, extent, and seriousness of the condition, despite a multitude of publications on the subject. For example, in the literature we reviewed in preparing this section, the percentage of women suffering from PMS is claimed to be anywhere from 3 to 95 percent. One problem in arriving at an accurate figure is the nebulous clinical definition of PMS and the wide range of symptoms which have been used to define it. Signs and symptoms reported to "diagnose" PMS include edema (water accumulation), breast swelling and tenderness, abdominal distension, constipation, skin eruptions, fatigue and lethargy, irritability, headaches, clumsiness, depression, anxiety, nervousness, uncontrollable crying, insomnia, hypersomnia, inability to concentrate, paranoid attitudes, backache, diarrhea, nausea, vomiting, hunger, thirst, increased craving for sweet or salty food, heightened sensory activity, rapid mood swings, and decreased sexual receptivity, among others (Dalton 1964; Janowsky, Gorney, and Kelley 1966; Sloane 1980; Muse et al. 1984; Rome 1986; Tortora and Evans 1986; Yen 1986; Marut 1987). Moos (1968) identifies over 150 symptoms falling into five sweeping categories: (1) affective symptoms, (2) neurovegetative symptoms, (3) central nervous system symptoms, (4) cognitive symptoms, and (5) behavioral symptoms. Needless to say, with this wide range of symptoms, virtually all women are likely to experience some of them, making all women "ill" on a monthly basis (see Zita 1988). The more physiological symptoms (e.g., water retention and breast swelling and tenderness) are indeed expected effects of decreased progesterone and increased estradiol concentrations occurring during the paramenstrum (the time just before and during the menses). Yet these symptoms, like most of the purported symptoms of PMS, pose no substantial threat to the ability of a woman to properly and effectively function in society generally or in positions of authority more particularly. As commonly treated in the medical literature, however, PMS resurrects the view of women as congenitally defective or diseased, simply clothing it in modern scientific dress (see Zita 1988).

Without question, there are very real changes within a woman's body during the premenstrual period, and discomfort during this phase is clearly physical in origin, not psychological. However, there are wide variations in how PMS affects women and in how they respond to the physiological changes their bodies undergo. Some women may pay little or no attention to the physical symptoms of edema, a pimple, breast tenderness, and so on. Other women may be more aware of and respond more negatively to these changes, and they may consequently experience and perhaps express some irritability and tenseness. But certainly these women in general are in no significant way incapacitated during this period.

However, a third group of women, some of whom do experience substantial physical discomfort and some of whom simply have a decreased ability to deal with the discomfort tolerated by others, demonstrate a greater emotional response to changes during their paramenstrum and exhibit more marked personality changes. Also clouding the issue are environmental conditioning and each individual woman's view concerning what constitutes permissible or expected behavior. As Zita (1988) points out, the social assumption that women will behave erratically or aggressively during the premenstrual period may lead some women to live up to the assumption by giving themselves permission to act as expected.

Over the years, numerous hypotheses have been proposed to explain the underlying physical causes of PMS (for a review, see Reid and Yen 1981). These include progesterone insufficiency or withdrawal, excessive estradiol retention, vitamin $B_6$ deficiency, hypoglycemia (low blood sugar), endogenous hormone allergy, excess prolactin (an anterior pituitary hormone), abnormalities of water- and salt-regulating hormones, and some psychosomatic influences. More recent evidence (Koob and Bloom 1983; Morley 1983) suggests that endogenous opiate peptides (i.e., natural opiumlike brain products that mediate pain) may also be involved. It has been suggested that these opioids increase in the central nervous system under the influence of high systemic concentrations of progesterone. With corpus luteum regression and progesterone removal from the system, opioid production likewise rapidly declines. This withdrawal of opioids may then trigger the subsequent psychoneuroendocrine manifestations of PMS.

As appropriately noted by Weideger (1976) and Sloane (1980), the various studies linking PMS to negative states and behaviors fail to link positive states and behaviors, such as creativity, increased self-confidence, and optimism, with the phases of the menstrual cycle. Koeske (1976, 1983) suggests that the changes a woman experiences during the premenstrual period might open her body to an undetermined arousability rather than to the particular negatively described emotional states commonly cited in the medical literature. Zita (1988) suggests we view these nonspecific, receptive states as "windows of sensitivity" which provide a woman with an opportunity to respond in a fine-tuned way to her environment. Such suggestions do not deny the reality of physiological changes during the premenstrual period. What they do deny is that we should accept as accurate the traditional categorization of these changes as negative and necessarily linked to negative states and behaviors. Indeed, Zita (1988) plausibly suggests that these changes, which can allow a woman to feel more deeply and experience her environment more keenly during certain regularly occurring periods, should be seen as a biological advantage, since, if properly understood, developed, and utilized, they can lead to considerable clarity and insight. It needs, then, to be made clear that many contemporary discussions of the changes women experience during the premenstrual period, as well as the collective name for these changes (*premenstrual syndrome*), medicalize women's bodies and experience and reassert the view that women are by their very nature diseased and therefore defective. And it needs to be emphasized that these discussions, despite their appearance of using objective, value-neutral descriptions, uncritically put forward an *interpretation* of the basic states women experience during the premenstrual period, an interpretation which reads malady into the very descriptions of these states and which has no special claim to being worthy of acceptance as objectively valid.

Finally, those who believe that women cannot be trusted in positions of high power because of the likelihood that they will make poor decisions can only feel justified if they simply ignore the many poor decisions made by men which have too frequently resulted in unjust and irrational wars, political scandals, and, in this age of insider trading, business activities based on incomprehensible greed.

GAMETE TRANSPORT

Following ejaculation by the male and ovulation by the female, a complex series of gamete-transporting events within the female reproductive tract must occur if fertilization is to be achieved. Interference with the effectiveness of these events is one way to prevent pregnancy.

*Sperm Transport*   Delivery of the ejaculate entails that previously the male experienced sexual excitement and there occurred erection of the penis and ejaculation. In contrast, ovulation is essentially disassociated from sexual excitement. The normal site of semen deposition in women (at least if pregnancy is likely to result from the deposition) is in the posterior portion of the vagina at or near the cervix. The ejaculate will normally contain approximately 200–500 million sperm. This population will immediately begin to undergo attrition, with a reducing number of sperm remaining alive as they move from the vagina into and through the cervix, through the uterus, out of the uterus and into the isthmus of the oviduct via the tubo–uterine junction, and finally into the lower ampullary region of the oviduct, where fertilization occurs. It is likely that only about 200 of the initial millions of sperm ever make it to the site of fertilization — an enormously wasteful system.

Sperm are ejaculated within seminal plasma that has a pH of 7.2–7.8; the vagina has an acidic pH of about 5.7 (Harper 1982). The sperm deteriorate rapidly in this hostile environment and within two to six hours most become nonmotile (Miller and Kurzrak 1932). Human semen coagulates almost immediately after ejaculation and liquefies within five to twenty minutes (Mastroianni and Zausner 1981). Sperm are released during liquefaction and the contractions of the vaginal wall can cause a proportion of them to come into contact with cervical mucus and thus ascend into the cervix. Some sperm are propelled directly into the cervix at ejaculation, as evidenced by the fact that living, motile sperm have been observed in the cervical mucus within one or two minutes after ejaculation (Sobrero and McLeod 1962) and found in the oviduct (Fallopian tube) within five minutes (Harper 1982). These sperm may undergo capacitation and later be transported to the normal site of fertilization in the oviducts, and this is why vaginal douches are such an unreliable method of contraception.

Three stages of sperm transport within the female tract have been described: (1) rapid, short transport; (2) colonization of cervical reservoirs; and (3) slow, prolonged release of sperm (Hafez 1978). Those sperm transported rapidly through the cervix and uterus are not likely to achieve fertilization, because they have not had sufficient time to undergo the process of capacitation. Sperm capacitation involves a series of morphological, physiological, and biochemical changes which a spermatozoon must undergo within the female reproductive tract before it is fully capable of fertilizing an egg. The cervical crypts and, secondarily, the tubo–uterine junction serve as the major sperm reservoirs. After adequate reservoirs are established, the sperm are released sequentially to the site of fertilization. This slow release, which relies (in small part) on the intrinsic motility of the sperm and (in large part) on the contractile activity of the muscles of the uterus and oviduct, continues for several hours after semen deposition until the reservoir is depleted.

It should be pointed out that, contrary to popular belief, sperm do not reach the egg by "swimming" there from the site of deposition. As we have already seen, some sperm appear in the oviducts within minutes and the majority within one to one and a half hours. Human sperm can swim at a rate of roughly one inch or less per hour (Forsyth 1986). Even assuming that sperm could maintain that pace indefinitely (which they cannot, because of inadequate energy reserves), it would take them six to eight hours or more to cover the anatomical distance between the sites of deposition and the site of fertilization. Additional evidence that inherent sperm motility plays (at most) a secondary role in sperm transport is that dead sperm and inert particles are transported from the vagina to the oviduct at roughly the same rate as are live sperm (Eli and Newton 1961; DeBoer 1972). It is the contractile activity of the female reproductive tract, perhaps aided by prostaglandin $F_{2\alpha}$ present in the semen, which is most responsible for sperm transport. Motility of sperm becomes crucial only after they reach the site of fertilization, since sperm must be motile in order to penetrate the various layers of the egg and achieve fertilization.

The cervix is a safe haven that the sperm must quickly arrive at following vaginal deposition. It provides protection for sperm from the hostile environment of the vagina and provides supplemental nutrients to meet their energy requirements. The endocrine changes just prior to ovulation create optimum conditions for sperm transport by increasing the quantity and decreasing the viscosity of cervical mucus. The cervical mucus tends to direct spermatozoa into the uterus and into the cervical crypts where they are stored. Conditions are less favorable at other times during the menstrual cycle, and hence sperm transport is most efficient at midcycle. (The cervix also serves as a filter for the removal of morphologically abnormal sperm, although it is not well understood how the filtering is accomplished.)

Sperm transport through the uterus is fairly rapid, due largely to the efficient contractions of the smooth muscles which compose the myometrium. This contractility is also dependent upon an estrogenic background (as exists at ovulation) and on direct stimulation by oxytocin (which is released from the posterior pituitary) and prostaglandin $F_{2a}$ (which is produced locally by the endometrium and is present in semen). Settlage et al. (1973) showed that between four and fifty-three spermatozoa per oviduct could be found in women within five to forty-five minutes after deposition of semen onto the external opening of the cervix by artificial insemination.

As we have seen, in comparison to the cervix, the uterine environment is relatively hostile to sperm. Large numbers of leukocytes appear in the uterus within ten to twenty-four hours after sperm enter, and sperm that have not been transported through the uterus to the oviducts begin to be removed by phagocytosis. Perhaps it should be mentioned that a woman's immunological system responds to sperm as a "foreign" protein. Thus, her body responds by killing these cells, much as it would respond to bacteria or a tissue graft from an unrelated individual. This is the main reason why although millions of sperm cells are released in an ejaculate, only a couple of hundred are able to arrive safely at the point of fertilization. Increasing the efficiency of sperm phagocytosis is thus another means of birth control, and it is one of several modes of action of IUDs.

The tubo-uterine junction acts as a selective barrier to sperm transport and prevents entry of nonmotile sperm. Once through the tubo-uterine junction, sperm may remain for several hours during the preovulatory phase, moving up to the site of fertilization about the time of ovulation. Sperm in the upper regions of the oviduct are much more active and have vigorously lashing tails, which is thought to be important in aiding sperm penetration through the various layers of the egg. Muscular activity of the myosalpinx (the oviduct muscle) aids in moving sperm upwards from the isthmus and ensures adequate mixing of tubal contents, thus enhancing the chances of a spermatozoon meeting the ovum (Harper 1982).

It is generally reported that human sperm are capable of fertilization 24 to 48 hours after intercourse; should ovulation occur at any time immediately preceding or during this interval, fertilization is likely (Hafez 1978; Harper 1982). However, as we mentioned in Chapter 1, motile sperm have been recovered from the cervix as long as 205 hours after insemination (Insler et al. 1980).

*Ovum Transport*    At ovulation, the fimbria of the oviduct is in close contact with the ovary to aid in "sweeping" or "picking up" the ovum from the surface of the ovary. When shed, the egg still has surrounding it two layers of granulosa cells: the corona radiata (immediately outside the zona pellucida) and the cumulus oophorus. The pickup of the egg is aided by the presence of these outer investments, since they provide a larger surface area for the cilia of the fimbria to grab. Vigorous contractions of the mesovarium and mesosalpinx, the supporting structures of the ovary and oviduct respectively, also aid the pickup of the egg. Once into the infundibular portion of the oviduct, the egg is rapidly funnelled into the ampulla and on down to the ampullary-isthmic junction. Both the infundibulum and ampulla are highly ciliated, with the cilia beating toward the site of fertilization. Movement is also aided by the wavelike contractions of the circular muscle of the ampulla. Following ovulation, the ovum has a finite fertilization life span of twelve to twenty-four hours (Hafez 1978).

FERTILIZATION

Fertilization, the union of the sperm nucleus and the nucleus of the ovum, involves three critical events: (1) passage of the sperm through the granulosa cell layers (cumulus oophorus and corona radiata) surrounding the ovum, (2) sperm attachment and migration through the zona pellucida, and (3) fusion of sperm and ovum plasma membranes.

During the course of sperm capacitation within the female tract, the plasma membrane and the outer acrosomal membrane (which covers the head of the sperm) fuse at a number of discrete points. Fusion leads rapidly to the formation of small apertures leading into the cavity of the acrosome, thus providing an exit for acrosomal contents. Contained within the acrosome and released by the sperm as it attempts to penetrate the egg is an enzyme called *hyaluronidase.* Hyaluronidase dissolves the jellylike substance holding together the cells which surround the ovum, thus allowing passage of the sperm through them and down to the zona pellucida. A second sperm enzyme, acrosin, which adheres to the inner portion of the acrosomal membrane, allows the sperm to penetrate through this thick glycoprotein membrane and reach the inner membrane of the egg, the vitelline membrane, to which the sperm then attaches. Membrane fusion between the two gametes is rapidly succeeded by perforation so that the membranes of the two cells become continuous and it is impossible to say where one begins and the other one ends. Soon after passage of the head of the sperm into the egg cytoplasm, the tail is shed and the nucleus in the head forms into a structure called the *male pronucleus*. The nucleus of the ovum develops into the corresponding female pronucleus. Each of these nuclei are haploid, containing twenty-three chromosomes bearing the genetic material of the corresponding parent. The nuclei rapidly move together and fuse (in a process termed *syngamy*) to restore the diploid number and the forty-six paired chromosomes characteristic of humans. The single-cell fertilized ovum is now referred to as a *zygote*.

Although any of the sperm which survived the trek to the site of fertilization may begin the process of fertilization, only one will succeed in completing the process. With passage of the first spermatozoon through the zona pellucida, the zona undergoes an immediate chemical change which renders it impenetrable to other spermatozoa. Although this change (the zona reaction) is usually highly effective in humans, there is a second line of defense, the vitelline block, which also minimizes the possibility that a second sperm could attach to the vitellus after the first one has done so.

EARLY DEVELOPMENT AND IMPLANTATION
OF THE CONCEPTUS

Immediately after fertilization, the zygote begins cleavage, a process of rapid cell division. Cleavage consists of cellular division without growth; thus with each progressive division, from two cells to four cells to eight cells, and so on, each of the cells (blastomeres) becomes smaller. The zona pellucida still surrounds the dividing cells and limits the size of the conceptus. Once the conceptus has reached the sixteen- to thirty-two-cell stage, it is referred to as a *morula* (because of its resemblance to a mulberry). In humans, the conceptus progresses to the morula stage while still within the oviduct, a process which requires approximately two or three days (McLauren 1982). Developmental requirements of the conceptus change as it progresses through these early stages. Therefore, either delaying or accelerating entry of the conceptus into the uterus is a potential means of birth control.

As the morula descends into the uterus on day 3 or 4, the blastomeres continue to divide and rearrange themselves into a hollow ball. The cavity which forms within the blastomeres is called a *blastocoel* and the conceptus is now called a *blastocyst*. Two distinct portions of the conceptus can now be identified: (1) an outer flattened layer of cells, the trophoblast, which will give rise to the chorionic portion of the placenta, and (2) an inner mass of tightly compacted cells, the inner cell mass, which will develop into the embryo.

Once the blastocyst stage has been reached, a sequence of changes begins in the uterus and in the conceptus that finally results in implantation. First, the blastocyst must "hatch" from the zona pellucida which surrounds it. The zona pellucida has been protecting the conceptus from leucocytic attack and premature attachment to the oviductal epithelium (Renfree 1982). While within the zona, the conceptus is electrostatically uncharged. Once the blastocyst emerges from the zona, it becomes negatively charged and very sticky. Recall that at this point in the menstrual cycle (about seven days postovulation or midluteal phase) the endometrium is a succulent, spongy bed awaiting the conceptus. Following shedding of the zona pellucida, the blastocyst adheres to the endometrium and the trophoblastic cells secrete an enzyme which enables the blastocyst to literally eat a hole in the luscious endometrium and become completely buried within it. The portion of the endometrium to which the blastocyst attaches and in which it becomes implanted, which is usually on the posterior wall of the fundus, is called the *decidua functionalis layer*. The erosive implantation allows the blastocyst to readily absorb nutrients from the endometrial glands and blood vessels. The trophoblastic cells of the conceptus also begin to secrete hCG almost immediately following implantation. As we have already seen, hCG serves to stimulate the corpus luteum to continue producing progesterone, which maintains the pregnancy.

Shortly after implantation, the inner cell mass differentiates into three specialized layers of cells (the primary germ layers): the ectoderm, endoderm, and mesoderm. The ectoderm will ultimately form all neural tissue, plus the epidermis of the skin and the receptor cells of sense organs; the endoderm will form the epithelium of various organs and glands; and the mesoderm will form bone, cartilage, and muscle.

## HORMONAL REQUIREMENTS FOR PREGNANCY MAINTENANCE

The corpus luteum is normally maintained until about the fourth month of pregnancy and continues to serve as the primary source of progesterone during most of this time. As already described, hCG is responsible for maintenance of the corpus luteum and the continuation of the progesterone (and estradiol) needed to maintain endometrial secretions. Production of hCG peaks during the middle of the third month of pregnancy and then declines as pregnancy continues (Tortora and Evans 1986). By the end of the second month of pregnancy, the placenta begins to secrete progesterone and estrogens (especially primate-specific estriol, $E_3$). The corpus luteum then regresses and hormones from the developing fetus and placenta assume a prominent role in preparing the woman's body for parturition (birth) and lactation.

.   .   .   .   .   .

Although much more could be said about human reproductive physiology and endocrinology, the information in this chapter and the previous one should be sufficient for a clear understanding of the birth control methodologies which concern us. We turn next to an account of those methodologies, which include true contraceptive techniques (Chapter 5) and techniques which involve birth control intervention after conception (Chapter 6).

# 5
# Contemporary Contraceptive Technologies for Women

## INTRODUCTION

The scientific and popular literature on the subject of birth control is a veritable jungle of semantical conflicts and confusions. For example, some reporters use the terms *birth control* and *contraception* interchangeably. Others describe "contraceptives" which work by preventing implantation—a contradiction in terms. Therefore, for the sake of general clarity and for a clear understanding of our use of the relevant language through the remainder of this book, we need to define a few terms.

In our vernacular, *birth control* is a generic term referring to any means of preventing birth; hence, it is appropriate for referring to any approach to preventing birth from abstinence to abortion.[1] *Contraceptive* (meaning against conception) refers to any method of birth control which has as its *primary* mode of action preventing fertilization. Contraceptives include the "natural" methods (e.g., abstinence, coitus interruptus, rhythm methods), barriers (e.g., condoms, diaphragms), spermicides, and chemical methods (e.g., oral contraceptives, long-acting steroidal implants, Gn-RH analogues). In contrast, other birth control methods routinely allow fertilization but prevent successful implantation of the conceptus. These methods are referred to by some medical practitioners as *interceptives*, since they are held to intercept, rather than terminate, a pregnancy. (We shall discuss this usage in a moment.) Still other methods act after implantation of the conceptus, though generally so early after conception that it is not known whether the woman using the method has conceived. These are universally called *abortifacient*

---

[1] See also the distinction between birth control and population control in Chapters 2 and 9.

techniques. Finally, there are methods which involve deliberate termination of a known pregnancy. These are commonly known as *induced abortion* techniques.

The distinction between so-called interceptive methods and abortifacient and induced abortion methods is taken by some to be a morally crucial one. In medical practice, it is common to understand pregnancy as commencing, not at conception, but at implantation. A fact we mentioned in Chapter 4 is taken to support the view that pregnancy begins at implantation rather than at fertilization, namely, that prior to implantation, the tissues of the conceptus are not yet differentiated into those that will give rise to the placenta and those that will give rise to the embryo. Thus, it is held that prior to implantation there is not yet even an early embryo. The moral implication of these considerations is taken to be that the effect of utilizing a birth control method which acts after conception but prior to implantation is not to be understood as abortion.

These biological facts and this line of reasoning are interesting. In particular, the fact that the very early conceptus does not contain even the differentiated precursor cells of an embryo may well explain the view of many people that what is commonly understood as very early abortion is morally acceptable but later abortion is not. It also needs to be emphasized, however, that people with this view do commonly understand pregnancy to commence with conception. And this ordinary understanding of pregnancy as beginning at fertilization informs the contemporary abortion debate, which cannot be settled by appealing to a technical definition of *pregnancy* or by simply pointing out that prior to implantation the embryo itself has not yet begun to develop. Those who oppose destroying at any point after conception what they understand to be a developing human being typically take as morally crucial the fact that the life of a unique human being begins at fertilization, and hence they hold that any intervention destructive of that life counts as aborting that life and, if done for reasons other than saving the life of the woman, is gravely morally wrong. We shall examine the central argument for this view in Chapter 7. For now, we mean merely to clarify the language we shall be using and our reason for adopting it.

Having acknowledged the factual distinction between so-called interceptives and other methods which act after implantation and also having acknowledged the distinction between the technical and ordinary notions of when pregnancy should be understood to mence, we nonetheless shall follow ordinary usage. That is, w take pregnancy to begin at conception, and we shall und abortifacients to include all those methods which act after conception, distinguishing these from contraceptive methods and from methods of induced abortion, as characterized earlier. We elect adoption of ordinary usage and the ordinary concept of pregnancy to avoid what might reasonably be interpreted as an attempt to dismiss the moral concerns of those who oppose destroying even the very early conceptus by appealing to technical language and to distinctions which they believe make no moral difference in the evaluation of birth control methods applied after conception.

Distinguishing between true contraceptive and abortifacient birth control methods is a matter of considerable importance to a large number of men and women. While many people have no moral objection to preventing conception, they find the termination of a human life,[2] once begun at fertilization, to be morally objectionable. Because of this, it is important to realize that even though the conceptual distinction between contraceptive and abortifacient methods is clear, in fact, for any individual in any given cycle effective birth control by use of a contraceptive may have been due to a secondary mode of action which allows conception rather than the primary mode of action of the method employed. For example, and as we shall see in more detail shortly, oral contraceptives generally prevent ovulation, but occasionally "breakthrough" ovulation may occur and fertilization may result. However, pregnancy may fail as a result of other alterations in the reproductive tract caused by the oral contraceptives. Likewise, IUDs may disrupt sperm transport and survival, thereby preventing fertilization. However, in many cycles fertilization does occur in IUD users, but survival and implantation of the conceptus is prevented by the hostile uterine environment created by the IUD. In each example, there is just no way for a woman to know which mode of action (i.e., contraceptive or abortifacient) was the effective one. She knows only that her menstrual cycle recurred when expected. No doubt, with the onset of menses many women assume that they did not conceive during the preceding month. However, it may be that conception indeed occurred but

---

[2] In Chapter 7, we shall point out some problems with using the term *human life* in this context.

that the conceptus was interfered with prior to implantation; as a result, the corpus luteum was not maintained to prevent the onset of the next menstrual period (see Chapter 4).

The physiological mechanisms underlying the effectiveness of commonly used methods such as the pill and the IUD are not always clear to women using them. Likewise, the physiological processes employed by some newly developed birth control methods, such as RU-486 and the "antipregnancy vaccine," may not be fully understood by many women considering using them. In this chapter and the next, we shall give a detailed description of the actions of existing and emerging birth control methods. As will become apparent, many of these are more appropriately classified as abortifacient methods than as contraceptive methods, and the moral acceptability of using these methods is an important but often-ignored component of the abortion issue, which we shall take up in Chapter 7.

ORAL CONTRACEPTIVES

The historical development of oral contraceptives (OCs) is briefly chronicled in Chapter 1. Previously approved for treatment of menstrual disorders and threatened spontaneous abortion, G. D. Searle's Enovid was the first product approved by the Food and Drug Administration (FDA) for contraceptive purposes (Diczfalusy 1979, 1982). This occurred in June 1960, and other pharmaceutical companies quickly rushed their products onto the market. Within two years, some two million American women were on the pill (Sloane 1980). By 1965, it was reported that nearly one-third of all American women who used contraception had at some time taken OCs (Westoff and Ryder 1967). Between 1965 and 1970, the number of American women using OCs doubled to almost nine million (Goldzieher 1970). Use of the pill peaked and leveled off in the early 1970s, and in response to increased reports about its potential hazards, use temporarily decreased in the mid-1970s. Accurate estimation of OC use is tricky, since overall figures can be misleading. For example, Westoff and Jones (1977) reported that in 1975, 34.3 percent of all married women practicing contraception used OCs. However, for women married less than five years, the pill was used by 64.8 percent. Sloane (1980) estimated that by 1980, between 10 and 15 million American women and between 80 and 100 million women worldwide were relying on OCs for birth control. Recent estimates suggest that OC use has again leveled off (Wilbur 1986).

In light of our earlier discussion of the limited contraceptive options available prior to 1960, it is easy to understand the rapid adoption of the pill and the role which it has played in the sexual liberation of women. With the advent of the pill, women finally had a simple, neat, tidy, and highly effective way to avoid unwanted pregnancy. No longer did women have to carry awkward and embarrassing birth control devices, such as diaphragms and tubes of jelly, or rely on the conscientiousness of their partners to provide protection. Especially for unmarried women, the previously unavailable freedom to enjoy a spontaneous sexual encounter without the usual fear of unwanted pregnancy gave women an approximation of procreational sexual equality with men, and it clearly contributed to the "sexual revolution." The pill has enriched the sex lives of millions of women and men in a measure which could not even be imagined three decades ago.

## Types of Oral Contraceptives

Perhaps partly because of the continued use of the term *the pill*, oral contraceptives tend to be erroneously thought of as being a single preparation. But there are actually dozens of different formulations which vary in type of synthetic steroid used, relative quantity of steroid, overall potency, potential side effects, and relative contraceptive effectiveness. Numerous pharmaceutical companies market OCs, and most distribute several formulations. A number of publications provide tables listing specific brand names, manufacturers, formulations, potency, and so on (e.g., Hafez 1978; Mishell 1979; Sloane 1980; Porter, Waife, and Haltrop 1983; Henzl 1986). Potential complications and adverse side effects of OC usage can be minimized if care is taken in selecting the pill formulation that is most suitable for each particular woman based on her age, overall medical history, menstrual history, physical condition, behavioral and health habits, and other individuating factors.

There are two major types of OCs currently in use: (1) the combination pill, which is by far the most widely used and most effective, and (2) the minipill, which contains only a low dose of progestagen taken daily, even during menstruation. Originally there was a third type of OC, the sequential pill, which consisted solely of estrogen taken for fourteen to sixteen days, followed by five or six days of an estrogen-progestagen combination. Sequential pills were removed from the U.S. and other markets in 1975 because of their relatively high failure rate and their link to an increased incidence of uterine cancer (Mishell 1979; Sloane 1980; Henzl 1986). Since combination pills are by far the most common type of OC, our discussion will focus on them.

Combination pills contain varying dosages of two main types of synthetic hormones, one that mimics progesterone (called a *progestagen*) and one that is a derivative of estrogen. Synthetic steroids are used rather than naturally occurring progesterone and estrogen, because the natural products would be rapidly inactivated by the body if taken orally. (Publications containing the tabular information on specific brands and formulations of OCs provide information on the specific synthetic hormones used in the various brands.) There are only two types of estrogen used in OCs, ethinyl estradiol and one of its derivatives, mestranol. There are over thirty formulations of combination pills, which use several different progestagens, the most common being norethindrone. All progestagens used in OCs have some degree of androgenic activity (see Chapter 4). Some progestagen derivatives may be weakly estrogenic and androgenic at low doses but can become relatively anti-estrogenic at high doses (Mishell 1979; Sloane 1980). Both so-called minor and major side effects are related to differences in various hormonal activities in different pills and their interactions within each individual woman.

When OCs were first introduced in 1960, it was thought that hormone levels had to be as high as those in pregnancy in order to provide maximum contraceptive effectiveness. While short-term effects of OCs were examined prior to marketing, it was not known what the long-term effects of these high levels of synthetic steroids might be. By 1970, evidence linking OCs with increased statistical risk of cardiovascular disease, stroke, and assorted other diseases began to accumulate. These links were initially made in women who began using the exceptionally high dose pills in the early 1960s. Soon after the first OCs began to be marketed, researchers began an investigative trend (which continues to the present day) of decreasing the hormonal components of the combination to make the pill safer. Today, OCs contain as little as 4 percent of the progestagen and 20 percent of the estrogen found in the original formulations

(Wilbur 1986). Thus women who begin using OCs today face far fewer health risks than did women who began using them in the 1960s.

The combination preparations in current use are commonly classified into two categories according to their daily estrogen content: (1) 50 $\mu$g, and (2) less than 50 $\mu$g. A third category, more than 50 $\mu$g, was removed from the U.S. market in early 1988. As a general rule, the lower-dose estrogen OCs decrease circulatory side effects, but breakthrough bleeding (i.e., intermenstrual bleeding or spotting) is more of a problem. Contraceptive efficacy does not appear to be significantly affected by reduction of the estrogen dose to as little as 35 $\mu$g (Henzl 1986).

The most recent development in the quest for a safer oral contraceptive which employs a minimal steroid dosage without sacrificing effectiveness is the triphasic pill. It is a sub-50 $\mu$g estrogen combination pill which contains 40 percent less progestagen than other pills. Triphasics contain the progestagens norgestrel or desogestrel, which are said to be more specific progestagens with less androgenic side effects (Schijf et al. 1984). The triphasic pill is so named because it employs three levels of steroids during the menstrual cycle, with an increasing level of hormones as the month progresses. For example, one commercially available product contains 50 $\mu$g norgestrel and 30 $\mu$g ethinyl estradiol (EE) for six days; 75 $\mu$g norgestrel and 40 $\mu$g EE for five days; and 125 $\mu$g norgestrel and 30 $\mu$g EE for the remaining ten days (Ratnam and Prasad 1984). The rationale behind this mixture is to mimic the hormonal changes of the normal cycle while providing the minimal effective dosage. While all types of OCs function best when taken regularly and according to schedule, it is especially critical that the sequence be followed precisely by women employing the triphasic pill, since, unlike regular combination pills, the dosage may vary from day to day.

Pills are normally provided in packages of twenty-one. With the exception of the triphasic pills mentioned above, all in the package are identical. Ordinarily, one pill is consumed daily from the fifth through the twenty-fifth day of the cycle. Some preparations are prepared in twenty-eight-day packages. The additional seven pills are placebo (blank) or iron pills, included so that one does not get out of the habit of taking a pill daily. It is recommended that the pill be taken each day at the same time (e.g., upon arising or before going to bed) to help minimize the fluctuations in the level of hormones in the systemic circulation. Generally, missing one pill does not increase the likelihood of conceiving, since the residual level of steroids remaining in the body is probably sufficient to continue a woman's protection. However, if a pill is missed, it is commonly recommended that two be taken the next day. If two or more pills are missed, it becomes much more of an "iffy" situation and prudence dictates employing an alternate form of contraception for the duration of that menstrual cycle. Most of the small percentage of pregnancies which have been reported to occur in users of OCs are not due to failure of the pill but rather to improper use.

### Mechanisms of Action of Oral Contraceptives

The extremely high rate of efficacy of the combination pill (a failure rate of only 0.3–0.5 percent, surpassed only by abstinence and sterilization) is due to its interference with reproductive processes on several levels. While the primary mode of action of OCs is the prevention of ovulation, they also provide backup systems which may effectively impair sperm transport, sperm capacitation, ovum transport, zygote transport, oviductal secretions, endometrial proliferation and secretory activity, and implantation. In short, the pill is highly effective because it covers all the bases.

The combination estrogen and progestagen pills suppress the production and release of Gn-RH by the hypothalamus and decrease the sensitivity of the anterior pituitary. The net result of these actions is the inhibition of FSH and LH synthesis and release by the anterior pituitary (see Chapter 4). The midcycle peak of gonadotropins that normally leads to ovulation in an unregulated menstrual cycle (see Figure 10 in Chapter 4) simply does not occur; therefore, no ovulation occurs. Although follicular growth does begin in a woman on the combination pill during her one-week break from daily consumption, when she resumes consumption of the pill on day 5, continued follicular development is blocked and the follicles undergo atresia. Generally, women on combination pills never develop mature Graafian follicles, never ovulate, and hence never form a corpus luteum or a corpus albicans (see Chapter 4). Endocrinologically, their ovaries resemble those of postmenopausal women. The progestagen-only minipills usually do not block ovulation; therefore, they are more dependent on the mechanisms described below for their contraceptive action. Predictably, the failure rate is greater for progestagen–only pills (2 percent) than for combination pills (0.5 percent) (Henzl, 1986).

Under normal conditions, it is ovarian production of estradiol and progesterone (see Chapter 4) and the ever–changing ratio of these two steroids that regulates the cyclical changes in the rest of the female reproductive tract and produces conditions optimal for conception. Due to the steady hormone level provided by the pill at a time which is "out of synch" with normal menstrual cycle events, assorted structural and biochemical changes are induced throughout the reproductive tract. For example, the physical and chemical characteristics of cervical mucus are altered by ocs. Rather than becoming watery and stringy to aid sperm transport, under the influence of ocs, cervical mucus remains thick, viscid, and difficult for sperm to penetrate. Furthermore, such alterations in reproductive tract secretions inhibit sperm capacitation. And if ovulation does occur, ovum transport from the oviduct into the uterus is also accelerated under the influence of ocs. This means that the ovum may be propelled into the uterus before it is fertilized or, if fertilized, transported into the uterus too soon for continued development of the conceptus. Additionally, altered oviductal secretions may be incapable of nourishing and sustaining early development of the conceptus even if it remains in the oviduct. Finally, even if ovulation, fertilization, and early development of the conceptus in the oviduct should have occurred, ocs also profoundly alter the structure of the endometrium such that continued development and implantation is highly unlikely. Under the influence of ocs, endometrial height is low and the glands are narrow, poorly developed, and incapable of producing the products required for nourishment and implantation of the conceptus.

Following completion of a twenty–one–day sequence of pills (day 25 of a cycle), similar physiological events transpire as normally occur following corpus luteum regression. As the steroids are cleared from the woman's system, endometrial shrinkage, sloughing, and bleeding occur in a fashion analogous to that described for a normal menstrual cycle (see Chapter 4). A major difference, however, is that the extent of endometrial proliferation and vascularization is considerably less under the influence of ocs. Therefore, the amount of blood loss and the duration of the menstrual period is considerably reduced in pill users. Menstrual cramps and symptoms of PMS (see Chapter 4) are also generally reduced by the pill (Sloane 1980; Porter, Waife, and Haltrop 1983; Henzl 1986).

There are no clearly established medical benefits derived from the menstruation induced by discontinuing ingestion of the pill for a week in the cycle. Some women, however, feel more natural and comfortable about pill usage by having a menstruation every twenty-eight days. If a woman should want to avoid menstruation for any particular reason, all she has to do is to continue to take active pills and menstruation will remain suspended, although some break-through bleeding may occur.

## Side Effects of Oral Contraceptives

The brochure insert which accompanies every package of OCs warns of more than 50 possible side effects. These range from the merely unpleasant to the downright fatal. However, to avoid undue alarm, several points need to be kept in mind.

As Djerassi (1981) points out, drug manufacturers and regulatory agencies often protect themselves by emphasizing the negative. One function of package inserts is providing legal protection for the manufacturer by letting a producer claim that every potential risk of a product has been pointed out to consumers. It is, of course, important that women be aware of the risks they assume in taking OCs. But if the concern is genuinely to allow informed consent, it would be far more helpful if statistics were included in these inserts, which would let women know the probabilities of their encountering some of the potential adverse effects mentioned. We shall see in Chapter 8 that some common warnings printed in package inserts have no sound scientific support.

Also, much of the warning is aimed toward women who have predisposing conditions that contraindicate OC usage, for example, a history of blood clotting disorders, coronary artery disease, estrogen-dependent malignancies, or liver damage. Additional precautions pertain to some women who probably should be advised not to use OCs because of their family histories, age, health, or behavioral habits (such as cigarette smoking). For women who do not fall into either of these categories, the risks of contemporary OC usage are really quite modest.

Additionally, many of the risk factors described are based on older studies that involved higher doses than are contained in many of the newer OCs (Astedt 1982). Realistic risk assessment is also complicated by the fact that many of the studies used to make recommendations concerning OC usage were conducted using various animal models and hence their results may or may not be appropriate to extrapolate to women (Holmes and Fox 1979).

With these caveats in mind, let's examine the potential side effects of the pill. So-called minor side effects may include weight gain, gum inflammation, nausea, headaches, breast tenderness, increased urinary tract infections, vaginitis, chloasma (facial skin pigmentation or "giant freckles"), menstrual spotting, and libido changes. Classifying these effects as "minor" is, of course, a relative matter. They may be minor to a physician or even to most women but may nevertheless be serious problems for certain individuals.

The association between OCs and these side effects is discussed in numerous reviews, including Connell (1978), Edwards (1980), Sloane (1980), Porter, Waife, and Haltrop (1983), Boston Women's Health Book Collective (1984), Henzl (1986), and Stadel (1986). There is no consensus as to the specific relationship between these maladies and OC usage. Since most of the so-called minor side effects may also be caused by myriad other factors, it is often difficult, if not impossible, to confidently attribute the occurrence of the malady to such usage.

Irritability, anxiety, depression, changes in libido, and headaches are symptoms often linked to OC usage. These symptoms may be due to the effects of OCs on metabolism of the amino acid tryptophan. Theurer and Vitale (1977) reported that Vitamin $B_6$ (pyridoxine), which is manufactured from tryptophan, is depleted in 80 percent of pill users and absolutely deficient in the other 20 percent. More recently, Henzl (1986) has theorized that the estrogenic component of the pill reduces the formation of the neurotransmitter serotonin in brain tissue. Tryptophan is the precursor for the production of serotonin. Serotonin has been associated with mood changes and depression. These effects may be eliminated, or at least reduced, by use of a vitamin-mineral supplement.

Although some sources (e.g., Boston Women's Health Book Collective 1984) have linked OCs with decreased libido, increased difficulty in achieving orgasm, and decreased sensation in the vulva, it should be noted, as pointed out by Masters, Johnson, and Kolodny (1986), that evaluating the effects of OCs on sexuality is tricky for a number of reasons. Older research on the negative sexual effects of the high-dose pill is not supported by more recent research examining lower-dose formulations (Porter, Waife, and Haltrop 1983; Henzl 1986; Masters, Johnson, and Kolodny 1986). Furthermore, in women and men sexual desire and fulfillment are more psychological than biological. For example, if a woman expects diminished sexual desire while on the pill, she is likely to experience diminished desire. Is she feels guilt because use of the pill conflicts with her religious beliefs or with her desire to become pregnant, she may attribute a negative sexual response to the pill. Also, there are at least as many women who ascribe to the pill improved sexual interest and enjoyment as women who ascribe to it reduced sexual interest and enjoyment. The psychological security of a very low pregnancy risk plus the sexual spontaneity afforded by the pill are likely to be the basis of this response. According to Masters, Johnson, and Kolodny (1986), most women using OCs today do not report any significant changes in sexual interest, behavior, or enjoyment. Approximately 10 percent report improved sexuality, with an equal percentage noting decreased sexual interest or responsiveness.

Side effects are most frequent in the first treatment cycle. Since OCs may provide a woman's body with a balance of estrogen and progestagen differing from what she was accustomed to from endogenous production, a brief period of adjustment to these new levels is required. Porter, Waife, and Haltrop (1983) indicated that one symptom or another usually occurs in about 25 percent of pill users during the first cycle, but the symptoms diminish rapidly so that only about 5 percent experience any side effects after three cycles of pill use. It is important to realize that in many cases, use of OCs may activate a latent condition — in much the same way that pregnancy may trigger a condition (e.g., diabetes) to which a woman is predisposed. Since OCs introduce a physical condition that is in many ways analogous to pregnancy, they challenge the body's physiological systems. In some women, some systems are unable to adapt to this challenge, others are only slightly affected, and still others are virtually unaffected.

The earliest and most serious side effects to be linked to the pill involve vascular problems. Oral contraceptives have been shown to affect clotting factors in blood and to produce alterations in blood vessel walls, creating an increased risk of pulmonary embolism, cerebral thrombotic stroke, and cerebral hemorrhagic stroke. OC users have been reported to be four to eleven times more likely to develop

these conditions (Sloane 1980). Hypertension, chances of a fatal myocardial infarction (heart attack), and high blood pressure have also
been linked to OC usage. Cigarette smoking greatly compounds the
risks of OC usage. For example, epidemiologist Howard Ory (1977)
reported that 1 of every 10,000 women between thirty and thirty-
nine years old who both used OCs and smoked will have a fatal
heart attack each year. For pill users of that age group who did not
smoke, the rate was 1 out of 50,000; in nonsmokers and nonpill users
it was 1 out of 100,000. Shapiro et al. (1979) estimated that smoking
enhances the risk of heart attack in OC users twenty- to fortyfold.
Risk of elevated blood pressure in OC users is also greatly enhanced
by cigarette smoking. There is more than adequate evidence indicating that smoking and OC usage is a potentially dangerous combination.

Additional side effects of OCs include the following: (1) alterations in carbohydrate metabolism, as evidenced by an impairment
of glucose tolerance and increased plasma insulin levels; (2) altered
lipid metabolism, as indicated by an elevation in certain serum lipids
(which could be a predisposing factor for heart disease); (3) increased
incidence of abnormalities of liver function; and (4) increased incidence of gallbladder inflammation and gallstones (e.g., Connell 1978;
Mishell 1979).

As we have just pointed out, OCs can precipitate conditions in
some women who have predispositions to those conditions, and
thus certain women should either not use OCs at all or should be
extremely cautious in using them and do so only under careful monitoring. Predisposing factors that militate against OC usage include
many circulatory or cardiovascular problems, for example, venous
thrombosis (an abnormal blood clot that forms in an unbroken blood
vessel), phlebitis (inflammation in a vein caused by a thrombus),
embolism (a "traveling blood clot" which can block blood flow to a
major organ), poor circulation (which may be exacerbated by smoking), high blood pressure, and a history of heart disease or a heart
defect. All of these conditions are further exacerbated by obesity.
Estrogen is generally blamed for venous complications, while arterial complications have been attributed to the progestagen component of OCs (Porter, Waife, and Haltrop 1983). Estrogens have also
specifically been shown to increase blood levels of several pro-
coagulant and fibrinolytic (blood clotting) system components
(Ambrus et al. 1970). Contemporary lower-steroid-dose formula-

tions substantially decrease these risk factors. Estrogens have also been shown to increase serum levels of high-density lipoproteins (HDL), while progestagens decrease them. Although an unequivocal link between the blood level of HDL, OC use, and cardiovascular disease has not been established, epidemiologic evidence indicates a general inverse relationship between HDL levels and coronary artery disease. Some estrogen regimens, such as those prescribed for postmenopausal women, *may* reduce the risk of coronary artery disease as a result of this salutary effect, but this has not been established. General statements concerning the effects of OCs on HDL levels cannot be made, because, as we have just seen, estrogens have been shown to increase HDL serum levels whereas progestagens decrease them. In users of various combination OCs, HDL levels varied with the type and level of the component steroids (Bradley et al. 1978; Henzl 1986). Hypertension is also an estrogen-induced side effect. Estrogen causes an increased secretion of renin substrate (angiotensinogen) that in some women leads to increased production of angiotensin II. The net result of these actions is vasoconstriction and an increase in blood pressure (Tortora and Evans 1986).

Other examples of predisposing medical conditions or a family history that may contraindicate use of OCs include diabetes and liver or gallbladder diseases. Glucose tolerance may be impaired in women predisposed to diabetes if they use OCs (Henzl 1986). Diabetic women on OCs do not invariably worsen or always need more insulin, but OCs do augment the already predisposing risk of diabetic women for cardiovascular diseases (Sloane 1980). Liver function tests, especially those measuring bile excretion (e.g., Bromsulphalein retention), are impaired in OC users (Henzl 1986). Active liver disease or a history of jaundice during pregnancy contraindicates use of OCs; however, a history of hepatitis with currently normal liver function is not a contraindication (Henzl 1986). Since OCs affect the composition of bile (produced in the liver, stored in the gallbladder, and used to break down fats), a history of gallbladder disease may contraindicate OC use (Sloane 1980; Henzl 1986). The likelihood of developing gallstones and cholecystitis (inflammation of the gallbladder) is twice as great in OC users and similar to the risk in postmenopausal women using estrogen substitution (Henzl 1986).

Prudent guidelines accepted by most family planning providers (see Porter, Waife, and Haltrop 1983) include the following: (1) women who take the pill should be advised not to smoke; (2) women who have conditions predisposing to circulatory system diseases should be aware of the risks attributable to OC use and women thirty-five to thirty-nine years old with these conditions should not take the pill unless no alternative method is acceptable; and (3) women over forty years old should not take OCs except in exceptional circumstances. Given the comparable risks associated with pregnancy at this age, tubal ligation may be the most prudent contraceptive recommendation for women over forty.

The most feared purported side effect of OCs is cancer. But much of the publicity on the potential for OC-induced cancer rests on extremely poor evidence. Simply stated, the existing evidence clearly suggests that contemporary OCs do not cause cancer. One major source of the belief that OCs cause cancer is a poorly conducted study using beagles reported by Finkel and Berliner (1973; see Djerassi 1981). The synthetic progestagen medroxyprogesterone acetate (MPA) was injected into beagle bitches and reportedly resulted in mammary tumors. Extrapolation of this finding to women was unjustified for several reasons, including these: beagle bitches are by nature highly prone to mammary tumors; bitches metabolize MPA in a different way than humans; bitches are enormously sensitive to sex hormones; and the semiannual heat cycle of a bitch is not comparable to a woman's monthly menstrual cycle.

Another probable cause of the scare was a 1968 study showing that cervical cancer was three to five times more common in women using OCs for at least four years than in women who had never used OCs. Closer examination of the statistics, however, clearly revealed that the critical factor was not OC use but the number of sexual partners and frequency of intercourse (Boston Women's Health Book Collective 1984). Similarly, an increased rate of malignant melanoma initially erroneously linked to OCs was found merely to reflect the fact that the affected population of OC users spent significantly more time sunbathing and were therefore exposed to more ultraviolet rays (Henzl 1986).

As reviewed by several researchers (Lipsett 1977, 1986; Connell 1978; Holmes and Fox 1979; Mishell 1979; Sloane 1980; Djerassi 1981; Harper 1983; Bromwich and Parsons 1984; Henzl 1986; Heywood 1986; Katzenellenbogen 1986; Sobel 1986; and Stadel 1986), the "evidence" often cited to implicate OC steroids as carcinogens is far from convincing and certainly not conclusive. Perhaps the strongest statement which can be made regarding this association is that steroids (especially estrogens) initiate proliferation of steroid-dependent tissues and that this action may then make these tissues available (or responsive) to the action of a carcinogen. It should, however, be strongly emphasized that there is a vast difference between promoting the normal (and essential) process of cell growth and tissue proliferation and *causing* cancer. In fact, there is evidence that the pill helps reduce the incidence of ovarian and endometrial cancer (see the references cited directly above), perhaps particularly in women over forty (Kaufman et al. 1980; Rosenberg et al. 1982; Cramer et al. 1982).

Although there are clearly serious risks involved in OC usage for some women, it also needs to be emphasized that pregnancy involves many of the same risks; thus there is a clear need for having a variety of birth control methods available. And although the negative side effects of the pill are often emphasized, the beneficial side effects are often ignored. As we mentioned previously, the pill was first approved for marketing because it is a highly effective gynecological tool for the treatment of irregular menstrual cycles and heavy blood loss during menstruation. Because it decreases blood loss, iron deficiency anemia is much less common in women on the pill. In regard to menstruation, there are also, as we have mentioned, the added benefits of decreased menstrual cramps and decreased incidence and severity of symptoms which sometimes precede menstruation (see Chapter 4). The pill can also decrease acne, rheumatoid arthritis, and protect against ovarian cysts and benign breast disease. Two potentially serious problems which also occur far less frequently in OC users are pelvic inflammatory disease (PID) and ectopic pregnancy (*ectopic* means out of normal place; ectopic pregnancies usually occur in the oviduct). Also, users of the pill are reported to have the added benefit of decreased ear wax! Finally, a very important noncontraceptive "side effect" for many women, one that is difficult to quantify, is the peace of mind and psychological security that comes from using a highly effective method of birth control; this reduces the fear of an unwanted pregnancy and therefore helps free the user to enjoy a more fulfilling sex life by being able to be a more enthusiastic and spontaneous sexual partner.

LONG-ACTING STEROIDAL CONTRACEPTIVE SYSTEMS

The synthetic steroids utilized in oral contraceptives induce an array of physiological effects that result in an extremely high degree of contraceptive effectiveness. However, a critical examination of the material just presented in our discussion of the pill reveals two major deficiencies which limit its acceptance and utilization.

The first of these limitations was quickly recognized when OCs were introduced into family planning practice in developing countries and even among the less educated segments of the U.S. population and other developed countries. As we've already emphasized, the effectiveness of OCs is totally dependent upon a rather strict adherence to a daily administration schedule. Despite a theoretical effectiveness of OCs approaching 100 percent, the actual effectiveness is no better than the conscientiousness of the user. Astounding stories of how the pill has been misused are legion (e.g., taking all 21 at once, taking only before or after intercourse, having the husband take it, using it as a vaginal depository, etc.). Undoubtedly, the greatest number of failures have been due to women simply forgetting to take it daily. Cultural factors may also be involved. For instance, many cultures object to taking any type of pill. And many women lack the privacy to effectively use the pill, privacy they need if other family members oppose the use of "artificial" birth control methods.

The second limitation stems from the physiological consequences of daily oral consumption and the resulting metabolic side effects which contraindicate use of the pill for some women. Since the pill is taken orally and daily, there are two unavoidable consequences: (1) Daily ingestion means that there will be some variation in the plasma concentration of active steroids over a twenty-four-hour period, even if directions for usage are followed. A peak in hormone level in the circulation will occur within one to two hours after consumption and a nadir will occur just prior to intake of the next pill. (2) Oral ingestion means that all the steroids have to pass through the liver during the first passage through the body. To ensure an adequate level of the steroid for twenty-four hours, the concentration within the liver cells during initial absorption of the steroids has been calculated to be 100 times above the minimum plasma concentration necessary for a contraceptive effect (Johansson 1981).

By 1963, only three years after the introduction of oral contraceptives, studies were already in progress to develop alternative methods of steroid delivery that eliminated daily pill taking. Administration of long-acting steroids in the form of injections or implants overcomes the two major disadvantages of oral contraceptives: (1) they do not rely on the woman's compliance with the administration schedule, with consequent reduction or elimination of user error; and (2) constant systemic release of the steroids decreases the daily fluctuations in hormone levels and avoids the daily "shock" to the liver. Using long-acting substances administered at infrequent intervals also means that women do not have to take any medication home, keep track of it, or store it. Further, in many societies that have been conditioned by years of exposure to vaccinations and antibiotics, injections are accepted medical interventions while pills are not.

As described by Djerassi (1981), there are several other advantages of injectable contraceptives which have made them attractive for use in various cultures. For example, injection avoids the need to expose one's genitals to medical personnel (as would be required for IUD insertion or diaphragm fitting) and the need to handle one's genitals (as would be required in the use of a diaphragm, foams, jellies, and condoms), both of which actions may be culturally taboo. Like the pill, injections are both coitus-independent and genitalia-independent, attributes highly desirable in cultures where privacy is rare and modesty is imperative. Also, an injection can be given in the village or even in the home by paramedical personnel, thus eliminating the need to visit an often distant hospital or clinic, which can be a threatening experience to persons in some cultures. Additionally, many women who would insist on a female physician for any procedure requiring genital exposure will readily accept an injection from either a male or female. Since long-acting steroid preparations are not dependent upon gastrointestinal functioning, they can also be utilized by women who cannot use the pill for various medical reasons, for example, by those with major bowel disorders. These preparations also do not suppress vitamin levels, as do OCs, and therefore are better suited for women who may have a limited nutritional intake. Finally, since long-acting steroid preparations eliminate or substantially reduce some of the potentially serious side effects associated with the pill, they may be appropriate contraceptives for millions of women who cannot use the pill because of such medical concerns and they may also be safer long-term alternatives for many other women currently on the pill.

Methods employed to achieve what has been termed *minimal intervention fertility control* using long-acting steroidal hormones can be classified into four major groups: (1) injectable depot formulations selected and used for their properties of injectability and slow release; (2) nonbiodegradable subdermal implants in the form of Silastic capsules or rods containing progestagens that diffuse slowly from the implant; (3) medicated devices placed within either the uterus, cervix, or vagina that release steroids locally; and (4) biodegradable systems that release steroids by diffusion or erosion of a biodegradable polymer. Injectables and implants are the two delivery systems that have received the greatest research attention over the past quarter century, and they are most widely utilized at present throughout the world (although not in the United States). Depending on the specific approach, form of preparation, steroid(s) used, dosage, and mode of administration, effective contraceptive protection may last from one month to five or more years. Specifics will be discussed for each system separately.

The extremely high degree of pregnancy prevention effectiveness of the long-acting steroid systems is due to the employment of multiple mechanisms of action similar to those described in the section on oral contraceptives. Minor dissimilarities will be pointed out in the discussion of each system. A comparison of long-acting formulations of steroids and daily oral administration is shown in Figure 11 (adapted from Beck, Cowsar, and Pope 1980).

*Injectables*

Initial research by Pincus and his colleagues in the 1950s (see Diczfalusy 1979, 1982) led to the development of synthetic progestagens which had to be administered at rather frequent intervals because of their short biologic half-lives. Continued research on the screening of already-synthesized progestagens and the synthesis of new compounds soon led to the discovery of structures which had longer durations of action and which made delivery by injection an attractive alternative to oral administration. Beginning with the study of Seigel (1963), numerous progestagens and estrogens (separately and in various combinations) have been investigated in regard to their efficacy as long-acting contraceptives (see the reviews

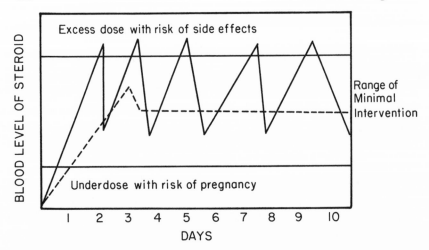

**Figure 11** Blood levels of steroids following oral or programmed release administration. (Adapted from Beck, Cowsar, and Pope 1980.)

by Benagiano 1977 and Fraser 1982). Ironically, the two formulations which have emerged as the most effective products after some 25 years of research are two of the initial progestagens synthesized, depot medroxyprogesterone acetate (DMPA or Depo-Provera) and norethindrone enanthate (NET-EN).

*DMPA or Depo-Provera*  Medroxyprogesterone acetate was first synthesized in 1958 and was initially used for treatment of habitual spontaneous abortion, threatened premature labor, and endometriosis (see the review by Fraser and Holck 1983). It was noticed that women who were treated with it were unable to become pregnant for a considerable time after their last injection. This led to its being investigated as a contraceptive beginning in 1963.

Evidence accumulated over the past twenty-five years leaves no doubt that DMPA is highly effective in preventing pregnancy. Because self-administration errors are eliminated, its use effectiveness (i.e., actual effectiveness) approaches its theoretical effectiveness. The most effective mode of administration appears to be by intramuscular injection of 150 mg of DMPA into the buttocks every three months. Pregnancy rates in large, multicentered studies have ranged from 0 to 1.2 pregnancies per 100 woman-years of use when this mode of administration is employed. A less common dosage schedule of 400 to 450 mg every six months has been tried with slightly higher pregnancy rates reported (0.45 to 3.8 pregnancies per 100 woman-years). Evidence used to support these conclusions and those which follow is reported in numerous sources, including reviews by Schwallie (1974), Nash (1975), Benagiano (1977), Mishell (1979), Beck, Cowsar, and Pope (1980), Ellinas (1980), Djerassi (1981), Fraser and Weisberg (1981), Johansson (1981), Fraser (1982), Fraser and Holck (1983), and Harper (1983).

DMPA's extremely high degree of effectiveness is a result of its multiple modes of action. At least for the three-month injection scheme, suppression of ovulation appears to be virtually absolute, ensuring that it is working as a true contraceptive. Additionally, none of the potentially serious side effects reported for OCs seems to occur in DMPA users. That is, DMPA seems to have no effect on blood clotting, blood pressure, carbohydrate or lipid metabolism, or liver function. DMPA is also economical. Harper (1983) reported that in 1980 the cost of one injection effective for a minimum of three months was only fifty cents.

There are two major side effects of DMPA. Indeed these two side effects are characteristic of all injectables and, to a varying degree, of all long-acting steroid systems. The major effect is a change in the menstrual cycle which is highly unpredictable; it may, though rarely, include very heavy periods, but it is usually manifested as oligomenorrhea (infrequent menstruation) or amenorrhea (no menstruation). These more common effects occur because the long-acting steroid preparations, by design and in contrast to OCs, are not abruptly removed from the system at periodic intervals to induce menstruation. Menstrual disturbances accompanying the use of DMPA have been extensively reviewed (see Gray 1980; Fraser 1981). Amenorrhea of greater than ninety days' duration occurs in at least 30–40 percent of women after twelve months of use. Most other women experience long and irregular cycles with scanty bleeding. It is appropriate to consider the physiological state of a woman using long-acting progestagens such as DMPA to be that of pseudo-pregnancy. While some women report oligomenorrhea or amenorrhea as undesirable side effects, others find DMPA use to be a convenient way of avoiding menstruation and view a reduction in or cessation of its occurrence as an added benefit rather than as a problem. One main reason many sexually active women welcome the onset of menstruation is that it is a monthly reassurance that their contraceptive (or good luck) has been effective for another month. Since amenorrhea is common with long-acting steroidal systems, it is not immediately clear to some women whether lack of menstruation is due to the nature of the contraceptive or to pregnancy. Only education and an understanding of the nature of a contraceptive's action is likely to alleviate that fear and convince such individuals that they should not worry about being pregnant when they don't have their menstrual periods. Other women are distressed at the loss of menstruation because menstruation reminds them that they still have the capacity to reproduce if they so choose. Loss of menstruation is a problem for these kinds of reasons but not because it is a medical problem as such.

It should also be noted that there is no relationship between the occurrence (or, in this case, the suppression) of the menstrual cycle and libido. Similarly, there is no consistent or clearly defined period of sexual receptivity (or lack thereof) during the human menstrual cycle. This is in sharp contrast to the case of other female mammals, which do have a clearly defined period of sexual receptivity (called *estrus* or, more commonly, *heat*) that is associated with the endocrine changes preceding ovulation (see Chapter 4). While it is tempting to extrapolate a similar hormonal explanation to human sexual behavior, in actuality human sexual response is far more complex and involves many more factors than simple hormonal control. For a detailed discussion of these and related points, see Hrdy (1981) and Forsyth (1986).

The second side effect, relative irreversibility, is actually related to the first and to the very nature of the contraceptive. Upon learning of the reason for their amenorrhea, the next main concern of users is that they will be permanently infertile. After discontinuation of DMPA use, there is a delay in return of normal ovulation and fertility. The length of this delay is highly unpredictable among individuals, since clearance of the steroid from the system is dependent upon a number of factors. In some women, uptake of DMPA from the depot injection site seems to be very slow. Most studies indicate that fertility resumes in approximately seven months from the presumed end of contraceptive protection (Fraser and Holck 1983). Studies summarized by Fraser and Weisberg (1981) indicate a re-establishment of menstruation and ovulation in 50 percent of women within 6 months after the last injection, in 75 percent within 12 months, and in 85 percent within 8 months. A comprehensive study in Thailand reported a median delay in fertility of 5.5 months;

after 12 months only 21.8 percent had not conceived and after 24 months only 7.9 percent (Pardthaisong, Gray, and McDaniel 1980). All reviewers on the subject conclude that DMPA does not cause permanent irreversible ovulation suppression, endometrial atrophy, amenorrhea, or sterility. However, the evidence also clearly indicates that a temporary and highly variable delay in return to fertility is to be expected in users of DMPA. For women to whom this delay is unacceptable, DMPA is not an appropriate contraceptive choice.

"Minor" side effects typically reported by users of OCs, such as weight gain, abdominal bloating, headaches, mood changes, nervousness, and fatigue, have also been reported in DMPA users (Benagiano 1977; Fraser and Weisberg 1981; Fraser and Holck 1983). Acne and hair loss may also be experienced; weight gains are sometimes extreme, and depression has also been reported (Boston Women's Health Book Collective 1984).

Depo-Provera is unquestionably the most controversial of the long-acting steroidal contraceptives. It has been the focus of much heated debate among scientists, feminists, consumers, government officials, and physicians and other health care workers. Adverse and strident criticism of DMPA has been widely disseminated in the popular press and the news media, and news stories are often filled with erroneous information about its development, use, safety, and side effects (e.g., Minkin 1980). Although such news stories have been extensively criticized by the scientific community (e.g., Benagiano and Fraser 1981), some governments have not approved its use or have refused to pay for its use (Fraser and Holck 1983; Hartmann 1987). This is bewildering, since, as we have just seen, virtually all the scientific assessments clearly indicate that DMPA is a highly effective contraceptive and has fewer serious side effects than other methods of similar efficacy (e.g., the pill and the IUD). Literally hundreds of valid scientific studies throughout the world have shown that there is no reason to believe that DMPA is carcinogenic. Yet, as in the case of OCs, the belief persists.

Of the two main issues of concern raised by opponents of using DMPA as a contraceptive, the easiest to deal with is the concern over its long-term effects, especially its purported carcinogenicity. The carcinogenicity charge is based on two misleading studies. The first (and the one which generated the greatest uproar) was the study that employed the unsuitable beagle bitch model, which was criticized above. The second involved a group of fifty-two monkeys which were given fifty times the normal dose of DMPA for 50 percent of their lives. Two DMPA-treated monkeys were reported to develop endometrial carcinomas. Data on these carcinomas were carefully reviewed on several occasions by World Health Organization researchers, who invariably concluded that the tumors were the effect of massive hyperdosage (World Health Organization 1982). Furthermore, the monkeys' endometrial lesions were found to have developed from an epithelial plaque, a structure unique to nonhuman primates which grows at the site of placental implantation under the influence of progesterone or develops in nonpregnant animals as a result of trauma (Benagiano and Primiero 1983a). These cells have never been found in women. Fraser and Holck (1983) indicate that only one case of endometrial carcinoma has been reported among the millions of women who have used DMPA, which is considerably less than would be expected in the untreated population as a whole. In fact, not only does it clearly seem that DMPA does not cause endometrial carcinomas in women, it is capable of completely reversing a well-known precancerous endometrial lesion, cystic hyperplasia, and has long been recognized as a potential therapy for treatment of this malignancy (Rozier and Underwood 1974; Bonte et al. 1978). While information on potential long-term side effects is still being amassed and a negative link may eventually be established, extensive investigations involving millions of women have to date failed to substantiate the concern about a link between DMPA and cancer.

The second concern raises thornier issues. While we have suggested that injectable long-acting steroids are highly effective contraceptives because they remove user error, they also remove user control. Any form of contraception over which a woman using it has no direct control is morally problematic. Since a woman using Depo-Provera cannot discontinue her contraceptive protection at will, her fertility is, at least for a fairly long period of time, out of her control. And unlike other easily reversible hormonal contraceptives, if a woman is adversely affected by DMPA, she faces what may be months of ill effects until the formulation is fully metabolized.

The method of application also raises concerns about abuses, since DMPA can easily be surreptitiously administered in certain contexts. Indeed, reports of alleged abuses have come from a number of places, including refugee camps and psychiatric institutions

(Fraser and Holck 1983). Bromwich and Parsons (1984) describe incidents in a London hospital involving the injection of a long-acting steroidal contraceptive into women without their knowledge or consent before hospital release following giving birth (see also Chapter 9).

Other worries are raised by how Depo-Provera has been studied. If, as has sometimes been the case with large-scale DMPA studies, the subjects are women of color and the investigators are white, concerns about racism and eugenicism enter the dispute. Because of rather rigid FDA restrictions on drug testing on human subjects in the United States, almost all developmental research is conducted in third world countries and utilizes women whose socioeconomic background inevitably raises concerns about genuine informed consent and exploitation.

None of these worries is to be taken lightly. And the kinds of abuses that have been mentioned are simply intolerable. At the same time, it is important to realize that virtually all technologies (reproductive or otherwise) have the potential for abuse, and such potential should not preclude being able to recognize a technology's merits. DMPA is available as a contraceptive option in numerous developed and developing countries, and where it is an option the World Health Organization (1982) has provided recommended guidelines for its use, including that there be a thorough discussion with potential users of its known potential effects, its mode of action, the contraindications for use, and the suggested management of potential problems. Although, as we shall see in Chapter 9, the emphasis on population control in some societies raises further worries about implementation of such guidelines, and although many people, including feminist activists, have rightly been made cautious by the premature marketing of high-dose estrogen OCs, at present DMPA holds out real hope of being the most appropriate hormonal contraceptive for many women. At this writing, arguments against FDA approval of Depo-Provera as a contraceptive continue to be successful. Physicians in the United States are, however, at legal liberty to prescribe it as a contraceptive provided they inform women of the currently known risks associated with its use and that the drug has not received FDA approval for contraceptive use.

*NET-EN* Norethindrone enanthate, first synthesized in 1957, is another of the older synthetic gestagens. Because it is a $C_{18}$ moiety rather than a member of the $C_{21}$ gestagen family used in the infamous beagle bitch tumor study of Finkel and Berliner (1973), investigation of its potential as an injectable contraceptive (which was already in progress) was given greater impetus by the FDA ban on some $C_{21}$ products (Benagiano and Primiero 1983a, 1983b).

Contraceptive trials with NET-EN began in 1966. Initial studies used a dose of 200 mg dissolved in 1 ml of oil and administered by injection every three months (Zanartu and Navarro 1968). It was found that contraceptive efficacy waned in the latter days of the postinjection interval. Shortening the interval to twelve weeks was still not completely satisfactory, and an injection scheme of NET-EN every sixty days during the first six months of use and every twelve weeks thereafter was finally proven to be the most effective (Benagiano and Primiero 1983a, 1983b). Prema et al. (1981) used a monthly injection of 20 mg.

Reports of contraceptive effectiveness of NET-EN vary depending on the investigators, regimen employed, and number of women examined. Data from multinational clinical trials sponsored by the World Health Organization involving 790 women (10,079 woman-months) who received NET-EN every sixty days for eighteen months indicated a pregnancy rate of 0.6 per 100 woman-years. A similar pregnancy rate of 0.7 per 100 woman-years was reported in 796 women (10,035 woman-months) who received NET-EN every sixty days for six months and then every twelve weeks for twelve months. Prema et al. (1981) tested 203 women, approximately half of whom were lactating, and based on 2,892 woman-months reported a pregnancy rate of 0.22 following his 20 mg per month treatment regimen. Therefore, although NET-EN must be administered more frequently than DMPA, its contraceptive effectiveness is similar.

The mechanism by which NET-EN inhibits fertility is apparently more complex than simply blocking ovulation (as does DMPA). Evidence suggests that ovulation is blocked in most subjects by NET-EN early in the drug's life span concomitant with high plasma concentrations of the drug within a week of injection. However, after this initial high concentration wanes, ovulation is restored. Kesseru-Koos, Noack, and Larranaga-Leguia (1971) reported a 50 percent incidence of ovulation after two months when using the twelve-week injection regimen. Interestingly, racial differences in the return to ovulation have been reported by several investigators, with non-Caucasian women ovulating sooner than Caucasians (Benagiano and

Primiero 1983a, 1983b). Even though ovulatory function is re-established comparably in Caucasian women, the assorted additional modes of action as described previously in our discussion of OCS apparently function effectively to prevent pregnancy somewhat longer in Caucasian women.

As with DMPA, the only major known side effects of NET-EN are those related to alterations in menstrual patterns. In all treatment regimens employed, bleeding irregularities and amenorrhea were the most common complaints. Incidence of amenorrhea is less for NET-EN users than for DMPA users. All investigators to date agree that menstrual-related problems are the only "major" ones associated with NET-EN administration (Benagiano and Primiero 1983a, 1983b). "Minor" side effects typical of OCS and DMPA (e.g., weight gain, abdominal bloating, headaches, nervousness) are also reported in NET-EN users.

One advantage of NET-EN as compared to DMPA is a more rapid return to fertility following discontinuation of treatment (Kesseru-Koos, Larranaga, and Parada 1973; Benagiano and Primiero 1983a, 1983b). As mentioned previously, follicular activity generally is resumed during the postinjection interval. Fertility is generally believed to be fully re-established by the end of the sixth postinjection month (Benagiano and Primiero 1983b). Kesseru-Koos, Larranaga, and Parada (1973) reported that of fifty-five women who discontinued NET-EN treatment because of their desire to get pregnant, fourteen conceived within six months postinjection and, except for one forty-three-year-old woman, all others had conceived within one year.

The situation regarding acceptability of NET-EN is analogous to that previously described for DMPA.

## Subdermal Implants

The use of subdermal (under the skin) implants for contraception is another "new" methodology with an old history. In the 1960s, work began on putting hormones into some type of capsule that would gradually release them into the body. Dziuk and Cook (1966) first described the passage of steroids through silicone rubber. Although numerous other products were tested, silicone rubber implants were found to be best suited for long-term delivery of contraceptive steroids. Clinical trials utilizing subdermal Silastic implants impregnated with the synthetic steroid megestrol acetate (MA) began in the late 1960s (Croxatto et al. 1969; Tejuja 1970). Given the promising results of these early studies, the International Committee for Contraceptive Research (ICCR) of the Population Council began a series of major studies in the early 1970s with the aim of identifying a combination of progestagen, carrier, and dosage in Silastic implants that would provide effective, reversible contraception lasting up to five years after a single implant (see Beck, Cowsar, and Pope 1980; Robertson 1983; Rabe, Kiesel, and Runnebaum 1985). Pilot studies, especially those of Coutinho and Da Silva (1974) and Croxatto et al. (1975), identified levonorgestrel, norgestrienone, and MA as the three progestagens with the greatest promise for use in subdermal implants. A large multinational ICCR-sponsored study which began in mid-1975 ultimately identified levonorgestrel as the most efficacious of the steroid choices (Diaz et al. 1982; Sivin et al. 1983). Before examining the specifics of the most commonly used system, we should consider the rationale behind the development and use of subdermal implants.

The efficacy of user-independent, long-acting steroid systems has already been pointed out. While maintaining all of the positive benefits described for injectables, implants have several additional attractive features. One advantage of implants over injectables is the duration of effectiveness — years as compared with months. For the user, this means greater convenience and less discomfort in administration, since the procedure needs to be repeated only every five years or so rather than every two or three months. Also, the release rate of the steroid from the Silastic capsules has been shown to be even more constant that the rate of absorption of steroids from the depot site following injection, thus providing more consistent circulating hormone levels over a longer period of time. Perhaps the greatest advantage of an implant system over an injection is that with implants contraception is almost immediately reversible. With injectables, there is no way to remove the hormone that still remains in the body if a woman should decide that she no longer wants contraceptive protection or if she suffers adverse effects from the drug. With implants, since the hormone not yet released is "trapped" in the implant, fertility returns as soon as the implant is removed, and there is no remaining compound to be metabolized.

Subsequent discussion will center on what are commonly known as *Norplant subdermal implants*. Norplant (a registered trademark of the manufacturer, Leiras Pharmaceuticals of Finland) is a system of six Silastic capsules, each 34 mm in length and 2.4 mm in diameter and containing 360 ng levonorgestrel (the total load is 216 mg).

The six Norplant capsules (also referred to as *rods*) are most commonly implanted inside the upper arm. Placement of the capsules is a quick and simple procedure. A local anesthetic is administered and the placement site is disinfected. The sterilized capsules are individually loaded into a sterile trocar (a device like a large hypodermic needle) and placed under the skin in a fanlike pattern through a very small incision (about 3–5 mm). Stitching of the incision is not required. A skilled practitioner requires only about two or three minutes for placement of the capsules and five to ten minutes to complete the procedure from start to finish. Removal of the capsules is effected by a similar simple procedure conducted under local anesthesia and requires only another 5 mm or so incision. Since fibrous tissue is probably surrounding the capsules by the time of removal, removal will generally require a bit longer than insertion, usually about twenty minutes (Sivin 1983). Once in place, the capsules are generally reported to be relatively inconspicuous and bother-free. (Various sites on the body, however, have been tested as potential places to put them, since some women are embarrassed by their visibility on the upper arm.)

Norplant is effective within about twenty-four hours after insertion. Daily release of levonorgestrel from Norplant has been shown to be about 60 – 70 μg per day immediately after implantation, gradually decreasing to 30 μg per day after six to twelve months and remaining at that level almost constantly for years (Johansson 1981; Johansson and Odlind 1983). The 30 μg per day is comparable to the daily dose of the progestagen-only minipill and is considerably less than the daily dose in combination ocs. Only about 10 percent of the contents of each capsule enters the body each year that the implants are in place, suggesting a theoretical duration of effectiveness approaching ten years rather than the commonly stated five years. Sivin et al. (1983) estimated a seven-year projected life span for the Norplant system, with a five-year "safe" usage period. It is really not known exactly how long it takes for the capsules to be completely depleted of hormone, since they have apparently never been left in place until this occurred.

All studies show the Norplant system to be a highly effective contraceptive for a minimum of five years following placement.

Overall figures indicate a failure rate of only about 0.5 per 100 woman-years, which is comparable to Depo-Provera and better than the pill or IUDs (Diaz et al. 1982; World Health Organization 1982, 1985; Sivin 1983; Sivin et al. 1983).

Like other steroidal contraceptives, the Norplant system works on several reproductive processes to achieve its high degree of effectiveness. Women do not ovulate in up to 80 percent of their cycles during the first year following implantation of the capsules and, on the average, in about 50 percent of their cycles in subsequent years (Diaz et al. 1982; Sivin 1983; World Health Organization 1985). It is not possible to predict which women will ovulate or how often. For some women, ovulation may be completely suppressed while the implants are in place; for others, ovulation is not suppressed at all. Levonorgestrel's ability to make the cervical mucus less penetrable to sperm and the uterine lining incapable of accepting a conceptus are probably the two most important "backup" systems responsible for the success of Norplant.

Norplant's actions are easily reversible, and it seems to have no adverse effects on fertility. Within one week after removal of the capsules, levonorgestrel is almost undetectable in the bloodstream. Within one month after Norplant removal in women who wished to become pregnant, 21.6 percent had conceived. Within three months, 43.1 percent were pregnant, 67.3 percent were pregnant within six months, 76.6 percent within a year, and 90 percent within two years (Sivin 1983). These figures are similar to natural fertility rates in women who had not previously been using any steroidal contraception. Without question, the Norplant system provides an unmatched combination of effectiveness, ease of use, and reversibility.

The one somewhat commonly reported adverse side effect of the Norplant system involves menstrual disorders. The chief complaint among the participants in clinical trials to date is excessive bleeding (either prolonged bleeding, numerous episodes of bleeding, or voluminous bleeding). Menstrual disorders, however, were far more common in the first year of Norplant usage than in subsequent years. Most studies show that the number of bleeding or spotting days tended to increase but that the actual volume of blood loss was not higher for individual women than before initiation of the contraceptive. Studies also show that actual blood loss decreases with length of use. A more regular bleeding pattern was established in most women after the first year of use. Roughly equal incidence of amenorrhea, irregular bleeding, and frequent bleeding have been reported by participants during the first year in trials. In the various clinical trials, such changes in bleeding pattern were most often cited by women as a reason for withdrawing from the study. Painful menses (dysmenorrhea) was not a common complaint (Sivin 1983; World Health Organization 1985). The menstrual disorder side effects associated with Norplant usage, therefore, tend to be those that might be classified as messy, inconvenient, or annoying but not ones that involve any serious physical discomfort or pose any health risks. Between 1 and 9 percent of participants have also reported various other side effects, including headaches (of varying severity, generally decreasing after the first year), dizziness, nausea, weight gain or loss (of up to 10 kg), pain at implant site, skin problems, and vaginitis. Norplant usage does not appear to be associated with the potentially life-threatening side effects described for ocs. No doubt this is because it is a progestagen-only product that is effective at a low systemic concentration.

Since Norplant, like DMPA and NET-EN, is not user controlled, there are also concerns about its potential for abuse. Women are dependent on practitioners for both insertion and removal of the capsules, and hence concerns about potential exploitation, involuntary infertility, and eugenic abuse have been raised. Once more the fact that most of the studies have been conducted utilizing poor and uneducated women of color helps give rise to such worries. The likelihood that many participants were not fully aware of what they were agreeing to and were not adequately informed as to what to expect, coupled with other concerns about long-term risks has again been among the primary issues. Especially considering the nature of the participants, clinics must be scrupulously vigilant in following up on the needs of the women who have received the implants, for example, to remind them to have them removed if they wish to become pregnant, to let them know when additional contraceptive protection is needed if they wish not to conceive, and so on.

Two recent variations of the Norplant system are currently under development: a two-capsule system, Norplant 2, and a biodegradable one-capsule system, Capronor (World Health Organization 1985). Both utilize the same progestagen as Norplant, levonorgestrel, and are intended to last for approximately eighteen months. Only the dosage and duration of protection make them different from the traditional Norplant system.

Norplant is already available as a contraceptive option in many countries, including several in Europe (Wilbur 1986). Its approval is currently pending in numerous countries throughout the world. Studies to date involving several thousands of women throughout the world (far more than preceded approval and marketing of the pill) overwhelmingly confirm its effectiveness, ease of use, reversibility, and lack of potentially life-threatening side effects. It is also extremely inexpensive. Harper (1983) estimated the cost of a six-capsule implant, effective for about five years, to be $8.50 (in 1980 dollars). Even allowing for inflation and considerable markup, five years of effective contraceptive protection should still cost no more than 10 percent of what oral contraceptives would run for a comparable period of protection.

Norplant is one of the most attractive of all the contemporary birth control technologies, because it is in many ways a nearly ideal birth control option. But it is not likely to be available to American women soon for several reasons. As Djerassi (1981) points out, existing FDA requirements for approval of a new drug for widespread marketing would involve investing ten and a half to seventeen and a half years and $15 to $46 million to get the drug approved. (Fraser [1988] has revised these estimates to range from $30 to $70 million.) And this assumes that everything goes well throughout the testing period. Although considerable information already exists on the Norplant system, information that is adequate to satisfy the licensing agencies of most countries, far more extensive testing would still be required for FDA approval. Further, it may not be cost-effective for potential manufacturers to undertake the enormous expense of producing the contraceptive, since the major group of Norplant users would likely be current users of OCs, which are already approved and which are probably considerably more profitable than Norplant would be. If one can sell a product that the consumer has to buy every month, why sell her a cheaper one that she has to buy only every five years? Additionally, the product liability crisis in America makes Norplant a gamble that U.S. manufacturers and distributors would be reluctant to undertake in the near future (see Chapter 10 for further discussion). As we shall see in Chapter 9, recent irregularities in testing Norplant involve just the kind of irresponsible behavior that has resulted in what many researchers believe are nonetheless inappropriately rigorous FDA requirements for approval of a new systemic contraceptive. Such irregularities also exacerbate the readiness to bring suit, and this, coupled with existing FDA standards, promises to preclude making Norplant a readily available contraceptive option for American women in the near future. What is unfortunate is that after being apprised of what the existing research has revealed about the safety and efficacy of Norplant, many of these women might well choose it as their contraceptive.

## Vaginal Rings

The medicated vaginal ring is a "new" method of contraception with a history of development spanning two decades. It is a contraceptive option designed to overcome the two primary disadvantages of injectables and implants, namely, lack of user control and menstrual irregularities. Vaginal rings, like subdermal implants, are devices made of a biocompatible polymer, usually Silastic, loaded with long-acting steroids that are slowly released at a predetermined rate. Hormones are absorbed directly into the bloodstream through the vaginal mucus membrane. Since the ring is placed in the vagina by the user, the woman maintains control. Vaginal rings can also be removed by the woman herself, washed, and reused. One scheme of usage, wearing the ring for three weeks and removing it for a week, ensures normal menstrual cycles and avoids the spotting, oligomenorrhea, and amenorrhea that results from continuous use of long-acting progestational steroids. In another scheme, the ring remains in place without removal for periods of time up to a year or more.

Initial studies, beginning in 1968, utilized a so-called Silastic 382 ring implanted with MPA. Mishell et al. (1970) reported no adverse effects after twenty-six days of use. Various refinements were made on the ring and a ten-month study utilizing twenty-four volunteers was initiated. Rings containing MPA were placed in the vagina on either day 5 or 10 of the cycle and removed on day 26. None of the women became discernibly pregnant during the trial, ovulation was inhibited, and little breakthrough bleeding occurred. Four women did suffer vaginal erosions (Mishell, Lumkin, and Stone 1972).

Fallout from the beagle bitch tumor report also affected work on the development of vaginal rings. Following the ban on 17-

acetoprogestins, the ICCR initiated studies utilizing rings containing various $C_{19}$ steroids, including trials reported by Johansson et al. (1975), Mishell, Lumkin, and Jackaniz (1975), Stanczyk et al. (1975), Victor et al. (1975), and Viinikka et al. (1975). The best results were obtained in studies employing rings containing 50 mg or 100 mg of norgestrel (Stanczyk et al. 1975; Victor et al. 1975). Although several steroids achieved contraceptive effectiveness, incidence of bleeding, ovulatory cycles, and vaginal irritation was least with norgestrel. The release rate of norgestrel was also slower and more constant than that for other steroids. Some women did report that their rings produced an objectionable odor.

It was concluded from these mid-1970s studies that although the concept was sound, the delivery system needed refinement. A new type of ring was developed consisting of an inner steroid-free core covered with a thin layer of Silastic impregnated with various amounts of norgestrel; this in turn was covered with Silastic tubing (diameter 60 mm, final thickness 9 mm). Studies in which a ring of this design was worn continuously, except for five days monthly when bleeding occurred, showed inhibition of ovulation in all cycles, no pregnancies, and reduced incidence of bleeding and spotting (Victor and Johansson 1977). However, four of sixteen women became amenorrheic.

The use of estrogen in combination with a progestagen was the next major modification to the system. Mishell et al. (1978) reported that combination devices delivering 200–300 $\mu$g per day of norgestrel and 175–245 $\mu$g per day of estradiol suppressed ovulation in 100 percent of the cases studied. Combination rings inserted for three weeks and removed for one week gave superior bleeding control compared with progestagen-only devices. However, the long-term effects of estrogen on the cervical and vaginal mucosa at this high release rate could constitute a serious problem.

Another modification was the development of a slightly smaller toroidal-shaped ring (diameter 55.6 mm) designed to be worn continuously and to release lower levels of progestagens (levonorgestrel or norethindrone). With this type of ring, ovulation is generally not inhibited and contraceptive effectiveness is due to the local effects of changing the consistency of cervical mucus, which prevents sperm transport and perhaps directly affects sperm motility. Burton et al. (1978, 1979), Gallegos (1980), and the World Health Organization (1980) found levonorgestrel to be the more effective steroid, and it is the one which continues to be used in this manner. While contraceptive effectiveness was similar to other vaginal ring alternatives (failure rate of 1–2 per 100 woman-years), menstrual bleeding irregularities were more common. Because they are transcutaneous and progestagen-only devices, one advantage of these rings is avoidance of the metabolic side effects (e.g., increased blood lipids) experienced with combination devices.

In summary, vaginal rings provide an effective alternative means of delivering long-acting steroids. There are several alternatives, allowing choices in duration of use, extent of menstrual disruption, and type of side effects one is most likely to experience. The primary advantage of the vaginal ring system over other means of administering long-acting steroids is that it is completely user controlled. This is also its primary disadvantage, since if it is positioned improperly, an insufficient release of steroid may occur and an undesired pregnancy may result. If removed and replaced on a monthly basis, menstrual irregularities are reduced but some convenience is sacrificed and the potential for improper placement is increased. Regardless of the type of ring, some women have reported trouble in retaining rings in their proper position in the posterior portion of the vagina. Although not a major problem with the more recently developed models, some women also experience local vaginal irritation. Vaginal microflora are also altered by the presence of the vaginal ring, and Roy, Wilkins, and Mishell (1981) reported an increase in pathogens in the vaginas of users, which raises concerns about potentially serious infections. Changes in the normal microflora may also result in a change in vaginal odor, and some women (and their partners) may find the new odor objectionable. Fewer clinical trials involving large numbers of women have been conducted with vaginal rings compared with other previously described long-acting steroid delivery systems.

Although generally considered a highly effective, inexpensive contraceptive with modest side effects and complete user control, vaginal rings are in the same situation as injectables and subdermal implants relative to FDA approval and the likelihood of being marketed in the United States.

### Medicated Intracervical Devices

A medicated device might also be placed into the cervix in an effort to effect contraception by local delivery of a drug to the cervical lumen. Local release of progestagens could be effected using a device similar to a vaginal ring. Relatively low doses released locally may sufficiently alter cervical mucus to prevent sperm penetration through the cervix, thereby disrupting sperm transport to the site of fertilization. Local delivery directly induces these changes without relying on systemic effects. Since low doses are released, ovulation is not inhibited and normal menstrual patterns are generally not disrupted. Thus the major advantage of this sytem is the minimal dose of steroids required, which results in minimal side effects and ready reversibility. Reservoirs with a drug release rate of 25 μg per day can have a lifetime of many years (Rabe, Kiesel, and Runnebaum 1985). Disadvantages are (1) the lower expected contraceptive efficacy compared with systems that exert both systemic and local effects and (2) the need for careful placement in the cervix by trained personnel. Inserting an intracervical device is easier than inserting an IUD, but these devices do require individual fitting, because the size of the cervical canal does vary among women (the variation is especially great among women who have had children).

Besides steroid delivery (norgestrel and norethindrone are currently under investigation), the intracervical pessary could also be used for release of drugs such as quinine and emetine, which are spermicidal. A 1978 World Health Organization report on intracervical devices indicated that a device releasing 20 μg per day of quinine sulfate showed inhibition of sperm migration in 80 percent of the postcoital tests. No side effects, either local or systemic, were recorded.

More recently, Gould and Ansari (1983) showed that the penetrability of the cervical mucus is increased by anions and lowered by cations. These effects apparently are due to the valence (i.e., chemical charge) of the ions. Therefore, a possibility that warrants continued investigation as a way of reducing or enhancing fertility is the use of electrolytes delivered by an intracervical device to alter the properties of cervical mucus. Such alteration would be safe, nonhormonal, and easily reversible.

Design problems have plagued the development of intracervical devices (Beck, Cowsar, and Pope 1980). The first attempt was made by Cohen, Pandya, and Scommegna (1970), who demonstrated that a Silastic capsule containing progesterone placed in the cervix altered human cervical mucus. However, the capsules were not well retained in the cervix. A successful intracervical device must remain in place for extended periods of time and not impede menstrual flow. Moghissi et al. (1977) designed and tested several prototypes. Most effective was the basic design currently utilized for continued study, a device consisting of a polypropylene spine supporting a cylinder of silicone rubber which serves as a drug reservoir. Branched arms at the end of the spine hold the device in place.

Considerable clinical study and development is required before the contraceptive effectiveness of this approach can be established. The possibility that an intracervical device might function as a conduit for infectious microorganisms from the vagina to the uterus and therefore cause some of the same problems associated with some IUDs also requires further investigation.

Long-acting progestagens may also be delivered via medicated IUDs. This approach will be discussed in Chapter 6.

*Biodegradable Systems*

Using biodegradable polymers as a delivery system for long-acting contraceptive steroids is the newest focus of study. Biodegradable systems have several theoretical advantages over injectables or non-biodegradable implants. The most obvious advantage compared with implant systems is that a biodegradable polymer drug delivery system eliminates the need for removal of delivery devices following depletion of the agent. Perhaps the most important advantages, however, are clinical: The controlled release afforded by biodegradable polymers minimizes side effects by augmenting the amount and persistence of the drug in the vicinity of the target cell and reduces the drug exposure of nontarget cells. The continuous nonfluctuating release of steroids that can be achieved using polymeric membranes allows for a superior control of drug release rate compared to any nonbiodegradable system. This makes possible the use of lower doses, thereby reducing dose-related side effects (Juliano 1980). Since steroids delivered directly into the systemic circulation do not pass through the gastrointestinal tract and hepatic portal system, first-pass clearance is avoided. Efficacy is also high, since user intervention is not required. Numerous biodegradable systems are now under development and being refined and tested. Systems differ with respect to the method of administration, polymer utilized, mechanisms of drug release, and duration of action (Beck, Cowsar, and

Pope 1980; Beck and Tice 1983). The rate of release can be adjusted to accommodate the potency of the steroid by selection of particle size. The daily dose can also be adjusted by changing the quantity of particles injected, an option not offered by large implants.

Polymers (i.e., high-molecular-weight compounds formed by a combination of simpler molecules) with hydrolytically unstable chemical structures (i.e., they are easily decomposed by taking up water) are potentially useful as biodegradable drug carriers in the form of implants (e.g., Capronor) or small particles. Since by design the degradation products of the polymers will pass directly into the systemic circulation along with the steroid which is released, polymers must be carefully selected to ensure that they are safe and nontoxic (Beck, Cowsar, and Pope 1980).

Lactic acid, an end product of carbohydrate metabolism, is a common body product. Two optical isopolymers of lactic acid, polylactic acid (PLA) and polyglycolic acid (PGA), have been the most commonly used polymeric matrices for controlled delivery of contraceptive steroids (Beck and Tice 1983). Excipients (inert components) of PLA and PGA have been combined with the long-acting progestagen norethindrone (NET) to form the so-called NET microcapsule delivery system (see Beck and Tice [1983] for an account of the procedure).

Extensive animal testing was conducted to establish the hormone release rate, and an injectable system providing a continuous controlled release for a precise period of six months following a single intramuscular injection was developed (Beck et al. 1979). Trials using female baboons show that this system inhibited ovulation completely during the six months of treatment (Beck, Cowsar, and Pope 1980). These investigators have also developed systems for other durations of efficacy and other rates of release by adjusting the size of the microspheres and composition of the polymer.

Trials in women using the NET microsphere six-month delivery system have also been promising. Trials reported by Beck and Pope (1984) and Rivera et al. (1984) indicate both a nonfluctuating level of steroid release at the rate predetermined by the investigators and, although based on limited numbers, 100 percent effectiveness in pregnancy prevention. Ovulation appears to be inhibited in about half of the women. There were practically no disruptions of normal menses and no major side effects.

Although research in this area is still in its early stages, results to date appear promising. Reversibility has not been adequately established, but since the duration of effective dosage can be rather accurately determined, infertility should not extend much beyond the projected period of contraceptive protection. Naturally, once the injection of the microspheres is performed, there is no way to remove them from the body, so the user is "stuck" with infertility for the effective life of the system employed. The lack of user control has the advantages and disadvantages discussed previously.

### Gn-RH Antagonists and Agonists

As we have seen in Chapter 4, the pulsatile release of gonadotropin releasing hormone (Gn-RH) from the hypothalamus is essential for the release from the anterior pituitary of the gonadotropins (FSH and LH) that cause follicular maturation. Shortly after Schally's laboratory (Matsuo et al. 1971) reported the structure of this small decapeptide (i.e., a peptide containing ten amino acids), it was synthesized and used for various experimental purposes. Modification of the Gn-RH molecule yielded analogues (i.e., similar compounds) 100–200 times more potent than the natural product (Henzl 1986).

The initial idea motivating continued research was that since inhibitors of Gn-RH (antagonists) could be used for contraceptive purposes, these "superactive" agonists might be usable in treating infertility. During the investigation of the potent new compounds, an interesting paradoxical effect of Gn-RH was discovered which subsequently changed the direction of the research. It was found that rather than stimulating reproductive functions, use of Gn-RH in doses higher than those needed for release of gonadotropins suppressed ovulation and induced luteolysis (corpus luteum breakdown) in women. In men, high doses of Gn-RH inhibited spermatogenesis and testosterone production.

Over 1,500 potent agonists and antagonists of Gn-RH have been synthesized (see Schally, Coy, and Arimura 1980; Clayton and Catt 1981; Harper 1983; Ratnam and Prasad 1984; Rabe, Kiesel, and Runnebaum 1985). Both agonists and antagonists of Gn-RH work by interfering with the normal action of Gn-RH and its membrane-bound receptor in target cells. The mode of this interference, however, is quite different: Whereas agonists inactivate the releasing hormone receptors in the pituitary by means of overstimulation of the receptor sites (a process referred to as *down regulation*), antagonists block the receptor competitively without provoking a biological response.

The most widely tested of the multitude of analogues is a compound referred to as *buserelin*. Originally, it was administered by subcutaneous injection, but this was found to be impractical for long-term treatment. Other delivery methods were explored and administration as an intranasal spray was found to be most effective. Several clinical studies have reported that daily intranasal administration of buserelin provides effective and safe contraception (Nillius, Berqquist, and Wide 1978; Berqquist, Nillius, and Wide 1979, 1982; Schmidt-Gollwitzer et al. 1981; Berqquist et al. 1981). Results of a one-year study indicated that daily doses of 200–600 $\mu$g of the Gn-RH agonist delivered once daily by nasal spray consistently suppressed ovulation and was 100 percent effective in preventing pregnancy (Berqquist, Nillius, and Wide 1982). No women experienced severe bleeding, although over 80 percent experienced either oligomenorrhea or amenorrhea (again, either an advantage or disadvantage depending on one's viewpoint). No serious side effects were reported in this study. After discontinuation of treatment, all women regained ovulatory menstrual cycles within an average of thirty-three days, including women who had been amenorrhic for up to a year during treatment. Volunteers in the study who later wanted to become pregnant had no difficulty in conceiving. All clinical trials to date suggest that long-term Gn-RH agonist treatment is effective and rapidly reversible. Since Gn-RH is not a steroidal product, all of the side effects and long-term potential risks associated with steroid usage are avoided. However, since its suppression of gonadotropin production tends to leave women estrogen deficient and men testosterone deficient, user acceptance is questionable.

To date, Gn-RH antagonists have been less well investigated than agonists. Clinical trials involving both types of products are currently in progress. Considerable further studies are required before widespread market approval is likely. Since Gn-RH agonists and antagonists are user controlled, readily reversible, and nonsteroidal, their potential for approval may be greater than that of the steroidal products described previously. However, approval is not likely in the foreseeable future for the reasons previously mentioned.

SURGICAL STERILIZATION

The popularity of voluntary sterilization as a birth control option has increased tremendously within the past two decades, and it is now the most widely employed method of contraception in the United States. In the 1970s, the number of people choosing sterilization increased fivefold, from 20 million to 100 million (Porter, Waife, and Haltrop 1983). Masters, Johnson, and Kolodny (1986) suggest that one-quarter of all American couples will undergo either male or female sterilization within two years of the birth of their last wanted child and that by ten years after their last child over one-half of the couples will opt for sterilization.

Reasons for the popularity of sterilization as a birth control option are readily apparent: It is effective, safe, and permanent. *Sterilization* is, of course, a generic term that may be applied to procedures designed to render either men or women infertile. Likewise, within both sexes there are numerous possible approaches to achieving sterility. For men, vasectomy is by far the most common technique utilized (see Chapters 1, 3, and 10). We shall limit our discussion in this chapter to sterilization in women.

Use of voluntary sterilization by women solely as a means of permanent contraception is almost entirely a twentieth-century practice. Prior to this century, sterilization of women was done almost exclusively for straightforward medical reasons. Even within this century, restrictive policies and societal attitudes precluded the widespread availability of contraceptive sterilization to American women until the 1970s. The standard rule of thumb employed by the medical profession was the so-called 120 Rule, which is essentially a pronatalist rule. Unless a woman's age multiplied by the number of her children equalled 120 (e.g., 30 years of age and 4 children), she generally was not granted her request for sterilization if it could not be justified for other reasons, such as pain, bleeding, severe health risk from an unwanted pregnancy, high likelihood of producing a genetically defective offspring, or psychiatric illness. It has been suggested that the dramatic increase in performance of hysterectomies during the 1960s may in part have been a result of attempts to provide sterilization to women who had no way to obtain it except by uterine removal (Sloane 1980), much as elective abortion was provided for specious medical reasons prior to its legalization.

No doubt the liberalization of voluntary sterilization was a general offshoot of the "sexual revolution" and an extension of the 1973 Supreme Court ruling on abortion (*Roe v. Wade* 1973; see also Chapter 7) to include voluntary sterilization as a woman's right implicit in her more general right to control her own body. However, even today state laws pertaining to criteria for obtaining contraceptive sterilization vary regarding age, family status, marital status, spousal consent, and other requirements (American College of Obstetricians and Gynecologists 1983). Such regulations raise concerns about paternalism and pronatalism in regulating access to sterilization. But sterilization abuses in the past (particularly eugenic sterilizations; see Chapters 1 and 2) raise other compelling concerns about obtaining a genuinely informed consent to sterilization (see Chapters 2 and 9). It is, therefore, absolutely imperative that a woman contemplating surgical sterilization elect it only after considering all other birth control choices and that she be provided adequate information upon which to base her choice. In order to protect against abuses, it is now required that written acknowledgment of informed consent be given by the woman—acknowledgment that indicates the physician has discussed with her the risks, benefits, and alternatives to sterilization—before the procedure can be performed (American College of Obstetricians and Gynecologists 1983).

One point which must be made exceedingly clear to individuals requesting surgical sterilization is that the procedure should be viewed as irreversible (American College or Obstetricians and Gynecologists 1983). Although progress is being made in reversing surgical sterilizations in both sexes (see also Chapter 10), the reversal procedures are expensive and success is not guaranteed. Thus, surgical sterilization should clearly be undertaken only by individuals who are unequivocal in the decision not to have children at any time in the future.[3]

For the vast majority of women, voluntary sterilization is a reasonable option for what may be considered the third phase or the end point of reproductive planning. For younger women whose objective is preventing an unwanted pregnancy, a highly effective but reversible method, such as an OC, is desirable. For women who

---

[3] Reanastomosis of Fallopian tubes following surgical sterilization currently has a success rate of roughly 85 percent for tubal potency and 65 percent for subsequent pregnancy.

want to have children but who also want to space their pregnancies, the pill or IUD or less effective but safer barrier methods (e.g., use of a diaphragm or condom) are nearly ideal. For women who have had as many children as desired or who are sure that they do not want to have children, surgical sterilization may be the best birth control option. For women approximately thirty-five years of age or older, consideration of the higher risk of pregnancy complications, higher potential risk of producing offspring with various birth defects, higher health risks associated with OC use, and greater cyclic variability as one approaches menopause (hence greater risk of unwanted pregnancy), makes surgical sterilization a reasonable choice.

Although most people associate female sterilization with tubal ligation, there are over 100 different types of operations to achieve female sterilization. Further, the classic operation of tubal ligation (literally tying the tubes) is rarely done today, since it has a considerably higher failure rate compared with more recent methods. Excluding ovariectomy (removal of the ovaries) and hysterectomy (removal of the uterus)—both are risky procedures and are generally not performed for the sole purpose of sterilization—almost all other sterilization methods are aimed at blocking the oviducts (Fallopian tubes) to prevent union of the sperm and egg. Given that all forms of female sterilization are basically variations upon the same theme, we will not attempt to summarize all the methods nor give the specifics of each. Instead, we will summarize the two primary methods of female sterilization. Additional details are available in several sources, including Edwards (1980), Sloane (1980), Porter, Waife, and Haltrop (1983), and Garcia (1987).

The oviducts are accessible from two directions—through the abdomen and through the vagina. The abdominal approach is by far the most common. Three techniques are employed for the abdominal approach, namely, laparoscopy, laparotomy, and minilaparotomy. Colpotomy (surgical cutting of the vagina) and culdoscopy (utilizing an endoscope inserted via the vagina) are the two techniques used in the vaginal approach. Complications, especially infections, are far greater in the vaginal approach. Because of its limited use, we shall not discuss the vaginal approach.

Sterilization by laparoscopy is by far the most common procedure today. *Laparoscopy* (meaning looking into the abdomen) refers to the surgical utilization of a laparoscope, which is an endoscope (a tubular instrument containing optical lenses and a light source to permit viewing of internal organs) inserted into the abdomen. Generally, laparoscopy is done through the navel and requires only about a one-inch incision. Because this small incision usually leaves no visible scar, this approach is often referred to as *Band-Aid sterilization*. In laparoscopy, the oviducts are occluded without bringing them outside the abdomen. The abdominal cavity is first filled with a gas (usually carbon dioxide) to make the abdomen taut and the oviducts easier to identify and grasp. In both laparotomies and minilaparotomies (which differ from one another primarily in the size of the incision), the oviducts are excised from the abdomen and occluded.

There are numerous ways of occluding the oviducts to make them incapable of transporting ova and preventing spermatozoa access. Rarely the entire tube is removed; usually it is simply interrupted. In classic tubal ligations, a suture was simply tied around a loop of the oviduct without cutting it. The tie often slipped off or did not completely block the tube. Today, surgeons sometimes use either a small silicone rubber band (called a *Falope Ring* or *Yoon band*) or a Silastic plug slipped over a loop or "knuckle" of the tube to occlude it and cause the formation of scar tissue. A more common method involves electrically cauterizing (sealing by burning) the tube at several places; another is the Pomeroy Technique, in which a loop of the tube is elevated, tied with absorbable suture, and then cut off. When the suture absorbs weeks later, there is a gap between the ends of the tube.

Laparoscopy can be performed under either local or, more commonly, under general anesthesia on an outpatient basis. The actual surgery generally requires only about twenty minutes. Most women are ready to leave the hospital within two to four hours after the procedure, even if a general anesthetic is used. Women may experience pain or discomfort for one to three days following the procedure. This includes pain from the incision in the abdominal wall, nausea from manipulation of internal structures during the procedure or as a result of anesthesia or other medication, residual discomfort from the gas used to inflate the abdomen, and menstrual-like cramps. Serious complications from laparoscopy sterilization are exceedingly rare (Porter, Waife, and Haltrop 1983; American College of Obstetricians and Gynecologists 1983).

Surgical sterilization provides the highest degree of contraceptive effectiveness short of absolute abstinence. All methods of tubal occlusion performed by laparoscopy are well over 99 percent effective. A failure rate of only 0.04 percent is the figure most commonly cited (Porter, Waife, and Haltrop 1983; Tortora and Evans 1986; Wilbur 1986). The U.S. Centers for Disease Control (CDC) have estimated that at least half of the rare sterilization "failures" in the United States are cases in which the woman has an unrecognized pregnancy at the time of the procedure (Porter, Waife, and Haltrop 1983). In the rare instance when a woman who has undergone tubal occlusion does become pregnant, the likelihood of an ectopic pregnancy is significantly greater — between 5 and 20 percent compared with the normal risk of 0.5 percent (De Stefano, Peterson, and Layde 1982). However, since pregnancy occurs so rarely following these procedures, overall risk of ectopic pregnancy is exceedingly low.

There are no long-term side effects of surgical sterilization. Some researchers have reported a so-called poststerilization syndrome that includes increased menstrual pain and irregular bleeding patterns (Bhiwandiwala, Mumford, and Feldblum 1982). However, other studies by the CDC and International Fertility Research Program (IFRP) indicate that number of days of menstruation, amount of flow, and frequency of spotting are unaffected by sterilization (see Porter, Waife, and Haltrop 1983). Especially in previous users of OCs, menstrual pattern changes following sterilization are more likely to be associated with the discontinuation of OCs (which minimize volume and duration of flow, menstrual cramps, and irregularity) than with the sterilization itself.

Just as some men report a reduced interest in sex following a vasectomy, some women report a decreased sex drive following sterilization. However, there is no physiological or endocrinological basis for this, since neither procedure affects hormone production. This is yet another example of a point made earlier: Human sexual response cannot be explained in simple hormonal terms. If a woman feels that she is "incomplete" or "less of a woman" following surgical sterilization or if she feels guilty for terminating her fertility or for "fixing herself" so that intercourse no longer has a reproductive potential for her, then these psychological factors may indeed cause a decreased interest in sex. This perspective is balanced by the perspective of other women who report increased sexual interest following sterilization because they no longer fear accidental pregnancy. For the majority of women, sterilization has no effect on sexual interest or response.

.    .    .    .    .    .

This concludes our discussion of birth control options for women that are truly contraceptive in nature. We now turn our attention to the more controversial abortifacient and induced abortion methodologies.

# 6

# Abortifacients and Induced Abortion Techniques

## INTRODUCTION

As we have seen in Chapter 5, even though the primary action of some birth control methods (e.g., oral contraceptives — OCs) is prevention of conception, a number of these techniques also have "backup systems" that can preclude continued development of an early conceptus if ovulation and conception should occur. In the present chapter, we shall look at some methods that are often thought to be contraceptive in nature but which are really primarily abortifacient techniques. That is, some of these methods have actions that impede fertilization, but they routinely involve interfering with the development of the conceptus, either before or after implantation. (See Chapter 5 for a discussion of the term *abortifacient*.)

## INTRAUTERINE DEVICES

Intrauterine devices (IUDs) have a storied and stormy history (see Chapter 1). The modern history of IUDs as pregnancy prevention devices dates from 1909, when German physician Richard Richter introduced his IUD, a ring made of dried silkworm gut. In the 1920s another German doctor, Karl Pust, combined Richter's silkworm ring with a glass disc fitted over the external cervical os. The use of IUDs in their present form dates from the late 1920s and early 1930s, when still another German physician, Ernst Graefenberg, introduced a ring of silkworm gut surrounded by a substance called *German silver*, an alloy of copper, nickel, and zinc. In Japan, T. Ota introduced a similar device composed of reinforced gold-plated silver (see Sloane 1980; Djerassi 1981; Porter, Waife, and Haltrop 1983; Bromwich and Parsons 1984).

Even though these IUDs reportedly provided good pregnancy protection in thousands of patients, by the mid-1930s they fell into

disrepute in the medical profession because of a partially substanti-
ated and partly theoretical fear that they caused uterine injury and
pelvic inflammations (Sloane 1980; Djerassi 1981; Corea 1985). Following the uproar, little was heard about the IUD for some twenty-
five years.

In 1959, W. Oppenheimer of Israel and Atsumi Ishihama of Japan
independently published articles detailing their experiences with
the IUD. Both reported low pregnancy rates and no serious side effects
following long-term use of the Graefenberg ring by their patients.
These reports, coupled with Malthusian worries about the worldwide increase in population, led to renewed interest in the IUD and
the initiation of clinical trials in many countries (Tietze 1973; Sloane
1980; Djerassi 1981; see also Chapter 1). Reports of these trials presented at two international conferences on IUDs shortly thereafter
(1962 and 1964) led to an overwhelming reversal of medical opinion
and the endorsement of the IUD as a medically acceptable birth control device. According to Tietze (1973), who was a major contribu-
tor to both of these international conferences on IUDs, this approval
was based on several considerations: (1) The new respectability of
contraceptive research led to the participation of highly qualified
scientists and physicians; (2) new methods of treating pelvic inflammatory disease (PID) made it a far less formidable complication than
previously; (3) new inert materials (especially plastics and stainless
steel) made IUD insertion and placement easier (because of improved
flexibility) and made it possible for IUDs to remain in the uterus for
an indefinite period; and (4) a sense of urgency had been created by
rapid population growth, especially in the less-developed regions
of the world.

Beginning with the Margulies Spiral, there was a rapid proliferation of second generation IUDs in the 1960s. This was facilitated
by innovations in plastic and stainless steel technologies that allowed
the development of IUDs that could be temporarily straightened or
flattened to fit into an inserter but that would spring back to their
original shape once in place inside the uterine cavity. The Lippes
Loop (named after Dr. Jack Lippe, who introduced it in 1962) became
the most famous and widely used IUD, and it is still the standard
against which all others are measured (Porter, Waife, and Haltrop
1983; Bromwich and Parsons 1984). The dozens of variations designed
and tried were all attempts to find the appropriate compromise
between surface area and effectiveness. It was realized that the larger

the device, the better it protected a woman against pregnancy. However, since the uterus naturally tends to reject foreign objects within it, the larger the device, the more the uterus contracts, making pain and bleeding more likely (Bromwich and Parsons 1984).

The third-generation IUDs were designed to solve these problems. Since they were much smaller in size, their insertion was easier and less painful, and they could also be used by women who had never been pregnant and had a smaller uterus. Their smaller size also caused less discomfort and bleeding while in place. Smaller IUDs were possible because they were medicated, which enhances their effectiveness. Although several chemicals were tried, the best early success was enjoyed by a plastic device in a T or 7 shape that was wrapped with copper wire. While working in Chile, Zipper, Medel, and Prager (1969) found that the release of copper ions into the uterus enhanced the effectiveness of the IUD. Several other copper-bearing devices were subsequently developed. Many other chemically enhanced IUDs have been tried, and currently the most prominent of these are IUDs impregnated with progesterone or progestagens. Among these devices, the Progestasert (Alza Pharmaceutical Co.), a T-shaped IUD delivering 65 $\mu$g per day of progesterone, has been the most widely tested and widely utilized. Such devices locally deliver progesterone to alter a number of physiological functions while also providing the disruptive actions of the IUD on the uterine lining to effect birth control (Newton and McEwan 1977; Beck, Cowsar, and Pope 1980; Bromwich and Parsons 1984).

One reason for the rapid proliferation in types, shapes, and designs of IUDs flooding markets in the late 1960s and early 1970s was that until the mid-1970s medical devices did not fall under the control of the FDA.[1] Therefore, unlike steroidal contraceptives, manufacturers could market their IUDs without extensive pre-introduction testing (Djerassi 1981). One innovative design introduced during this period (in 1971) substituted a metal stem threaded through two openings for the plastic tubular inserter and added five pair of little "legs" along the edge of the device to keep it from being pulled out when the stem was withdrawn (Davis 1971; Tietze

---

[1] Although the FDA cannot control what drugs or devices will be made available in non-U.S. markets, a number of nations rely heavily on FDA regulations and rulings in formulating their own drug policies.

1973). This crab-shaped IUD, marketed by A. H. Robins Company, was the now infamous Dalkon Shield. (As we mentioned in Chapter 1 and shall discuss shortly in more detail, this product has wreaked havoc in the American IUD market.)

*Mechanisms of Action of IUDs*   Like steroidal contraceptives, IUDs employ multiple modes of action to achieve their high degree of effectiveness. Unlike steroidal contraceptives, these effects are exerted locally rather than systemically. IUDs have no effect on ovulation or circulating hormones. But, to state the obvious, an IUD is a foreign body within the uterus. The natural response of the woman's body to the presence of this foreign object is to try to neutralize and eliminate it. Thus, the IUD evokes the release of large numbers of phagocytic (destructive) white blood cells. The endometrium is maintained in a chronic state of low-grade inflammation resulting from the mechanical trauma induced by an IUD's presence (Mehrotra and Srivatava 1985). Also, as we saw in Chapter 1, since the IUD is inserted by passing through a nonsterile structure, the cervix, bacteria not normally present in the uterus may be introduced into it with the IUD. This potentiates and intensifies the inflammatory process, creating a transient endometritis. The net result of these effects is that the uterus becomes a very inhospitable location. In its inflamed state, the endometrium is no longer an acceptable site for implantation. The increased numbers of phagocytic leukocytes present in the uterus of an IUD user make it difficult for sperm to successfully traverse the uterus. Certainly the number of sperm which do survive is reduced. However, it is quite likely that in most IUD users, especially long-term users, a considerable number of sperm do succeed in traversing the uterus and in reaching the oviduct, there achieving fertilization. Indeed, Moyer and Shaw (1973) report that fertilization is generally not prevented by the presence of an IUD. In such cases, the abortifacient properties of the IUD prevent the continued development of the conceptus.

If fertilization does occur, the increased production of prostaglandin $F_{2\alpha}$ stimulated by the presence of the IUD is likely to alter tubal motility so that the fertilized ovum is prematurely forced into the uterus. Even if the conceptus does enter the uterus at an appropriate time, it is likely to be either destroyed by the large population of leukocytes present or die because the inflamed uterine lining either will not allow it to implant or will not allow it to continue development following initiation of implantation. There are indications that implantation does occur in some IUD users. Beling, Cederqvist, and Fuchs (1976) and Landesman, Coutinho, and Saxena (1976) reported detecting elevated levels of urinary human chorionic gonadotropin (hCG) in over 40 percent of IUD users they examined. Hodgen et al. (1978) reported elevation of urinary hCG for a brief period of one or two days late in the cycle of 25 percent of the IUD users they examined. These results clearly suggest that implantation followed by early abortion occurs fairly frequently in IUD users (see Chapter 4). (For those who believe that pregnancy or a right to life of the conceptus commences, not at fertilization, but at implantation [see Chapter 5], this knowledge may muddy the waters regarding the moral acceptability of IUD usage even further.) Perhaps it should also be mentioned that a positive hCG test followed by a spontaneous abortion is also commonly observed in women who use no birth control protection.

The uterine environment is even more altered when a medicated IUD is used. Copper enhances the inflammatory response and may affect the carbohydrate metabolism of endometrial cells (Hsu et al. 1976). Copper also appears to be toxic to sperm and may inhibit sperm transport (Sloane 1980).

For any individual IUD user during any particular cycle, it is impossible to assess whether pregnancy prevention was due to prevention of fertilization, prevention of implantation after fertilization, or an early abortion after implantation. In each case, intercycle length is likely to fall within what would generally be accepted as a normal range.

*Advantages of IUDs*    When the IUD was "rediscovered" in the early 1960s, it was hailed as the ideal contraceptive. Since the explosion of IUD usage worldwide coincided with the introduction and widespread adoption of the pill, the IUD shares some of the praise and the blame for women's sexual liberation and for reducing birthrates throughout the world. In regard to its efficacy, the IUD has often been compared with the pill, since the two are acknowledged to be the most effective of the more widely used reversible birth control methods. Some consider the IUD to be the ideal birth control technology, at least in theory, for several reasons. (1) It is highly effective. The theoretical effectiveness of the IUD is generally reported to be in the range of 97–99 percent (Tietze 1973; Sloane 1980; Harper

1983; Porter, Waife, and Haltrop 1983; Bromwich and Parsons 1984; Wilbur 1986). The estimated failure rate of 1–3 percent is second only to the pill among widely approved and widely utilized birth control products. In actual practice, efficacy of the IUD often exceeds that of the pill, since the effectiveness of the IUD, unlike the pill, is not subject to user error. (2) IUDs require only one insertion for prolonged protection. Not only does this make them more highly effective, it adds an element of convenience not offered by the pill. (3) The birth control effects of IUDs are not directly related to each act of intercourse. Like the pill and unlike some barrier methods, they allow sexual spontaneity by not requiring genital handling in preparation for intercourse. (4) Their contraceptive effect is readily reversible. In theory, as soon as the IUD is removed from the uterus, fertility should return. Since there has been no suppression of "higher centers" of endocrine control or of ovarian function, fertility should return as soon as the disruptive influence on endometrial activity is removed. (5) IUDs lack serious systemic side effects. Especially in light of the potential side effects of alterations in cardiovascular function linked to the pill, the IUD has been viewed by many as safer than OCs because of the absence of such long-term, systemic side effects. (6) The IUD is inexpensive. Cost to U.S. users of the Copper-T device in 1980 was about $6.00 per device (Harper 1983). In third world countries, its cost was estimated to be between $0.20 and $1.20, depending on bulk and individual packaging. Similarly, the Lippes Loop D was priced at $0.08 to $5.00 per device. In 1980 dollars, the Progestasert IUD was priced at $18.00 per device in the United States and $6.00 per device in less developed countries (Harper 1983). Considering that IUDs may provide effective protection for one to ten years following a single clinical insertion procedure (depending on the particular device and other variables), they are indeed inexpensive.

*Disadvantages and Side Effects of IUDs*   A re-evaluation of IUDs some two decades after they were hailed as the "ideal" contraceptive indicates that they are far from perfect. Many serious problems have been linked to IUDs, problems which raise legitimate doubts about the wisdom of encouraging their widespread use. While these problems and potential hazards certainly merit concern, negative points have generally been emphasized to the exclusion of benefits, as has been the case with the pill.

Before discussing the disadvantages and side effects associated with the IUD, two points should be emphasized. First of all, *intrauterine device* is a generic term for any of the many devices that have been placed in the uterus for birth control purposes. As we indicated previously, IUDs vary greatly according to size, shape, design, material composition, whether they are medicated or nonmedicated, type of medication, and so on. Likewise, they vary in regard to extent of testing, number of individuals who use each type, intended duration of use, actual duration of use, effectiveness, and general and specific side effects associated with each type. For example, while the Dalkon Shield was clearly a faulty product and the serious adverse effects of using it are unacceptable, other IUDs, such as the Copper-7 and Copper-T (Tatum-T), have not been associated with significant health risks and should not be unfairly indicted for the devastating effects on women of the Dalkon Shield.[2]

Second, although they are not the most appropriate birth control choice for all women, IUDs may still be the ideal choice for some. As with the pill, there are individual variations regarding tolerance of an IUD and its associated side effects. Some women do not experience any of the problems ascribed to IUD usage. Overall, the women best suited to IUD usage are those who are over thirty years of age, multiparous (i.e., have had more than one child), and involved in a monogamous relationship with a monogamous partner. Least suited to IUD usage (and likely to have far more of the problems described below) are younger women (i.e., those in their teens and early twenties) who are nulliparous and have multiple sex partners.

The most common side effects associated with IUD insertion and use are pain and bleeding. While most women do not report the actual insertion procedure to be especially painful, virtually all women experience some cramping pain immediately following insertion. This pain is generally minimal in women who have had children, and the pain may last a few minutes to an hour. In younger and nulliparous women, moderate to severe menstrual-like cramps probably will last several hours to several days. After insertion,

---

[2]Information relative to specific IUDs is available in several sources, including Tietze (1973), Moyer and Shaw (1973), Edelman, Berger, and Keith (1980), Hatcher et al. (1980), Harper (1983), and Porter, Waife, and Haltrop (1983).

almost all women experience some vaginal bleeding accompanying the pelvic pain. The extent and duration of this bleeding also varies among individuals. Both pain and bleeding are a greater problem during the first three months following insertion. If a woman can tolerate them for that long, these problems usually decline thereafter. Approximately 15 percent of women have their IUDs removed because of bleeding, spotting, or pain (Hatcher et al. 1980).

Most women will also experience an adverse change in their menstrual periods. Menses are likely to start earlier, last longer, and have a heavier flow. In many incidences, severity and duration of menstrual cramps is greater with an IUD present, and dysmenorrhea is much more likely to occur. The Lippes Loop has been reported to increase menstrual blood loss by 90 percent, the Copper-7 and Copper-T devices by 42 percent (Harper 1983). Usually, the length of the menstrual period is extended to include two to three days of a brownish discharge both before and after the true bleeding. Intermittent spotting might also occur during the intermenstrual period. While only slightly annoying to some women, in cultures that associate vaginal bleeding with various taboos (see Chapter 4), this is a major point of concern. Increased blood loss also makes a woman more likely to develop anemia. Since anemia is a common health problem in many third world countries where the IUD has been introduced, this can create serious problems for women who do not have access to mineral supplements. In contrast to all other types of IUDs, the Progestasert, because of its local release of progesterone, actually reduces blood loss, menstrual cramps, and dysmenorrhea (Hatcher et al. 1980; Sloane 1980; Tyrer 1980; Harper 1983; Bromwich and Parsons 1984).

The cramping following IUD insertion is, of course, an expected response of the uterus to this foreign object. Mechanical disruption of the endometrium by the IUD, resulting in local release of prostaglandin $F_{2\alpha}$, is the actual biological cause of the cramps. (Release of prostaglandin $F_{2\alpha}$ is also the cause of normal menstrual cramps; see Chapter 4.) Sometimes the uterus succeeds in its attempt to expel the device. Expulsion rates of 5–20 percent within the first year of IUD use have been reported (Hatcher et al. 1980; Sloane 1980). Risk of expulsion is greatest during the first month of use and is greater in young and nulliparous women. Some types of IUDs are more easily expelled than others. Initially, one of the advantages attributed to the Dalkon Shield was that its design prevented easy expulsion (Tietze 1973). However, while vaginal expulsion was reduced, this same design trait made it more likely to perforate the uterus and cause very serious problems following entry into the peritoneal cavity (Kirkpatrick, Schneider, and Patterson 1975; Simcock 1985). About 50 percent of women who undergo reinsertion following expulsion ultimately retain the IUD (Tietze 1973; Sloane 1980; Tyrer 1980). If a woman does not detect that her IUD has been expelled, a serious undesired side effect may occur — pregnancy. The attached string that extends through the cervix and into the vagina should be palpated regularly to assure that the IUD is still in place. Tampons or pads worn during menstruation should be checked to be sure that the device has not been expelled. If the string cannot be palpated but the woman is sure that her IUD has not been expelled vaginally, she needs to immediately consult her physician to determine if it has become embedded in the uterine wall or has perforated through the uterus into the peritoneal cavity. Given the dangers of infection associated with uterine embedding and perforation, this cannot be emphasized strongly enough.

While IUDs are highly effective devices, they are not perfect, and, as we have already pointed out, conceptions and implantations with an IUD in place do occur. Two problems far more common with an IUD in situ than with other birth control methods are ectopic pregnancies (i.e., pregnancies outside the uterus) and pregnancies which end in abortion as a result of infection. Both conditions are medically hazardous.

If pregnancy should occur with an IUD in place, there is a tenfold greater risk that the pregnancy will be ectopic (usually occurring in the oviduct). Approximately 5 percent of all pregnancies among IUD users are ectopic compared with 0.5 percent in the general population (Vessey 1979; Edelman, Berger, and Keith 1980; Porter, Waife, and Haltrop 1983; Simcock 1985). However, since the overall pregnancy rate in IUD users is only about 2 percent, the risk of ectopic pregnancy is actually less than for women using no birth control product.

Over 50 percent of the known pregnancies that occur when a woman is wearing an IUD will terminate in abortion should she decide to continue the pregnancy with the IUD in place. If the IUD is removed as soon as the woman realizes that she is pregnant, the rate of abortion is reduced to about 25 percent (Edelman, Berger, and Keith 1980; Sloane 1980; Porter, Waife, and Haltrop 1983; Simcock 1985).

This latter rate is comparable to the rate of spontaneous abortion in all pregnancies which have progressed far enough to be recognized.

Ignoring possible ethical considerations, one may wonder why it wouldn't be reasonable to leave the IUD in place and enhance the odds of miscarriage (assuming the pregnancy is unwanted). The answer is that doing this is extremely dangerous to the woman. Of the 50 percent of known pregnancies in IUD wearers that are aborted, 50 percent of these (i.e., 25 percent of all known pregnancies occurring with an IUD left in place) are what are termed *septic abortions*. These abortions are accompanied by infection and high fever. Infection originates in the uterus but can spread rapidly throughout the body and may be fatal. Over 90 percent of IUD users who abort as a result of the device show some signs of infection (Tortora and Evans 1986). Rates of IUD-induced abortion and the resultant complications are very much dependent on the type of IUD. Rates were far greater in Dalkon Shield users than with any other type of IUD. The highly serious septic abortions were also particularly linked to the Dalkon Shield. First, the "legs" of the Dalkon Shield were perfect for harboring bacteria and "injecting" them into the uterine lining if the IUD perforated through the wall of the uterus. Second, the tail of the Dalkon Shield (located in the vagina) was composed of multifilaments contained within a nylon or polypropylene sheath. Tatum et al. (1975) found that the interior of the Dalkon Shield thread provided a potential reservoir for bacteria and hence was a source of intrauterine infection. Before being withdrawn from the market, the Dalkon Shield was implicated in 14 deaths and 223 septic abortions (Sloane 1980).

In those pregnancies which go full term despite the presence of an IUD, premature labor, excessive bleeding, and stillbirths have been reported (Dreishpoon 1975). If a pregnancy is maintained and premature delivery is avoided,[3] there do not appear to be adverse effects of the IUD on fetal growth, development, or survival (Bromwich and Parsons 1984; see also Chapter 8).

As we pointed out in Chapter 1, another very serious side effect linked to IUD usage is pelvic inflammatory disease (PID). The term *pelvic inflammatory disease* is used to refer to any bacterial infection

---

[3] See the discussion of low birth weights and attendant problems in Chapter 9.

involving the uterus, oviducts, or ovaries. Widespread, acute PID usually involves a salpingitis (infection in the oviducts) which has spilled over into the peritoneum. Lower abdominal tenderness and pain, generally accompanied by a fever and often by nausea and vomiting, are the common symptoms of PID. A urinary tract infection may also be present. PID tends to occur more frequently following a menstrual period, because the sloughed off endometrial tissue provides a good growth medium for bacteria (Sloane 1980).

According to Soderstrom (1980), women using an IUD have a five times greater risk of PID than non-IUD users. Certain women are statistically at particular risk, namely, nulliparous women under twenty-five, women with a previous history of PID, and women who have multiple concurrent sex partners or who change sex partners frequently. An interaction of these risk factors may increase the risk tenfold.

An increased risk of PID seems unavoidable based upon the nature of IUDs. Regardless of how careful and aseptic an insertion technique, it is inevitable that some cervicovaginal bacteria will be introduced into the uterus. Indeed, a transient endometritis is an expected result of IUD insertion. In most cases this infection is temporary and the uterus returns to a relatively sterile state in a fairly short time. However, in some cases infection may persist, intensify, and develop into PID. Numerous factors determine the extent to which the normal defense systems of the body can counteract this initial infection. These include (1) the extent to which the insertion procedure was aseptic; (2) the type, size, and design of the IUD inserted; (3) the type, number, and virulence of the bacteria introduced into the uterus; (4) the inherent resistance of the woman; (5) the general health status of the woman; and (6) the possible presence of a pre-existing infection which is aggravated by the insertion (Sloane 1980). Even following successful accommodation of the initial bacterial contamination caused by IUD insertion, the thread hanging from the IUD through the cervix and into the vagina will constantly be covered in whatever secretions may be present in the area and provide a "ladder" for the bacteria to climb up from the vagina into the uterus. This is true both for bacteria inherently present within the woman's vagina and for bacteria which may be introduced into her vagina by a sexual partner. Also probably contributing to the increased incidence of PID in IUD users is that the tissue damage and trauma inflicted upon the endometrium by the IUD creates a favorable environment for bacterial growth. Since some types of IUDs (e.g., the Dalkon Shield) inflict more severe tissue damage than do others, incidence and severity of PID varies according to the IUD used. A large percentage of the thousands of lawsuits filed against the A. H. Robins Company allege that the Dalkon Shield induced PID resulting in infertility.

According to Tietze and Lewit (1970), rates of PID are substantially higher (7.7 percent) during the first fifteen days following IUD insertion than at any subsequent period. They report that 2–3 percent of women had PID in the first year of IUD usage. Vessey et al. (1976) provide convincing evidence that the greater rate of PID in IUD users (3.5 times higher based on their data) is in fact caused by the IUD.

PID is a serious condition which can be life-threatening without immediate antibiotic treatment. It is a more serious problem among third world users of IUDs, since access to appropriate and immediate medical care is likely to be limited. Besides the pain and discomfort associated with PID, it may result in infertility or subfertility even when successfully treated. This is especially true regarding infections within the oviduct, for these may cause the development of scar tissue or adhesions that impair gamete transport (Sloane 1980; Bromwich and Parsons 1984). Soderstrom (1980) reports FDA estimates of the probability of infertility following PID as 12 percent after one episode, 40 percent after two episodes, and 75 percent after three episodes.

*Current and Future Status of IUD Availability*  In a word, the IUD may be doomed on the American market. In retrospect, it appears that the Dalkon Shield, an ill-designed product, not only placed the future of its manufacturer, A. H. Robins Company, in peril, but it also imperiled the future availability of IUDs in the United States. Robins, faced with thousands of lawsuits from women who were injured and the families of some who died allegedly because of the Dalkon Shield, filed for Chapter 11 bankruptcy protection in August 1985. As we write this chapter just over two years later, the bankruptcy case is still in litigation. Under appeal is an order signed by a federal judge in the spring of 1985 creating a $15 million emergency fund to finance surgery, in vitro fertilization, or both for women who allege that the Dalkon Shield made them infertile.

A predictable consequence of the justified outrage initially directed against Robins and the Dalkon Shield was the surge in lawsuits against other manufacturers of IUDs. Equally predictable was the consequent business decision made by the manufacturers of IUDs to remove their products from the American market. In January 1986, the G. D. Searle Company withdrew its popular Copper-7 and Tatum-T models from the market, leaving only the Progestasert (Women's Global Network on Reproductive Rights 1986c). Ortho Pharmaceutical had already halted production of its Lippes Loop because of falling sales and increasing lawsuits. The Searle devices have traditionally been considered to be the safest IUDs available. Searle has successfully defended the devices in several lawsuits, but hundreds of cases are still pending. Searle emphasized that withdrawal of its IUDs from the U.S. market (it still sells them in other countries) was a purely economic decision. While Searle considered its devices safe and effective, they were relatively low-profit items that cost more in liability insurance premiums and legal defense costs than was justified by their sales (Wilbur 1986; Women's Global Network on Reproductive Rights 1986a, 1986c). In early 1986, 775 lawsuits had been filed against Searle and 305 were pending (Women's Global Network on Reproductive Rights 1986a). More suits may be forthcoming, since concerns are being raised about copper IUDs. For example, Knowles (cited in Hartmann 1987) reports that copper migrates away from these devices into the body, leaving most of the device devoid of copper after two years. Since it is not yet clear how much copper the body can safely tolerate, the number of potential suits cannot be known. By way of example, Knowles raises a concern about the devices' possible potential for activating Wilson's disease, which adversely affects the brain, liver, and kidneys (cited in Hartmann 1987). The Progestasert, too, may soon be gone, since reports are emerging that British physicians now rarely prescribe it because of its association with a higher incidence of ectopic pregnancy than other IUDs (Women's Global Network on Reproductive Rights 1987b).

In light of the removal of IUDs from the U.S. market in particular and the more general liability crunch which currently overwhelms the entire birth control industry (Wilbur 1986; Fraser 1988), it is important to distinguish between a corporate financial decision to withdraw a product from the market and a decision voluntarily made or mandated on the grounds of medical safety. Medical evidence regarding the safety and efficacy of IUDs has not changed. IUDs have not been removed from the U.S. market by government mandate. Voluntary withdrawal of the Dalkon Shield by A. H. Robins in 1975 was morally appropriate, given its implication in the deaths and serious injuries of a number of users from septic abortions and PID. In contrast, voluntary withdrawal of the Copper-7 and Tatum-T IUDs by G. D. Searle in 1986 was fiscally appropriate based upon the fact that they were not bottom-line money-makers for their company. It is far from clear, however, that the Searle devices in any way approximate the injuriousness of the Dalkon Shield.

The reactions of women and of members of various groups particularly concerned about questions of reproductive rights to the withdrawal of IUDs from the marketplace has been mixed. Some feel that all IUDs are dangerous devices which have been forced upon unsuspecting women and that women are better off now that they are no longer available. Others, particularly representatives of the Planned Parenthood Federation, lament the reduced choice of birth control options available to women (e.g., Women's Global Network on Reproductive Rights 1986a, 1986c). Clearly, the IUD is not an appropriate birth control device for all women. However, depriving women for whom it is an appropriate option of its availability is troubling insofar as maximizing reproductive choice is a good. Further, given that other reversible, nonsteroidal birth control options are less effective, more unintended pregnancies and greater reliance on abortion are possible consequences of the withdrawal of IUDs.

Today, there are still some 2–3 million women in the United States with IUDs in place. Since some devices may have an effective life of up to ten years (e.g., the Copper-T220), many current users will continue to rely upon this method for some time to come. Also, since IUDs have not been banned—they are, as we have seen, merely no longer produced and sold—IUDs in the inventory of clinics, hospitals, and physicians will continue to be utilized until the existing supply has been exhausted. According to Wilbur (1986), most of the devices in stock have already been reserved and many women are reportedly already going to other countries to have IUDs inserted. The costs of liability insurance and the dread of lawsuits have so overwhelmed the U.S. birth control industry that not only has research on many new products been slowed to a crawl but previously available options are being eliminated. It seems ironic that there are far more birth control options available to women in third world countries than in the United States. Although worries about abuses, exploitation, and genuine informed consent arise here as they do with other birth control methods (see Chapters 5 and 9), many American women who are capable of giving genuine informed consent to the assumption of the risks that are known to be or might possibly be associated with particular IUDs are unable to choose to use them. But once all has been done that reasonably can be to minimize potential risks of a birth control method, respect for individual autonomy would seem to require that women should be free to waive their rights to bring actions for nonnegligent harms from a method if its known and theoretical potential risks are made clear to them and they decide that those risks are worth the value to them of using it. (We shall make a similar suggestion in Chapter 9 when we discuss mutagenic and teratogenic harms in the workplace.) We do believe that the information provided must include the past history of techniques (e.g., the first generation of pills, the Dalkon Shield), along with the potential of the method to involve similar problems. At a time when the spectre of AIDS increasingly threatens those who are sexually active, we would agree that condoms should be employed where there is any potential for transmission of the AIDS virus. But given the dangers associated with OCs and with pregnancy itself, and also given the failure rates of condoms (and other barrier methods) in regard to preventing pregnancy, it is not unreasonable for many women to choose a birth control methodology that holds out certain *theoretical* risks as opposed to *known* ones. Thus, despite the known risks of IUDs in general, it is not clear that having virtually none available for informed women who might choose them and be willing to waive their right to bring suit for nonnegligent harms resulting from their use is the most desirable state of affairs if reproductive choice is to be most effectively preserved.

As we go to press with this book, there are reports which indicate that an improved IUD may be available on the U.S. market soon (Weiss 1987). According to reports from the Population Council, Gyno Med Pharmaceutical of Somerville, New Jersey, has been approved to market a new copper-containing IUD called the *Copper T 380A*. This device was approved by the FDA in 1984. It has been used in other countries, including Canada, since 1982, but has never been sold in the United States. It will be explicitly marketed as a contraceptive option *only* for those women who fit the profile of an "ideal IUD user" described earlier in this section.

## POSTCOITAL METHODS OF BIRTH CONTROL

Postcoital birth control interventions are designed to act after conception. Despite the fact that the approaches to be described in this section are not aimed primarily at preventing the ovum from being fertilized (and indeed assume that fertilization has or may have already occurred), they are still erroneously and misleadingly referred to as *postcoital contraceptives*.

Postcoital birth control is aimed at the interception and destruction of the conceptus. Even if they do not subscribe to the view that an early conceptus has moral rights, many people simply object to the use of birth control "after the fact." They may view planned intercourse with planned protection as acceptable but feel that if a woman engages in unprotected intercourse she should have to pay for her transgression. Some people also disapprove of postcoital birth control because they believe that its availability as a backup to luck or contraception will encourage what they take to be irresponsible sexual behavior. (Compare some of the views discussed in Chapter 2.)

Administering some product or performing some ritual following each act of coitus is reminiscent of some of the earliest attempts at preventing unwanted birth (see Chapter 1). Physical gyrations (e.g., assuming unusual body positions, jumping up and down after intercourse) are ineffective but harmless. Vaginal douches with any of a wide array of products are also ineffective, since spermatozoa reach the cervix and uterus before they can be applied (see Chapters 1 and 4); furthermore, they can often be harmful and painful as a result of the astringent properties of many of the products used.

A bit of categorizing and explaining is in order before we proceed with a discussion of postcoital birth control. While we shall consider the physiological rationales for all major postcoital approaches to birth control, there are two general reasons why a woman may choose to employ a postcoital birth control method. The first of these is to provide "emergency" protection following unprotected intercourse. There are numerous reasons why women may seek emergency postcoital protection against an unwanted pregnancy, including condom breakage, a forgotten diaphragm, mul-

tiple missed pills, and rape. Some women may desire postcoital intervention simply because they engage in sexual activity very
infrequently and it is more convenient (and often safer) to seek protection as needed rather than constant protection. While one may
argue about the relative merits of the reasons for seeking postcoital
protection, and while some individuals may view some reasons (e.g.,
rape) as more meritorious than others (e.g., a decision to have intercourse despite lack of a contraceptive), the fact remains that there is
a need and demand for so-called morning-after birth control intervention. Some of the methods which we shall describe (e.g., various steroid pills, pre-emptive endometrial aspiration) are basically
"one-shot deals," utilized solely as measures following isolated incidents. They are not regular methods of birth control. Since many
emergency approaches also tend to include some unpleasant temporary side effects (e.g., nausea, vomiting, headaches, dizziness,
cramps), most women are unlikely to want to utilize them on a regular basis.

The second general reason for selection of a postcoital method
is to provide routine birth control. Some postcoital approaches usually allow fertilization and some degree of subsequent development
of a conceptus but then intrude at some point (usually prior to or
during implantation) to halt the continuation of development. Such
approaches include some of the antisteroidal products, such as RU-
486, and the "antipregnancy vaccine" (anti-hCG) described below.
These types of postcoital techniques have been referred to as *retrospective methods of birth control* and *contragestives*. Perhaps calling them
*postcoital* approaches is somewhat misleading, since their application has no necessary relationship to coitus. However, like the more
traditionally defined postcoital methods, their mode of action is to
intercept and eliminate a fertilized ovum. Also like the other
postcoital methods, it is generally never known whether fertilization did actually occur. Complicating the neat categorization of
approaches into the two categories of emergency and routine use is
the fact that some products (RU-486 is a good example) may be used
either as a one-time emergency measure or as a routine monthly
birth control method.

One final point should also be made before considering
postcoital methods, especially those that we have categorized as emergency measures, namely, that despite the impression one might get
from television and movies, humans, in general are relatively infer-

tile when compared to other species. Because of the large number of variables involved, most of which are related to individual traits of the man and woman involved, it is impossible to determine the probability of conception following unprotected midcycle intercourse. However, based on figures for the entire population, on the "most fertile" day of her cycle, a woman seems to have only about a 25 percent chance of conceiving if she has intercourse with a fertile man (Tietze 1960; Marshall 1971; Hatcher et al. 1980; Sloane 1980; Bromwich and Parsons 1984). In theory, this means that the odds of "getting away with it just this once" are three to one. This should not be taken as an endorsement of "risking it," since, among other things, statistics cannot be used to determine the risk in individual cases. It does suggest, however, that before resorting immediately to emergency postcoital birth control methods, particularly ones involving considerable expense and health hazards, one may want to wait and be sure that pregnancy has resulted from coitus. If unprotected intercourse occurs at any time other than just prior to ovulation, the odds of not becoming pregnant are even greater. It may also be helpful to keep in mind that any form of treatment (or nothing at all) is likely to work, on average, three times out of four. No doubt this fact has also helped to perpetuate a lot of the inadequate birth control methods that continue to be considered effective despite lack of scientific evidence.

## POSTCOITAL INTERVENTION WITH STEROIDS

*Estrogens* Various natural, synthetic, and conjugated forms of estrogens have been administered as postcoital interventions (Morris and van Wagenen 1973; Bennett 1974; Kuchera 1974; Haspels 1976; Aref and Hafez 1977; Schindler et al. 1980; Yuzpe 1980). Diethylstilbestrol (DES) has been used most frequently. DES is a nonsteroidal synthetic estrogen which was approved by the FDA in 1975 as a postcoital agent for use in certain instances, such as "rape, incest, or where unprotected coitus had occurred and continued pregnancy would be undesirable" (Djerassi 1981). It has been colloquially referred to as the *morning-after pill.* If used appropriately, DES has been shown to be a quite effective intervention, with reported failure rates of 0–2.4 percent (Kuchera 1974; Yupze 1980). Numerous variables affect its efficacy, however, the most important being the interval between conception and initiation of treatment. Treatment should begin no later than seventy-two hours following intercourse. Usual dosage is 50 mg per day taken orally for five days. Since intense and unpleasant side effects usually occur (including nausea, vomiting, headaches, and breast tenderness), continuing treatment for five days is often a problem, as is regurgitation of a dose already taken.

Another point of concern is that DES has been alleged to cause vaginal adenocarcinomas in the daughters of women who were given this drug in the mistaken belief that it would prevent miscarriage. While DES is not as likely to have the same effect on daughters when taken briefly just after conception, the FDA recommends that a therapeutic abortion be considered when a pregnancy supervenes despite DES treatment because of this possible teratogenic effect on daughters that survive postcoital DES treatment (Hatcher et al. 1980; Yupze 1980; Djerassi 1981).[4]

Various other synthetic estrogens (e.g., ethinyl estradiol) and conjugated estrogens (e.g., Premarin) have also been investigated using a regimen similar to DES treatment (Crist and Farrington 1973; Haspels and Andriesse 1973; Lehfeldt 1973; Morris and van Wagenen 1973). Pregnancy rates in all studies were 1.5 percent or less, but side effects similar to those following DES treatment were common. Injectable estrogen preparations (e.g., estradiol benzoate) have also been explored as postcoital products and have been shown to be effective (failure rate of 3 percent) and to have fewer side effects than oral estrogens (Schindler et al. 1980).

While effective, their adverse side effects surely limit the desirability and use of all of these products, especially since other approaches are at least as effective and cause fewer problems.

*Progestagens* Most of the progestagens mentioned in Chapter 5 in the discussion of ocs, injectables, implants, and medicated devices may also be used as postcoital products. However, if so utilized, considerably higher dosages must be administered. A number of clinical studies (in South America especially) show that progestagens administered at high dosages have a failure rate approaching 0 per-

---

[4] DES has been manufactured under many brand names. A partial list can be obtained from The National Cancer Institute, National Institutes of Health Publication No. 81–118 (March 1980). For another partial list, see Boston Women's Health Book Collective (1984). See Chapter 8 for a further discussion of DES and teratogenicity.

cent (Kesseru et al. 1973; Mischler et al. 1974; Garmendia et al. 1976; Yuzpe 1980; Bromwich and Parsons 1984; Ratnam and Prasad 1980; Rabe, Kiesel, and Runnebaum 1985). While the severity appears to be less than with the estrogen preparations, side effects of nausea and vomiting are again commonly reported. Alteration of the menstrual cycle also usually results. The modes of action of these products employ all of the potential postovulatory progestational effects previously described.

*Estrogen-Progestagen Combinations*   Of the steroidal choices, combinations of estrogens and progestagens are clearly the most effective. Combinations of ethinyl estradiol and dl-norgestrel have proven particularly effective (Yuzpe 1980; Bromwich and Parsons 1984). A dose of four tablets of what is referred to as *Ovral* or *Eugynon 50* taken within 3 days of unprotected intercourse has been shown to be effective in nearly all cases reported. The usual intervention is two doses of two tablets taken twelve hours apart. While nausea is experienced by some women taking the tablets, it is not as common or as severe as in the preparations previously described, and vomiting is commonly alleviated by concomitant administration of an antiemetic (i.e., an antivomiting preparation).

The primary mode of action of these combination products is the induction of endometrial changes incompatible with implantation. A marked asynchrony between endometrial glandular and stromal maturation is induced, with the glands lagging behind the stroma. LH production by the anterior pituitary may also be suppressed, in turn affecting ovarian steroidogenesis (Yuzpe 1980; see Chapter 4).

POSTCOITAL INTERVENTION WITH ANTISTEROIDS

The normal functions of both estrogen and progesterone during the menstrual cycle and in preparation for implantation were described in Chapter 4. Since both play crucial roles in numerous reproductive processes, including gamete transport and endometrial function, interfering with either steroid and altering the ratio between the two is likely to result in failure of pregnancy.

In order for all hormones to work, they must interact with receptors located in the cells of their target tissue (e.g., the endometrium).

Hormones normally act on cells in a manner analogous to keys unlocking a door. If a lock has been jammed by putting a very similar key into it—that is, a key that will fit into the lock but that will not turn to open the door—then the appropriate key cannot be inserted to open the door. Likewise, if a steroid hormone receptor site is occupied by a look-alike interloper (i.e., an antisteroid), then even though the "true" steroid is present, it is unable to exert its usual effect. Both anti-estrogens and, even more effectively, antiprogestins have been successfully used to disrupt the normal events leading to implantation.

*Antiestrogen Agents*    The most widely utilized anti-estrogen is a product called *Anordin*. Also known as the "Chinese vacation pill," it has been investigated and utilized quite extensively in China since the early 1970s. It was developed in China for use as a postcoital pill for married couples who live apart for extensive periods and who meet only a few times a year for vacation (Lei and Hu 1981). According to instructions, the vacation pill should first be taken immediately after coitus and then again the following morning. While it may interfere with normal oviductal motility and egg transport, its more probable mode of action is blockage of the normally estrogen-dependent synthesis of progesterone receptors during the proliferative phase of the endometrium (Aitken 1979; Mehta, Jenco, and Chatterton 1981; see Chapter 4). The consequence of this treatment is a failure to develop an adequate endometrium to support implantation.

One problem with Anordin (and the reason why it is never likely to gain FDA approval) is the potentially large amount of the active steroid ingredient that may be consumed by women engaging in intercourse frequently during a relatively brief time. Since each tablet contains 7.5 mg of active steroid (Djerassi 1981) and since taking a tablet is "event related," a woman who had coitus daily during a four-week vacation would consume over 200 mg of active estrogenic steroid during that period. This would be considered a potentially unsafe dosage.

There are other anti-estrogenic products which have been investigated (e.g., Dinordin I, Dinordin II, Centchroman), again primarily in China. But these products appear even less suitable than Anordin (Harper 1983; Ratnam and Prasad 1984). Also under investigation is the use of Anordin in a modified regimen which would require one pill monthly rather than daily and with a dose sufficient to suppress ovulation.

*Antiprogesterone Agents*   As we saw in Chapter 4, progesterone is an absolute requisite for the establishment and maintenance of pregnancy. Logically, then, a product which interferes with the usual roles of progesterone (i.e., an antiprogesterone agent) has potential as a postcoital agent. While several products have been investigated for this purpose (see Harper 1983; Rabe, Kiesel, and Runnebaum 1985), we shall concentrate on the one product shown to be most effective, RU-486, which has recently received considerable international attention.

Not since the controversy surrounding the introduction of the pill has there been a birth control option that has caused the degree of excitement and optimism and outrage and condemnation created by RU-486. Elements of the controversy are apparent in some of the monickers used in reference to this preparation, which include *the NEW pill, the abortion pill, the antifetus pill,* and *the French death pill.* This last appellation is apparently inspired by the fact that the drug was developed by Roussel-Uclaf (hence the *RU*), which is a French affiliate of Hoechst-Roussel Pharmaceuticals, based in Geneva, Switzerland. Although perhaps more commonly recognized by its in-house designation, *RU-486,* it has also been given the name *mifepristone.* Before considering the controversial aspects of this product, we need first to examine its basic properties.

RU-486 is classified biochemically as a norsteroid. The substituents at the C-17 and C-11 positions on the steroid structure cause it to resemble a progestin in structure, but its full structure more closely resembles some anti-estrogenic products. It has a unique capacity to bind with very high affinity to the progesterone receptor (a five-times greater affinity for the progesterone receptor than progesterone itself), but it lacks progestin activity. Despite its general structural similarity to anti-estrogens, it also has no estrogenic or anti-estrogenic action (Harper 1983; Rabe, Kiesel, and Runnebaum 1983; Philibert et al. 1985). If we briefly reconsider the normal role of progesterone, it will be easy to see how RU-486 works and why it is creating (and is likely to continue creating) such an intense controversy.

As we described in detail in Chapter 4, progesterone is needed to cause the endometrial proliferation and secretion essential to allow implantation and continued development of the fertilized egg. To exert this effect at the level of the cell, progesterone must first bind with a specific receptor located within each endometrial cell. RU-486, because of its greater binding affinity for the receptors normally bound by progesterone, simply blocks the cells of the endometrium from responding to progesterone. In the absence of progesterone support, the uterus is "tricked" into doing exactly what happens at the end of every menstrual cycle—sloughing off and expelling the uterine lining. Within forty-eight hours after taking a single 600 mg RU-486 pill, uterine bleeding begins. Thus, RU-486 simply induces, at the time decided upon by the woman taking it, the shedding of the uterine lining and the onset of menses. The potential difference here, however, is that if a conceptus was present in the uterus—either free-floating prior to implantation or implanted in the superficial layer of the endometrium, which dies and is sloughed off without progesterone support—that conceptus is also expelled. If the woman has not conceived, RU-486 has merely induced a menstruation like any other. If she has conceived within the previous week (i.e., prior to implantation), then RU-486 has blocked implantation. If she conceived earlier, perhaps up to as much as two months earlier, then RU-486 has induced what is universally recognized as an abortion of an established pregnancy (see Chapter 5).

Thus, it is clear why RU-486 is such a revolutionary and controversial drug. There are numerous options for its use. Which, if any, of these uses is morally acceptable depends on one's moral positions on contraception and elective abortion.

How effective is RU-486? As reported by Etienne Baulieu, the University of Paris-Sud biochemist credited with pioneering the development of RU-486, and cited by Baulieu (1985, 1987), Clark, Springen, and Alderman (1986), Franklin (1987), and Halpren (1987), when Baulieu administered RU-486 to 100 women within the first three weeks of an unwanted pregnancy, 85 women experienced a relatively painless onset of a menstrual period at home within four to fourteen days. The most serious side effect was prolonged bleeding, which was experienced by eighteen of the women. The fifteen women who did not abort reported some degree of bleeding without embryo expulsion and they subsequently underwent conventional suction abortions. Baulieu claims that by adding a "touch" of prostaglandins (to induce uterine contractions) the success rate of RU-486 is 95 percent. Based on tests of RU-486 in about 4,000 women in various stages of pregnancy in fifteen countries over the past five years, scientists involved in the studies conclude that a single 600 mg dose taken within roughly a month after conception will usually terminate pregnancy with few side effects. By adding supplemental injected or intravaginal prostaglandins, Baulieu (1987) suggests that the effective period may be extended by an extra month or perhaps more.

What about its use as a drug for terminating known pregnancies following implantation? Again, the value of RU-486 depends on one's view concerning whether the means to elective abortion should be available to women. According to John Willke of the National Right to Life Committee (quoted by Clark et al. 1987), RU-486 is "chemical warfare on the unborn . . . you have a direct killing of the baby already implanted."[5] However, proponents of RU-486 argue that it offers to women who desire abortions an alternative which is safer and far less emotionally and physically traumatic than the currently available options (which we shall discuss shortly). Baulieu (see Franklin 1987) points out that botched abortions in developing countries claim the lives of an estimated 125,000 women each year. Thus, many supporters of allowing elective abortion are quick to note that since RU-486 is a far safer abortion alternative, it may literally be a lifesaver for many of the women who use it.

What of its use as a more traditional postcoital birth control drug (i.e., a drug employed following coitus and potential pregnancy but where there is no confirmation whether pregnancy did result)? In comparison with older morning-after approaches such as DES, RU-486 is vastly superior. Should it be made available for use in the emergency situations described earlier but not for use as an elective abortative? Not only does it avoid the harsh side effects associated with most of the previously mentioned products (e.g., nausea, vomiting, cramps, heavy bleeding), but it also provides women with a longer time interval after unprotected intercourse within which to take a postcoital preparation. With RU-486 as an option, women could avoid the side effects of the early intervention products, wait until pregnancy could be accurately determined by an hCG test (days 7–9), and then, if they so choose, terminate the

---

[5] For a discussion of the implications of the use of terms like *baby* and *parasite* in the abortion debate, see Chapter 7.

pregnancy at basically the same time and with basically the same effects as their normal menstrual period.

Should RU-486 be available to women for use as their primary means of birth control? In theory, RU-486 could be taken once every four weeks approximately forty-eight hours prior to a woman's expected date of menstruation. Menstruation would simply occur at its expected time, with the woman unaware of whether or not an early embryo was being expelled with the menstrual flow (analogous to the situation of IUD users). A one-pill-a-month regimen is convenient and avoids the long-term and potentially serious side effects of OCs and IUDs. At present, Baulieu (see Baulieu 1987) does not recommend that RU-486 be used as a repeated menstrual inducer, since, at the currently used dosage, it interferes with the next cycle, causing a delay of follicular maturation and thereby disturbing periodicity. He hastens to point out that while the potential to use an antiprogestin in this manner is quite possible in the future, one with a shorter half-life is needed to avoid spillover into the next ovulation. He suggests that with the knowledge that has already come out of the development of RU-486, a second generation of products will be developed that will effectively counter any action of the progesterone needed in order to achieve fertility control.

It is interesting to note which potential use of RU-486 is seized upon by proponents and opponents of the drug in an attempt to "sell" their views to the public. Those who oppose elective abortion label it as a "chemical inducer of abortion" or, even more magniloquently, "a chemical death pill for killing unborn babies." People who hold this moral position are clearly concerned that the public perceive RU-486 as an abortative and not as a contraceptive. At the same time, those who support keeping abortion as an option for all women want RU-486 to be identified as a once-a-month rather than a once-a-day contraceptive pill that has fewer side effects and long-term health risks than already accepted OCs. Since more people support the routine use of what they perceive to be contraception than advocate the routine choice of abortion as a method of birth control, the public relations approach of the two sides in the debate is understandable. Also, since RU-486 is applied only very early in the gestation process, opponents of elective abortion cannot utilize the emotionally powerful, often effective, but invalid technique of showing graphic evidence of the remains of aborted late-term fetuses to marshall supporters to their cause. (This technique was employed in *The Silent Scream*; see Chapter 7; Callahan 1986c.) As pointed out by Halpren (1987), "there is no public relations value in a menstruating woman." Opponents of elective abortion fear that the availability of a product which allows women to abort in the privacy of their homes by merely swallowing a pill would lead to even more women choosing abortion. And they may well be correct.

At present, even the supporters of RU-486 are divided regarding the manner and extent to which the drug should be utilized. Perhaps the major concern among most members of the scientific community is the long-term safety of repeated or continuous use of RU-486. The question of safety cannot be answered at present, or in the near future for that matter, since RU-486 has been tested in women for only five years. A constant dilemma arises from the desire to have adequate information to assess possible long-term risks of any new technology while not inordinately delaying the availability of that technology to the individuals who need and desire it. Clearly RU-486, based only on an assessment of the short-term side effects reported to date, is not totally risk-free. Prolonged uterine bleeding has been reported to accompany its usage in some women. Dizziness, nausea, and painful contractions have also been reported. In assessing the severity and acceptability of side effects, it must be kept in mind that such assessments are always relative to a potential benefit. In regard to its use as a postcoital agent, which is the use of RU-486 that appears to have the widest support at present, its side effects appear to be far less severe than those associated with any other currently available method. As an early-gestation abortative, its complications likewise appear to be less common and less severe than currently utilized procedures. Prolonged bleeding is also the most common side effect of all other abortion methods, as we shall see shortly. It might be prudent to require that RU-486 be used as an abortative only under the care of a physician (not by a woman at home); this would ensure that excessive bleeding does not occur and that the abortion was successfully completed. Unexpelled tissue remaining in the uterus (from any type of abortion procedure) can lead to infection and serious complications. Also, a woman using RU-486 must be completely sure that she does want to abort, since if the abortion should be unsuccessful, the drug may cause fetal damage. Possible teratogenic effects of RU-486 have not been assessed yet, because the drug is so new (teratogenic effects of conventional birth control methods are discussed in Chapter 8).

While we have to this point limited our discussion of RU-486 to a consideration of its potential birth control implications, we should also point out that as an antiprogesterone agent it has several other potential applications which are less controversial and vitally important to women's health (see Franklin 1987). For example, it may in the future prove to be a valuable treatment for breast cancer. As many as 33 percent of breast cancers in women contain an abundance of progesterone receptors and the tumors require progesterone to survive. Laboratory studies indicate that RU-486 can block these progesterone receptors in cancer cells in the same way they block endometrial progesterone receptors. By so doing, the drug would prevent the growth of a tumor. Since RU-486 also has a strong affinity for receptors of glucocorticoid (a product of the adrenal gland structurally similar to progesterone), it may also turn out to be effective in the treatment of conditions such as Cushing's syndrome (a condition of excess glucocorticoid production leading to skeletal, metabolic, and skin abnormalities). Traditional drugs used to treat Cushing's syndrome have often caused total destruction of the adrenal tissue and have other side effects of a very serious nature. Early studies have suggested that RU-486 can block the effects of excess glucocorticoids and reverse the symptoms of Cushing's syndrome without damaging the adrenal gland. Preliminary findings reported by Franklin (1987) also indicate that RU-486 may successfully treat endometriosis, an aberrant growth of the endometrium which is quite painful and often leads to infertility. Finally, when used at parturition, RU-486 has been shown to aid in cervical dilation to widen the birth canal and allow vaginal deliveries in cases where the process of cesarean delivery (which is riskier to women) might otherwise be necessary.

Although these potential uses of RU-486 are not directly germane to the issue of birth control, those who oppose research funding for investigation of RU-486 and other antiprogesterone agents because of their potential use as abortatives should also be aware of their other potential applications. Ironically, two of these potential applications (i.e., decreasing infertility resulting from endometriosis and aiding vaginal childbirth) actually aid the cause of producing healthy and wanted babies.

Research still in its initial stages suggests yet another way in which RU-486 may be utilized for birth control. Preliminary findings by Gary Hodgen at the Jones Institute for Reproductive Medicine in Norfolk, Virginia, reported by Franklin (1987), indicate that a lower dose of RU-486 given two to three days prior to ovulation blocks release of the egg; thus, the drug may be capable of being used as a true contraceptive (see Chapter 5) without disrupting the menstrual cycle.

From the viewpoint of American women who may want this drug available, our discussion of the potential merits of RU-486 is purely academic. For the reasons pointed out in our discussion of other promising birth control technologies, RU-486 is not likely to be available in the foreseeable future. This is again because of the lengthy and costly process necessary for FDA approval, the prohibitive cost of liability insurance, and risk of lawsuits, which function as disincentives to pharmaceutical companies. Further, because of its clear potential use as an abortative, the political controversy surrounding RU-486 makes approval even more of a long shot than in the case of other contemporary methods.

By June 1988, RU-486 was approved for use in five countries, namely, France, Great Britain, the Netherlands, Sweden, and China (Fraser 1988). In the fall of 1988, at the annual conference of the International Federation of Obstetricians and Gynaecologists, it was announced that Rousell-Uclaf had decided to withdraw RU-486 from the market, apparently in response to threats of boycotts of all its products by American and European antiabortion groups. The French minister of health subsequently ordered the company to reverse its decision, allowing it to claim that it had no choice in putting the product on the French market (Women's Global Network on Reproductive Rights 1988). Other similar political actions are not unlikely as the drug moves onto international markets. The future is difficult to predict, but safe and successful clinical experiences and public acceptance in other countries is sure to lead to increased pressure on the FDA to approve experimental use in the United States by informed women who believe that RU-486 is the most appropriate birth control method for them.

POSTCOITAL IUD INSERTION

Morning-after insertion of an IUD is the oldest of the modern methods of postcoital intervention. Little more on IUDs needs to be said at this point, since we have already discussed the modes of action and relative merits and disadvantages of the IUD. Even if pregnancy results from unprotected intercourse, insertion of an IUD any time prior to implantation (from the perspective of efficacy, the sooner after the event the better) is likely to inhibit implantation and cause the conceptus to be expelled. Copper IUDs, no doubt because they immediately interfere with endometrial activity, are the best choice for postcoital interception. Naturally, all the discomforts previously described as accompanying initial IUD insertion discourage many women who request postcoital intervention from choosing this option. Psychologically, a woman who has not made a conscious decision to choose the IUD as a birth control method and who is upset because of the "accident" or rape that resulted in her needing postcoital protection is likely to be less able to tolerate the pain and discomfort which accompanies initial IUD insertion. On the positive side, of course, the IUD would provide continued future protection, which is not afforded by other methods.

## PRE-EMPTIVE ENDOMETRIAL ASPIRATION

It is really a matter of semantics whether to consider this a postcoital intervention abortifacient method or a method of abortion proper. It is, in essence, the same procedure as the vacuum aspiration or suction abortion described later in this chapter. Theoretically, one need only wait a sufficient time after intercourse to ensure that, if pregnancy did result, the conceptus has had time to reach the uterus (i.e., a week or so). Usually the procedure is performed within a day or two after a missed or expected period. A small cannula (tube) can be passed into the uterus, usually without the need for using a local anesthetic; it is attached to a syringe that provides minimal but sufficient suction pressure to evacuate endometrial tissue and blood from the uterus (Hatcher et al. 1980; Sloane 1980). The procedure is quick, relatively painless, and has a very low rate of complication. Since it is generally performed at a time when it is possible to discern whether the woman is pregnant, one would think that most women would want to know if they were pregnant and avoid this procedure if they were not. However, some women apparently choose to have it performed as soon as possible and without a confirmation of pregnancy in order to avoid the ethical dilemma that would arise if they knew they were pregnant. But this approach is troubling, not only because it is a "head in the sand" way of dealing with a question of moral import, but also because it is important for a woman's psychological well-being that she be clear that she accepts abortion as morally permissible before using any birth control method which might result in what is commonly considered abortion. And, as we have suggested previously, many contemporary birth control technologies can have abortifacient actions not known to be such by women using them. Some women who were not clear on their positions and have had abortions or have used abortifacient methods have spend a lifetime dealing with guilt and anger. This is among the several reasons why we shall, in Chapter 7, undertake a careful discussion of the morality of elective abortion. The points discussed there will apply equally to the use of abortifacient methods of birth control.

ANTIPREGNANCY VACCINES

It has been proposed that a woman who does not wish to become pregnant could simply be "vaccinated" against pregnancy (i.e., given a vaccine for the purpose of protection), just as one is immunized against measles or smallpox. This concept is very simple and based on the most fundamental immunological principle: The antigen-antibody reaction. An antigen is any foreign (non-self) protein (in this case the "vaccine"), and an antibody is a protective protein (or globulin) made by the body's immune system in response to an antigen. Generally speaking, except in the case of so-called autoimmune diseases, self-antigens (i.e., proteins normally present in the body) that are specific to the reproductive process do not cause any immunological interference with reproduction. However, reproductive-specific antigens can be altered or modified so that a woman's immune system no longer recognizes them as proteins to be tolerated but rather perceives them as foreign proteins to make antibodies against. The basis of an antipregnancy or birth control vaccine, therefore, is to utilize a pregnancy-specific antigen (i.e., a protein produced only when pregnancy occurs), modify it so that it would not be tolerated by the woman's immune system, and stimulate the production of antibodies so they are present in the woman's circulation to combat the antigen if it reappears. Thus, when pregnancy occurs and the pregnancy-specific antigen is detected by the body, the circulating antibodies will combine with the antigen, neutralize it, prevent it from performing its normal function, and cause pregnancy to fail. Before addressing the specific case of antipregnancy vaccines, let's very briefly consider immunological approaches to birth control in general.

In theory, any protein specific to the reproductive process is a possible target for immunological control of fertility. This suggests that this approach could be utilized in men as well as women, the obvious male target being the proteins specific to spermatozoa. Unfortunately, research on men has indicated that this approach is not feasible as a reversible method of fertility control (although it is a possible approach to sterilization), since irreversible destruction of spermatogonia has been the usual result (Bahl and Muralidhar 1980; Jones 1980; O'Rand 1980; Fawcett 1982; Harper 1983; Goldberg 1983; Zatuchni 1985). For women, antibodies against the zona pellucida (the outer glycoprotein membrane covering the ovum) have been investigated as a means of disrupting the ovum (Aitken and Richardson 1980; Bahl and Muralidhar 1980; Shivers and Sieg 1980; Sacco et al. 1981; Wood, Liu, and Dunbar 1981; Zatuchni 1985). Research in this area appears to be suspended at present (as a result of restraints and the complexity of the zona pellucida antigens) in order to concentrate on a more promising immunological target – placental proteins. Several placental-specific proteins are produced during pregnancy and many have been investigated for potential immunological control of fertility (Edwards 1980; Heyner 1980; Johnson, Brown, and Faulk 1980; Stevens 1980; Harper 1983; Ratnam and Prasad 1984; Rabe, Kiesel, and Runnebaum 1985). By far the most promising placental antigen for developing an antipregnancy vaccine is derived from the beta-subunit of hCG (Talwar 1980). We shall concentrate the remainder of our discussion on the anti-hCG vaccine.

As we saw in Chapter 4, hCG is a pregnancy-specific glyco-protein hormone (protein with a carbohydrate group attached) that is produced by the trophoblastic cells of the early embryo beginning about the time of implantation (days 6–8 after fertilization). Detection of hCG is the basis of pregnancy testing. The major role of hCG is to stimulate the corpus luteum to continue to produce the progesterone necessary to maintain pregnancy. Conversely, if the normal effects of hCG are negated, progesterone levels decline, implantation is disrupted, and pregnancy fails.

In women, hCG does not normally produce an immunological response. However, if modified and linked to other molecules (e.g., tetanus toxoid, the source of vaccines against tetanus), antibodies are produced against hCG. If a woman so immunized should subsequently conceive, the antibodies in her system would counteract the normally stimulatory actions of hCG as soon as it appeared, and her pregnancy would not be maintained. Therefore, this approach to birth control involves using a potentially continuous abortifacient agent that acts after implantation.

Like several other glycoprotein hormones, hCG consists of two subunits or "chains" linked together. In general, the first of these two subunits, the alpha-subunit, is structurally similar to several hormones and to the same hormone in different species. The second, or beta-subunit, is both hormone- and species-specific. Since hCG has the same basic biological properties as does luteinizing hormone (LH — see Chapter 4), it is not surprising that their structure (specifically, their amino acid sequence) is very similar. This fact caused some of the early attempts to develop an antibody against hCG to fail, since the antibody developed against the entire beta-subunit cross-reacted with LH (also with follicle-stimulating hormone [FSH] — see Chapter 4 — and with the thyroid-stimulating hormone, TSH). Since the most critical requirement of an hCG vaccine was that it be highly specific towards the embryo and its product and not interfere with the maternal hormones, it was back to the drawing board. Subsequent attempts concentrated on developing antibodies against a series of thirty amino acids located on the "tail" of the beta-subunit of hCG but which do not appear on the beta-subunit of LH. This allowed the development of antibodies which are highly specific to hCG and do not cross-react with LH or any other hormone. In order to increase its antigenicity (potency as an antigen), the beta-subunit is commonly linked to a "carrier," such as tetanus toxoid. Details of the studies which have led to development of the antipregnancy vaccine and details regarding its preparation can be found in the reports of Bahl and Muralidhar (1980), Hearn (1979), Stevens (1980), and Talwar (1980).

One problem in testing the immunological approach to birth control is the availability of a suitable model. For most other birth control technologies, there have been several animal models which were appropriate for designing initial testing, a common prerequisite to testing in humans. However, since only primates produce hCG during pregnancy, possible test subjects are limited. Tests utilizing baboons and monkeys indicate about a 95 percent success rate (Hearn 1978, 1979; Hingorani and Kumar 1979; Thanavala et al. 1979;

Harper 1983; Wilbur 1986). The rate may be even higher when purer preparations are utilized in women.

Human testing is now under way, primarily in Australia (Wilbur 1986). Initial trials to verify the production of antibodies against hCG following administration of the vaccine have been highly successful. For ethical reasons, these early trials were conducted with women who had already been voluntarily sterilized, since reversibility was unknown. It is, therefore, impossible to assess the actual birth control effectiveness of the vaccine on the basis of these trials.

Reports to date, however, do suggest that this immunological approach will prove to be effective. Since it was strictly to counteract a product of pregnancy, if should not produce any of the long- or short-term side effects or health risks common to some of the birth control approaches discussed earlier. It does not appear to disrupt normal menstrual cycles, and women have no way of knowing if conception did occur. It is convenient, and initial studies suggest that a single vaccination is good for about a year (Wilbur 1986).

Despite its positive features, it is unlikely that an antipregnancy vaccine will gain widespread acceptance. In reconsidering the points of disquietude mentioned in our discussion of other birth control methodologies, it is obvious that this approach raises several of the same issues. Unlike some other products which *may* have an abortifacient mode of action, this product depends solely on that mode. This makes it highly controversial and would in itself be reason enough for many people to choose not to use it and to launch a major protest against it should serious consideration ever be given to making it available as a birth control method. The very idea of a vaccination that would immunize women against babies is a horrifying prospect to many people. Not only is it perceived as a futuristic technology; but it also has a serious potential for abuse, including possible eugenic uses which exceed those of other products objected to on similar grounds. At present, we do not have reliable data regarding the reversibility of this vaccine or the homogeneity of response among individuals. From a purely scientific point of view, lack of reversibility and variations in response may prove to be the major drawbacks of this approach. If the antibodies last too long, a woman may not be able to regain fertility when she so desires, and certainly the potential exists for protracted or even permanent infertility. On the other hand, if the antibody protection does not last as long as expected, an unwanted pregnancy may occur while a woman thinks that she is still protected. This leads to the other reason why it is not likely to be approved, at least in the United States — the likelihood of lawsuits resulting from such potential failures.

MISCELLANEOUS POSTCOITAL METHODS

As we have already seen, there are numerous kinds of postcoital pregnancy interventions. Before leaving this subject and concluding the chapter with a look at induced abortion techniques, for the sake of completeness we briefly list some of the other approaches which we have chosen not to discuss in detail, primarily because of limits to their use. Reviews of the methods listed below are available in several sources, including Bennett (1974), Hahn, McGuire, and Chang (1980), Harper (1983), and Rabe, Kiesel, and Runnebaum (1985).

*Inhibitors of Egg Transport*    Products such as reserpine, chlorpromazine, and tetrabenazine have been investigated because of their capacity to interfere with smooth muscle activity and to consequently alter the rate of egg transport and cause the failure of pregnancy (especially see Bennett 1974).

*Enzyme Inhibitors*    Since the establishment and maintenance of pregnancy is dependent on many biochemical pathways, products which interfere with the normal function of the enzymes controlling biochemical conversions have the potential for pregnancy intervention. To date, the area examined most extensively is the inhibition of enzymes involved in the steroidogenic pathway. By inhibiting steps in the pathway required to produce the steroid hormones needed to maintain pregnancy, some success has been achieved in causing pregnancy failure.

*Plant Toxins*    Although of relatively little applicability to women in the United States, the use of toxins extracted from plants indigenous to various regions is still one of the most common methods of inducing abortions worldwide. This ancient approach (see Chapter 1) has been refined by scientists working in several programs; they have collected the plants traditionally used for this purpose, isolated and tested the active ingredients, and undertaken studies to examine their potential as abortifacients. Among the hundreds of plants so examined are the "Chinese motherwort" and a plant indigenous to Mexico, Zoapatle, both of which have been extensively investigated. Trichosanthin, a compound obtained from the roots of a plant common in China, has been used in Chinese medicine for centuries to induce menstruation and expel fetal membranes. As might be expected, the toxic nature of several plants that make them effective abortifacients also tends to produce other toxic effects which can cause serious illness and even death to women consuming them.

*Prostaglandins* We shall discuss the abortifacient use of prostaglandins and their analogues in the next section. However, they could also be used postcoitally to induce menstruation prior to confirmation of pregnancy. Since prostaglandins (especially prostaglandin $F_{2\alpha}$) cause strong uterine contractions, they could be used to expel the pre-implantation conceptus, to trigger endometrial sloughing, and to cause regression of the corpus luteum and lack of progesterone support. For reviews of the use of prostaglandins as both abortifacients and induced abortion technologies, see Lauersen (1979), World Health Organization (1981), and Harper (1983).

INDUCED ABORTION TECHNIQUES

The methods we are about to discuss, which involve deliberate termination of a known pregnancy, differ from the preceding insofar as there is virtually universal agreement that they are not appropriate for use as routine forms of birth control. Even those who stridently support a policy of elective abortion almost universally agree that these methods (which are commonly categorized as *induced abortion methods*) should be used only as a last resort when other methods have failed or other methods were not used or could not be used (see Chapter 7). No type of induced abortion is completely devoid of pain and trauma, both physical and emotional. Those who oppose the availability of medically safe induced abortion as a choice for women on the grounds that its availability discourages the use of contraceptives and that abortion would be routinely used as a form of birth control fail to understand the reluctance of women to resort to induced abortion (see Chapter 7).

While we readily acknowledge that the distinction between abortifacient birth control techniques and induced abortion techniques may be viewed by many as a mere conceptual distinction of no moral importance, it can also be argued that the physiological differences accompanying use of these two kinds of methods are significant enough to make for a moral difference between the methods, much as early term physiological differences were once held by Roman Catholic theologians and secular courts to be grounds for distinguishing between morally acceptable and morally unacceptable induced abortions (see Chapter 7).

Reproductive physiologists refer to the event of hCG production which accompanies implantation and facilitates the "rescue" of the corpus luteum (i.e., hCG prevents the corpus luteum from regressing and a new cycle from occurring by stimulating maintenance of the corpus luteum and continued progesterone production to support pregnancy) as *maternal recognition of pregnancy*. The term is meant to acknowledge that there is a narrow "window in time" in the menstrual cycle during which the corpus luteum must be "signalled" that it should continue to function (if conception has occurred) or, in the absence of this signal, regress to allow another cycle to occur, thereby providing another opportunity for pregnancy. In a scientific context, *maternal recognition of pregnancy* means that the maternal endocrine system "recognizes" that conception has occurred (due to the hCG signal from the embryo) and that the endocrine system (through its hormonal production) should in turn cause appropriate modifications to occur in other systems to accommodate the embryo. Until these signals are sent, received, and acted upon, a woman is not yet in a full state of pregnancy, since the conditions necessary for support of the embryo do not yet exist. The embryo may fail to send the proper signals, the woman's systems may fail to recognize (or "read") the signals sent, or the woman's body may refuse to recognize (or "obey") the signals, rejecting the "order" to move into a state of full pregnancy. Since the actions of the products we have discussed take place during the period before a woman's body has made a commitment to pregnancy, it can be argued that, even though they allow conception and implantation, these methods *preclude* rather than *terminate* pregnancy and are therefore more like contraceptive techniques than they are like induced abortion techniques.

Rather than taking conception or implantation as the morally crucial physiological event (see Chapters 5 and 7), such arguments take the commitment of the woman's body to pregnancy as the crucial event, an event that distinguishes as morally acceptable true contraceptive techniques and techniques that intervene prior to maternal recognition of pregnancy from unacceptable induced abortion techniques.

But this argument from the way the natural world is to what is morally required or permitted is closely related to another argument which condones induced abortion. This latter argument also turns on the physiological fact that a woman's body must "accept" a pregnancy for that pregnancy to become established and continue. The argument then holds that, although chronologically later than physiological recognition (i.e., "knowledge") of pregnancy, an event that might be called *phenomenological maternal recognition of pregnancy* occurs which is analogous to physiological recognition. This event occurs when a woman receives confirmation that (i.e., comes to know that) conception has taken place. Generally, this event is preceded by a woman's realization that she has not begun menstruating, and cognitive recognition (i.e., knowledge) of pregnancy is reached when physiological pregnancy is confirmed by a medical test. But, as in the case of physiological maternal recognition of pregnancy, it can be argued by analogy that full recognition also involves *commitment* to pregnancy, and (again as in physiological recognition) a full maternal state is not achieved until that commitment is made—that is, until the woman consciously accepts and commits to supporting the developing embryo. The argument contends that just as there is no moral wrong involved when a woman's body declines to commit to sustaining an embryo, there is no moral wrong involved in a woman's consciously declining to sustain an embryo or a fetus.

It might be objected at this point that the most this analogical argument can establish is that a woman is morally permitted to terminate a pregnancy immediately upon having it confirmed. Thus, only very early abortions could be justified by the argument. In reply, the argument's proponent can now point out that 15–25 percent of all physiologically recognized pregnancies end in spontaneous (i.e., natural as opposed to willful) abortion (French and Bierman 1972; Ahmad 1979; Edmonds et al. 1982; Benirschke 1986) and that it has been estimated, although it is impossible to prove, that up to 75 percent of *all* human conceptions are aborted spontaneously (Lauritsen 1982). Of spontaneous abortions, some 50 percent (Boué et al. 1975) are reportedly due to "cytogenetic errors" (i.e., problems in development due to genetic causes). Lauritsen (1982) estimates that "Mother Nature" eliminates about 95 percent of "her cytogenetic errors" through spontaneous abortions prior to the twenty-eighth week of gestation, and he suggests that this should be regarded as an important selective mechanism. On the basis of the analogy, it can be argued that elective induced abortion is morally acceptable through at least the end of the second trimester, which, as we shall see in Chapter 7, is where contemporary U.S. policy draws the line, guaranteeing a woman the right to have an abortion for any reason whatever up to this point in pregnancy (though procedures may be regulated to protect her health). That policy, however, is argued for on other grounds, as we shall see.

We do not find either of the analogical arguments for morally distinguishing abortifacient from induced abortion methods or the analogical argument for classifying these methods together convincing, since all arguments which proceed immediately from the way nature is to the way persons may or may not function share two crucial problems. First, there are many occurrences in nature that we think ought not be imitated by rational beings, for example, certain aggressive interactions between animals. Thus, the fact that something occurs "in nature" does not in itself entail anything about the moral acceptability of actions or practices of moral agents. Second, natural occurrences are so varied that virtually *any* conclusion can be "justified" by appealing to some selected set of them. There are also arguments from natural events which conclude that "artificially" assisted contraception is never morally justified, just as there are arguments from natural occurrences for and against the moral acceptability of genetic engineering, homosexual interaction, in vitro fertilization, artificial insemination, surrogate motherhood, and a host of other things. What has been established is that there are arguments from nature *for* the moral acceptability of routine use of abortifacients and for electing induced abortion to counteract the arguments from nature against these practices. Thus, the arguments given above help to show that arguments from natural events are just not helpful in answering hard moral questions. (For additional problems with arguments from nature to the morality or immorality of actions, see, e.g., Gorovitz 1982, chap. 10; de Sousa 1985; Leiser 1986, chap. 3; Callahan 1988b, chap. 1.) In the next chapter we shall outline and evaluate what we take to be the strongest argument against the use of abortifacients and induced abortion. Before doing that, however, we need to describe existing methods of induced abortion (hereafter referred to simply as *abortion*).

As we have implied, abortion is generally sought because a failure has occurred. This may be a failure to use any form of contraception—it is estimated that up to 80 percent of all women seeking abortion were using no birth control method at the time of conception (Ahmad 1979)—or a failure of the method of birth control being used. As we have indicated previously, most method failures occur because of improper usage, but one must also keep in mind that no method except total abstinence is 100 percent effective. In an ideal world, unwanted pregnancies would not occur and there would be little demand for abortion. However, ours is not an ideal world, and we often must deal with undesirable realities. One of those realities is that accidents will happen, for neither people nor products are perfect. Birth control methods having a failure rate of only 1 percent are certainly considered to be highly effective. Yet, even if all women faithfully and appropriately used methods having such a low failure rate, there would still be millions of women who would become pregnant when they did not want to be. Thus, the demand for abortion will continue to exist, even with relatively safe and effective contraceptives and abortifacients readily available to all women.

For women considering any induced abortion procedure, appropriate pre-abortion testing, which should include a pregnancy test, assorted blood tests (hemoglobin and hematocrit determination, clotting time, blood typing, etc.), a pap smear, a gonorrhea culture, and a urinalysis, should be conducted prior to the performance of the procedure. Nonjudgmental professional counseling regarding the attending risks and the expected effects of the abortion should also be provided.

*Menstrual Extraction* We have already discussed this technique as a potential method of postcoital intervention. As a postcoital technique, it is usually referred to as *pre-emptive endometrial aspiration*, indicating that the endometrium can be aspirated and menstruation induced before it is known whether pregnancy occurred. Once the presence of a conceptus has been established, the term pre-emptive is no longer appropriate; however, the technique of utilizing a thin tube (or cannula) passed into the uterus and applying minimal suction via a syringe attached to the tube removes the endometrium (and the early embryo) in an identical fashion. Other terms used for this procedure include *menstrual regulation* and *endometrial extraction*, although they are really euphemisms, since they imply that this procedure is being used merely to "regulate" an irregular cycle or "extract" menstrual products that for some reason are trapped. (The terms linger on from the days when elective abortion was illegal.)

This procedure is used only in the very early stages of pregnancy, specifically within two weeks of a missed menstrual period (approximately four weeks into pregnancy). The approximate equivalent of a menstrual period follows endometrial aspiration. The initial advantage of this procedure was felt to be that, since it was conducted very early in pregnancy, a small tube and minimal suction could be used and anesthesia could be avoided. However, many women have reported significant discomfort and in many places this procedure has been discontinued in favor of the more traditional vacuum aspiration technique (Potts and Diggory 1973; Fortney and Laufe 1978; Ahmad 1979; Brenner and Edelman 1980; Sloane 1980; Porter, Waife, and Haltrop 1983; Bromwich and Parsons 1984).

*Vacuum Aspiration*   A variety of terms are used to refer to this same basic technique, including *uterine aspiration, vaginal evacuation, vacuum curettage, suction curettage,* and *suction abortion.* This is by far the most commonly used abortion technique and, at least in developed countries, the one now used almost exclusively in the first trimester (twelve weeks) of pregnancy. The technique was introduced in the United States by Kerslake and Casey in 1967.

Like the menstrual extraction procedure previously described, vacuum aspiration employs a tube or cannula that is passed through the cervix into the uterus and attached to a suction device. However, there are several differences which make this procedure a bit more complex than menstrual extraction.

Preliminary to vacuum aspiration, a bimanual pelvic exam is performed to ascertain uterine size and position, and a speculum is inserted vaginally to visualize the cervix. The cervix and vagina are then swabbed with an antiseptic solution and the upper portion of the cervix is grasped with a hooklike instrument, a tenaculum, to hold it steady. A local anesthetic, usually lidocaine, is injected into each side of the cervix. The cervix is then dilated by progressively introducing larger and larger sizes of tapered metal dilators into the cervix until it has widened enough to permit passage of the appro-

priate sized cannula, a vacurette. The further into the first t
weeks of pregnancy a woman is, the larger the tube that is rec
(since a more powerful suction is necessary) and the greater th
tion that must be achieved. For this reason, the basic procedure of
curettage is not very safe or practical much beyond twelve weeks of
pregnancy.

After the cannula has been passed into the uterus, it is attached
to an electric suction machine. Once the vacuum is applied, the
cannula is gently and systematically rotated around the entire uterine cavity, moving from the fundus to the cervix. The operator must
be sure that the entire endometrial surface has been cleaned of all
products of conception, since failure to do so can result in serious
infection or bleeding.

As the uterus empties, the myometrium contracts, preventing
hemorrhage and reducing the uterus to its original size. These contractions cause rather severe cramps for a short time; but they generally subside within thirty minutes or less.

During the first trimester, this procedure is generally performed
on an outpatient basis, with the woman free to leave after a short
period of recovery. As a general rule, the shorter the time of gestation when the abortion is performed, the quicker the recovery and
the fewer the complications. Most women will experience some
cramps and bleeding for up to two weeks after this type of abortion, and spotting may occur for two weeks after that. The next
normal menstrual period usually occurs within four to six weeks of
the abortion.

Additional procedural details are available in many sources
including Potts and Diggory (1973), Van der Vlugt (1973), Potts, Diggory, and Peel (1977), Ahmad (1979), Zatuchni, Sciarra, and Spiedel
(1979), Hatcher et al. (1980), Sloane (1980), Tietze (1981), and Porter,
Waife, and Haltrop (1983).

*Dilation and Curettage*   Prior to the introduction of vacuum aspiration, the major surgical abortion method was the dilation and curettage (D and C) procedure. This procedure was also generally performed in the first trimester of pregnancy. Compared with vacuum
aspiration, D and C is outdated and rather barbaric. The dilation of
the cervix is required to insert a sharp metal curette used to literally
scrape the uterine cavity free of the conceptus so that the parts can
be removed with forceps. In comparison with vacuum aspiration, a

D and C requires a greater degree of cervical dilation, is more painful, results in a greater loss of blood, requires a longer time to perform, requires general rather than local anesthetic, is more likely to
necessitate a hospital stay, and is not as effective in completely evac-
uating the uterus (Potts and Diggory 1973; Edelman, Brenner, and
Berger 1974; Potts, Diggory, and Peel 1977; Zatuchni, Sciarra, and
Spiedel 1979; Hatcher et al. 1980; Sloane 1980). Other than the fact
that some older doctors may be more familiar with this procedure
than with vacuum aspiration, it has nothing to recommend it as an
abortion procedure. If a physician recommends a D and C to a
woman seeking a first trimester abortion, she should run, not walk,
to a more up-to-date professional.

*Dilation and Evacuation* We now will consider abortion techniques employed after the first trimester. Before describing this procedure, it should be pointed out that all forms of second trimester
abortions are far more hazardous and considerably less desirable, on
both medical and psychological grounds, than earlier interventions.
Once a woman has moved beyond the point in gestation where a
vacuum aspiration can be performed, which is a procedure with an
outstanding record of safety and effectiveness, her risk of complications is enormously increased.

A simple suction procedure cannot be performed much beyond
twelve weeks of pregnancy, because the products of conception are
simply too large to pass intact through the bore of the largest uti-
lizable suction cannula. Insertion of a larger cannula is not possible
because of potential damage to the cervix. Hence, an abortion procedure which can be used between the thirteenth and sixteenth weeks
of pregnancy is, in essence, a combination of vacuum aspiration and
traditional D and C, namely, dilation and evacuation (D and E).

The D and E procedure requires a greater cervical dilation than
the D and C and suction methods. Since this cannot be easily accomplished using metal dilators without causing pain and risking cervical
injury or laceration, gentle and gradual enlargement of the cervix is
often achieved through the use of sterilized Laminaria tents.
Laminaria tents are made from two species of seaweeds having the
unique property of being extremely hygroscopic (having the ability to attract, absorb, and retain water in a moist environment).
Stems from these seaweeds are dried, cut, and shaped into smooth
cylindrical sticks about 6 cm long and in varying diameters. A plas-

tic disc is attached to one end to keep them from migrating into the uterus and a string is attached for retrieval. After the dry Laminaria stick is placed in the moist environment of the cervical canal, it gradually swells to up to five times its original diameter, slowly and painlessly dilating the cervix. Sufficient dilation is generally achieved in about six hours (Sloane 1980).

After dilation has been accomplished, the woman is put under general anesthesia, and crushing forceps are inserted into the uterus to grasp and remove the products of conception. (Since the fetus is too large to remove intact, it is crushed and removed in pieces, thus the name *crushing forceps*.) Usually oxytocin, the hormone which normally stimulates uterine contractions at birth, is administered to aid contractions and the expulsion of the conceptus. Vacuum suction is used to complete the procedure and to ensure that all products of conception have been removed; as noted before, failure to remove all products can lead to a serious infection or hemorrhage.

Despite the obvious points that the thought of crushing and removing the products of conception in pieces may be psychologically disturbing and that a D and E is a more complicated and riskier procedure than a vacuum aspiration, it is still a relatively safe procedure if it is performed by a skilled surgeon under appropriate conditions. The rate of major complications following second trimester D and E has been reported to be 0.69 per 100 abortions (Grimes et al. 1980). After describing the other approaches, we shall return to the D and E procedure to compare it with other second trimester abortion techniques.

*Intra-amniotic Infusion*   The most widely employed second trimester technique (and the only abortion technique usable in the latter half of the second trimester) involves the direct infusion of some product into the amniotic cavity. Recall that the fetus develops in a fluid-filled environment — the amniotic cavity (i.e., the space between the fetus and its surrounding placental membrane, the amnion), which is filled with amniotic fluid. Intra-amniotic infusion cannot be readily utilized until about the sixteenth week of gestation, since insufficient amniotic fluid is present prior to that time. Like several of the other abortion procedures, a variety of terms can be found in the literature referring to this technique, including *intra-amniotic instillation, amnioinfusion, amnioinstillation,* and *intra-amniotic injection*. Reference is also often made to the particular product being infused, instilled, or injected (e.g., *saline infusion*). We shall first examine the general technique and then consider the solutions which can be successfully used for infusion.

From a medical perspective, the technique is extremely simple. After urinating to assure an empty bladder, the woman assumes a supine position and her abdomen is disinfected. Under local anesthetic, a large-gauge needle is inserted through the abdominal wall and the uterus and into the amniotic cavity. Up to this point, the procedure is identical to the commonly performed diagnostic procedure of amniocentesis, which is often utilized to screen for various possible fetal chromosomal abnormalities and hereditary metabolic defects and to determine the sex of a fetus. In the abortion procedure, some of the amniotic fluid is aspirated with a syringe attached to the needle, and the abortative product is then infused. The amount of amniotic fluid withdrawn depends upon the solution to be infused, as we shall see shortly. Many clinicians insert a Laminaria tent into the cervix at the time of amniocentesis to facilitate cervical dilation and to aid the subsequent "delivery" of the fetus and placenta. Following infusion, the woman is simply returned to her hospital bed to await the onset of labor induced by the infusion. The extent of this wait is highly variable, usually ranging from twelve to forty-eight hours (Grimes et al. 1980; Sloane 1980). Also variable among women is the degree of pain which will accompany the expulsion of the fetus and other conceptus products. Since the delivery is totally analogous to childbirth, the ease with which it may be accomplished also varies among individuals. As in natural childbirth, the cervix dilates and effaces, the uterus contracts, and the fetus and placenta are expelled. Appropriate drugs are sometimes given to aid dilation of the cervix and contraction of the uterus. In almost all cases, the fetus is dead at the time of delivery, death being caused by the product infused.

Certainly there are many products which could trigger abortion if infused into the amnion. Numerous toxic agents have been used in illegal and self-induced abortions. The three products most widely and successfully employed for intra-amniotic infusion are hypertonic saline, hypertonic urea, and prostaglandins.

Hypertonic saline (in essence, a very concentrated salt solution, usually 20 percent) is a highly toxic solution which must be used carefully, since accidental placement into a blood vessel would seriously disrupt the woman's electrolyte balance and could cause cardiovascular collapse, killing her. This is just one reason why illegal abortions are so very dangerous. However, when used properly, hypertonic saline has been proven to be a rapid and reliable abortative. If it is to be used for infusion, 150–250 ml of amniotic fluid is withdrawn following the placement of the needle into the amniotic cavity. Aspiration of the amniotic fluid also ensures that the needle has been properly placed (correct placement must be ascertained with 100 percent accuracy before infusing the hypertonic saline). A volume of the saline solution equivalent to the volume of amniotic fluid removed is then infused. Following saline induction, fetal death (monitored by following the fetal heartbeat) usually occurs within one to three hours (Kovacs et al. 1970). Death of or damage to the placenta also begins quite quickly, and decreased placental production of progesterone can be seen during the interval between infusion and onset of labor (Csapo, Sanvage, and Weist 1970). This is quite important, since the placenta is the primary source of progesterone at this stage of gestation and a decline in progesterone production helps lead to the onset of parturition.

Another hypertonic solution which has been employed in a similar fashion is urea. Urea is a high-nitrogen waste product of protein breakdown. When infused in high concentrations, it is always feticidal. An accidental intravascular injection of hypertonic urea is not likely to result in the dire consequences associated with the same error in the use of hypertonic saline; thus, infusion of hypertonic urea is safer than infusion of hypertonic saline from the standpoint of the woman's health. The major problem with its usage is that when used alone it often fails to succeed in aborting or, if abortion does occur, the interval from infusion to abortion is considerably longer than for other products. Combining hypertonic urea with oxytocin or prostaglandins alleviates some of these problems. Hypertonic urea is apparently rarely used in the United States but is employed fairly commonly in England and Europe (Sloane 1980).

Prostaglandins have also been extensively investigated and utilized, for induction of abortion via intra-amniotic infusion, especially during the past decade. Prostaglandins make up a family of structurally related compounds that are involved in numerous reproductive and other physiological phenomena. We have previously mentioned their roles in several reproductive events (see especially Chapter 4). The two members of the prostaglandin family investigated for use in abortion induction are prostaglandin $F_2$ and prostaglandin $E_2$. Since all naturally occurring prostaglandins have a very short biological half-life (ranging from a few seconds to a few minutes), synthetic analogues of these two prostaglandins ($F_{2\alpha}$ and $E_{2\alpha}$) have been used to a greater extent than have the natural products.

As indicated earlier in this chapter, prostaglandins have also been investigated as potential postcoital agents. Additionally, they have been investigated for their potential for inducing first-trimester abortions. Reviews of these investigations are available in Lauersen (1979, 1980), World Health Organization (1981), and Harper (1983). We shall concentrate on the use of prostaglandins in second-trimester abortions.

In November 1973, the FDA approved the use of prostaglandin $F_{2\alpha}$ for second-trimester abortions. Since that time, prostaglandins have replaced hypertonic saline as the primary product utilized in the United States. The routine method of usage is to inject a single 40 mg, low-volume (8 ml) infusion into the amniotic cavity. Unlike saline infusion, only a small volume of amniotic fluid is aspirated (mainly to assure correct placement of needle) prior to introduction of the prostaglandin infusion. Use of prostaglandin $F_{2\alpha}$ in this manner was shown by Cates et al. (1977) to be associated with a considerably lower maternal mortality rate than hypertonic saline infusion. Grimes et al. (1980) conclude, however, that hypertonic saline infusion results in lower rates of hemorrhage, infection, and retained placental tissue than does prostaglandin infusion. An advantage of prostaglandin $F_{2\alpha}$ is the shorter interval between infusion and delivery. Disadvantages are that sometimes a single infusion is not sufficient to induce abortion in some women and a second infusion is required. Also, immediate short-term side effects (e.g., vomiting and diarrhea) are more common. Because of the more powerful contractions directly induced by prostaglandin $F_{2\alpha}$, the uterus tends to be more quickly and completely emptied, but cervical trauma is also more likely. Of even greater concern to many are reports, such as that of Stroh and Hinman (1976), that the fetus is more likely to be delivered still showing some fleeting signs of life, since prostaglandins are considerably less feticidal than either hypertonic saline or hypertonic urea.

A second mode of employing prostaglandins was approved by the FDA in 1977, namely, the use of a prostaglandin $E_2$ analogue as a vaginal depository. This procedure is safer for the woman, since it does not require uterine invasion. However, it has often been associated with even more violent episodes of diarrhea and vomiting. If vaginal bleeding occurs, the uptake of the prostaglandin is impaired. However, another advantage of this route of administration is that it can be employed earlier in gestation, since the mode of administration does not depend upon the presence of amniotic fluid. If used early in pregnancy, complications are minimized.

A third mode of prostaglandin administration which has also been shown to be quite effective is serial intramuscular injection (every two to three hours) of a prostaglandin $F_2$ analogue. An increased incidence of placental retention is the major drawback of this approach (Lauersen 1979, 1980).

*Hysterotomy and Hysterectomy*   We shall mention these final two techniques only briefly, since they are rarely applicable. A hysterotomy is, in essence, a less-than-full-term cesarean section. It is a major operation that entails surgically opening the uterus and removing the contents. Because of its invasiveness and the attendant risks to the woman, it should be utilized only late in gestation and only in special situations in which the life of the woman may be in peril.

Hysterectomy (surgical removal of the uterus and its contents) might be considered as a possible option by a woman who finds herself with an unwanted pregnancy and is sure that she desires permanent sterilization. However, because of the risks of the procedure, practitioners today are unlikely to be willing to perform a hysterectomy unless it is also justified by the presence of a uterine disease appropriately treated by uterine removal.

*Assessment of Safety Risks*   As might be expected, the rule of thumb regarding abortion safety is to have the abortion performed as soon as possible. Abortions by vacuum aspiration (which can be done only during the first twelve weeks or so of gestation) are exceedingly safe and generally free of complications. As reported by Porter, Waife, and Haltrop (1983), CDC statistics indicate that the risk of maternal mortality due to a vacuum aspiration abortion is less than the risk following a tonsillectomy. Unquestionably, a woman with a known pregnancy who desires abortion should have it performed as early as possible and certainly within the first twelve weeks if possible.

Women who may delay their decision beyond the first trimester for whatever reason (e.g., irregular cycles or amenorrhea that kept her from realizing she might be pregnant, ambivalence about the decision, fear, financial concerns, nonavailability of service) may find themselves in what has sometimes been called the "gray zone." This is the period between thirteen and sixteen weeks of pregnancy when the conceptus is too large to be removed by suction and the uterus is too small and the amniotic fluid too meager to perform intra-amniotic infusion. As we indicated previously, this is the period during which the D and E procedure is usually performed.

However, some physicians (perhaps because of misinformation regarding the relative risks of D and E as compared to infusion techniques, perhaps because of an inability to perform a D and E themselves, or perhaps because of a reluctance to perform a procedure that they find distasteful) recommend that their patients in this stage wait an additional month or so to have their pregnancies terminated. This despite very convincing evidence (Tietze and Lewit 1972; Brenner and Edelman 1974; Rooks and Cates 1977) that there is a substantially greater health risk to the woman if the abortion is delayed for an additional month. All data indicate that although it is a messier and a more aesthetically offensive procedure, a D and E performed between the thirteenth and sixteenth week involves a far lower health risk to a woman than an amniotic infusion (regardless of the product used) at week 16 and beyond. As emphasized by Rooks and Cates (1977) and Sloane (1980), while it is easier, cleaner, and possibly less disturbing for the physician to administer an intra-amniotic infusion and avoid manually extracting fetal parts as demanded in a D and E, by having a woman wait for an infusion, the physician is subjecting her to a more painful and more dangerous procedure. In addition, a woman told to wait is being forced to endure the psychological burden of an additional month of an unwanted pregnancy.

Finally, the risks of abortion, even including riskier latter second-trimester abortions, is, from a purely objective health-risk assessment, safer than childbirth. As shown by Cates (1982), from the standpoint of a woman's health-risk, induced abortions in the first 20 weeks of pregnancy (all types combined), are approximately five times safer than pregnancy continued to full term. As we shall see in the next chapter, this fact played a crucial role in the American legalization of elective abortion in 1973.

.　.　.　.　.　.

Despite the intrinsic undesirability of abortion, it has been used since antiquity and will continue to be sought by women. Outlawing abortion has proved futile and dangerous to women determined not to have a child (and they are legion). Reports show that in countries where abortions are illegal or highly restricted, 85 percent of women denied legal abortions still find ways to terminate their unwanted pregnancies (Ahmad 1979). Back room abortion "mills" and self-induced kitchen table abortions using coat hangers, broom straws, and toxic chemicals are not figments of anyone's imagination—they are horrible realities. Those who favor retaining a public policy allowing elective abortion argue that to deny women the option of choosing to terminate an unwanted pregnancy under conditions that are safe and nonjudgmental is to deny women not only their rights but also their humanity. In response, those who favor reversing U.S. policy on elective abortion and establishing a prohibition on the use of abortifacients argue that allowing such practices is to deny fetuses not only their rights but also their humanity. We now turn to this debate.

# 7
# Elective Abortion: The Moral Debate

## INTRODUCTION

As we explained in Chapter 5, we shall classify as abortifacient birth control methods those having among their primary actions interventions designed to be effective after conception. As we saw in Chapter 6, a number of contemporary birth control technologies are not appropriately classified as contraceptives, since, rather than acting primarily to prevent fertilization, their primary actions involve interfering with the conceptus in ways that prevent its successful implantation or its continued development if implantation occurs. We have also seen that some widely used methods, particularly oral contraceptives (OCs), that have preventing conception as their primary action can also act as abortifacients if ovulation and fertilization should occur. Thus, many contemporary birth control methods either routinely or occasionally work not as contraceptives but by intervening after conception or implantation.

The central moral position of those who have been most active in the movement against allowing elective abortion is that the human being must be recognized as a person with a full-fledged right to life from the moment of conception onward. The implication of this position for a number of contemporary birth control methods is very clear. If a public policy permitting elective abortion is not morally acceptable because conception marks the beginning of personhood (with its attendant moral rights), then elective use of those methods having abortifacient actions is equally unacceptable and must be outlawed. Our central question in this chapter is

Portions of this chapter appeared in Callahan (1986a,1986c). We are grateful to the publishers of *Commonweal* and to the Philosophy Documentation Center for permission to adapt this material.

whether public policies permitting elective induced abortion and elective use of abortifacient birth control technologies is morally justifiable.

Abortion has always been practiced as a variant of birth control, and it may even be the preferred method for avoiding birth in some societies, for example, in societies where safe and reliable contraception is not readily available. Further, abortion may be the preferred method for some women under some circumstances (e.g., in rigorously pronatalist societies or when a husband is opposed to birth control), since abortion, whether self-induced or surreptitiously performed by someone else, puts birth control in the hands of women (e.g., pills and devices need not be hidden), and it can be disguised as illness (Van de Warker 1872; Himes 1936; Wrigley 1969; Deveraux 1976; Degler 1980; Tietze 1981; Harrison 1983; Petchesky 1984).

Primitive methods of self-induced abortion include jumping from great heights, having others jump up and down on the abdomen, ingesting emetic and toxic substances, and using invasive probes (e.g., sticks, knitting needles, and, more recently, wire hangers). These obviously dangerous kinds of techniques have been employed by women for centuries and, as we saw at the end of Chapter 6, in spite of public policies and public attitudes condemning abortion (e.g., Green 1971; Mohr 1978; Ahmad 1979; Degler 1980). For example, the dramatic increase in self-induced abortion in the nineteenth century despite restrictive abortion laws is well documented (e.g., Steward 1867; Storer and Heard 1868; Christine 1890; Mohr 1978).

As medical practice was professionalized in the nineteenth century, physicians campaigned to make morally and medically appropriate decisions on abortion a matter of technical judgment. The emerging profession of medicine claimed the expertise to decide when a pregnancy was threatening to a woman's health and could therefore be justifiably terminated (e.g., Mohr 1978; McLaren 1983; Luker 1984). Social acceptance of this position gave individual physicians authority to use their discretion in deciding who would receive a legal abortion. In the United States, the use of physician discretion to decide when abortions would and would not be performed resulted in stark contrasts in the numbers of "therapeutic" abortions performed in liberal and conservative settings, with legal abortions in the most liberal settings being performed as much as fifty-five times more frequently than in the most conservative settings

(Luker 1984). Needless to say, such figures raise questions about the sincerity of the profession's moral argument against elective abortion and for physician control of abortion (for discussions of the profession's moral campaign against elective abortion, see below and, e.g., Mohr 1978; Luker 1984; Petchesky 1984). But perhaps what is most interesting about these statistics is what they reveal about the "demand" for abortion in the United States prior to the required liberalization of state policies on elective abortion that came with *Roe v. Wade* (1973). Indeed, it seems that despite restrictive abortion laws, between one in four and one in five married women in the late nineteenth century aborted at least one pregnancy, and almost 90 percent of premarital pregnancies were aborted, most of them illegally (e.g., Gebhard et al. 1958). Estimates commonly put the occurrence of abortion prior to liberalization of laws in the same range as postliberalization (e.g., American Medical Association 1871; Calhoun 1919; Luker 1984), suggesting that legalization of elective abortion merely legitimizes actual practices. *Roe v. Wade* (1973), for example, legitimized a trend to relax restrictions on abortions that had already begun in the states as a result of popular support for elective abortion. By the time of the decision, nearly a third of the states had already liberalized their abortion laws, making them more coherent with the demand for abortion reflected in actual practices, including attempts to self-abort, the use of abortionists acting illegally, and the spurious use of "therapeutic" abortion (e.g., Luker 1984; Petchesky 1984).

The use of abortion to avoid unwanted births, then, seems not to be significantly affected by public policy restricting or permitting it. Rather, the legal protection of elective abortion seems not to increase the occurrence of abortion so much as it increases the safety of abortion for women. For example, when abortion laws were made less restrictive in Czechoslovakia in the 1950s, abortion-related deaths dropped by 56 percent between 1953 and 1957 and by an additional 38 percent between 1958 and 1962. Romania, on the other hand, enacted a restrictive abortion law in 1966. There followed a sevenfold increase in abortion-related deaths. Specifically, abortion-related deaths of Romanian women aged fifteen to forty-four rose from 14.3 per million in 1965 to 97.5 per million by 1978 (Henshaw 1987a). Despite the fact that public policies making abortion more accessible to women seem to have an insignificant impact on how many abortions actually occur and a great impact on the health of women, much of the effort of those who oppose elective abortion in the United States is expended on seeking the reversal of *Roe v. Wade* (1973).

ROE V. WADE

The majority decision in *Roe*, written by Justice Harry Blackmun, contains three major conclusions.

1. Abortion decisions during the first trimester of pregnancy must be left up to the woman and her physician. The Court argues to this conclusion by pointing out that prior to the development of antiseptic techniques, surgical abortion at any stage was a seriously dangerous procedure for a woman. But with the development of antisepsis, early abortion became safer for a woman than continuing a pregnancy to term. Since a crucial part of the rationale for the earliest statutes prohibiting abortion pertained to protecting the health of pregnant women, prohibiting early abortion can no longer be justified by appeal to such considerations.[1] Combined with this, the Court leans on a series of decisions going back to *Union Pacific R. Co. v. Botsford* (1891) that recognize a constitutional right of citizens to make decisions within certain areas or "zones of personal privacy," including decisions regarding reproduction. Thus, the Court takes the health of a woman and her right to privacy to be the overriding interests to be protected during the first trimester of pregnancy.

2. During the second trimester, the same interests remain overriding. But because of the increased risk to women as pregnancies proceed, the Court allows that states may regulate abortions by requiring that they be performed in certain kinds of facilities by personnel with certain kinds of licenses or credentials.

3. After the second trimester, the woman's health is still taken to be an overriding interest to be protected. But since abortion is now more dangerous for the woman, this interest is taken by the

---

[1] In 1800, no American jurisdictions had statutes proscribing abortion. The earliest U.S. laws appeared between 1821 and 1841 and were enacted to protect women from (initially) poisoning and (a bit later) surgical injury as a result of the "rashness of young practitioners" attempting to distinguish themselves (*Revised Statutes of New York* 1836). See also Means (1968) and Mohr (1978).

Court to justify disallowing elective abortion in the third trimester. Thus, it is concluded that states *may* prohibit elective abortion in the third trimester to protect the health of pregnant women. What is more, jurisdictions need no longer recognize privacy in reproductive decisions as an overriding interest to be protected. That is, jurisdictions may (but need not) recognize the state's interest in protecting the fetus as overriding (or what the Court calls "the potentiality of human life," using language that ought to be rejected because it obscures one of the central questions in the abortion debate, as we shall see in a moment). In the third trimester, then, states may refuse to permit abortion unless the life or health of the woman is threatened by continuing the pregnancy.

The *Roe* decision makes elective abortion during the first and second trimesters a freedom protected by law. And it leaves open the possibility of a jurisdiction's allowing elective abortion into the third trimester. Further, given that *health* is a vague term that can easily be interpreted to refer to mental or emotional health as well as physical health,[2] the decision, in principle at least, extends the option of abortion into the third trimester for any woman who is sufficiently emotionally distressed by a pregnancy late in term even in those jurisdictions disallowing elective abortion in the third trimester. In fact, however, performing an abortion during the third trimester subjects a woman to risks more serious than those involved in bringing the pregnancy to term — unless she has a special physical condition (e.g., uterine cancer, toxicity from the fetus) making continuation of the pregnancy a special risk to her. Absent such special circumstances, performing a third trimester abortion would be unsound medical practice. Thus, elective abortion in the third trimester is virtually unheard of.

There are a number of problems with the specifics of the Court's argument in *Roe*. For example, problems with clarifying the con-

---

[2]The World Health Organization (1958) in fact, defines *health* as "a state of complete physical, mental and social well-being and not merely the absence of disease or infirmity." This definition has been subjected to some serious criticism. See, e.g., Callahan (1973) and Gorovitz (1982). For other discussions of the concept of health, see, e.g., Feinberg (1970), Macklin (1972), Hastings Center (1973), Boorse (1977), Clouser, Culver, and Gert (1981), and Culver and Gert (1982).

cept of privacy, justifying the claim that there is a constitutional right of privacy, and defending viability as a dividing line (since it shifts) have been raised by various authors, including Blackmun's colleagues on the Court (see, e.g., Noonan 1970; White 1973; O'Connor 1983).[3]

An additional problem lies in the Court's "argument" for accepting viability as the point at which the state's interest in the life of the fetus becomes compelling. Blackmun writes, "With respect to the State's important interest in potential life, the 'compelling' point is viability. This is so *because* the fetus then presumably has the capability of meaningful life outside the mother's womb" (emphasis added). But this is no argument for viability as the "compelling point," since "has the capability of meaningful life outside the mother's womb" is simply the *definition* of "viable." Schematically, the argument is as follows: "X is the point of compelling interest because at X the fetus is X." It would be equally invalid to assert as an argument "birth is the compelling point because at birth the fetus is born" or "conception is the compelling point because at conception the fetus is conceived." What the Court needed to do—but failed to do—was make clear why the fetus's capacity for existence independent of its biological mother might make it legitimate to prevent a woman from obtaining an abortion. We shall take up the question of independent existence below, and we shall suggest a way to understand how independent existence is morally relevant to setting policy on when very young human beings are to be recognized by the law as persons. Blackmun, however, makes explicit the Court's unwillingness to consider the question of the moral status of the prenatal human being. But it is precisely this question that continues to haunt the contemporary debate on the morality of elective abortion.

PRENATAL MORAL STANDING:
UNDERSTANDING THE DEBATE

In Chapter 2, we supported Luker's (1984) suggestion that the contemporary abortion debate is so intractable because it involves a

---

[3] Judge Robert Bork's disagreement with the Supreme Court's argument from a constitutional right to privacy used in *Roe* was a significant cause of the successful opposition to his nomination to the Supreme Court in 1987.

clash of complex worldviews. Embedded in these worldviews are opposing positions on the moral status of the prenatal human being.[4] Unhappily, the debate between those opposed to allowing elective abortion and those in favor all too often degenerates into mere assertion and the use of language which is "loaded" in a way that begs the question of the moral status of the prenatal human being. But it is not enough for those who oppose allowing elective abortion to call themselves "pro-life" and to call conceptuses, embryos, and fetuses "babies" and take the matter to be settled. Nor is it enough for those who believe we must retain abortion as an option for women to call conceptuses, embryos, and fetuses "parasites" or to merely assert that women have a right to use their bodies as they see fit and take the matter to be settled. Trying to decide public policy responsibly must involve refusing to use language which implies that the opposition is against something any morally reasonable person would support or which simply begs the question. To call a prenatal human being a "baby" is already to assert that it has the moral standing and should therefore have the legal standing of a child. And to call a fetus a "parasite" is already to assert that it has no more moral standing and hence should have no more legal standing than a tumor. Such language on either side of the debate simply begs the question on the moral status of the prenatal human being and prevents rational discussion from proceeding.

Most opponents of elective abortion concede that women do have the important moral right to use their bodies as they see fit. But they argue that this right is limited when using one's body as one sees fit necessitates killing an innocent person. Thus, those who oppose permitting elective abortion hold that the argument based on this right of women also begs the question by simply assuming

---

[4] We shall use the term *prenatal* to refer to the full period of development from conception to birth. Calculating from conception, we shall use the term *conceptus* to refer to the developing human organism through the first two weeks of gestation, *embryo* to refer to the organism between weeks 2 and 6 of gestation, and *fetus* to refer to the organism from week 6 of gestation through birth. These stages are also commonly calculated from the first day of the last menstrual period, which adds roughly two weeks to their calculation (i.e., the conceptus stage is weeks 1–4, the embryonic stage is weeks 4–8, and the fetal stage is week 8 through birth).

that prenatal human beings do not have the moral standing of persons. Most opponents of elective abortion insist that all human beings are persons from the moment of conception and that they must be treated as such from that moment.[5]

If prenatal human beings *are* persons, then moral consistency requires that we recognize that they have the same range of fundamental moral rights as persons generally, including the right not to be killed except for the most compelling moral reasons. Ordinarily, we believe that individual persons may not kill other persons except in cases of self-defense.[6] Thus, if prenatal human beings are persons, allowing elective abortion will not bear moral scrutiny. Further, our laws must be changed to preclude the elective use of induced abortion techniques, abortifacient birth control technologies, and contraceptives which might act as abortifacients, since only the moral reasons which justify killing persons generally will be sufficient to justify interfering with the establishment of even the earliest pregnancy. The crucial question, then, is whether we must accept that developing human beings are persons from conception onward and have the full range of fundamental moral rights possessed by all other persons.[7]

---

[5] Although in the clearest cases, persons are beings which are understood to possess moral rights and have moral duties, it is customary in the abortion debate to discuss personhood exclusively in terms of prenatal rights and to put aside the question of duties. We follow this custom.

[6] There may be other cases where killing is also justified, for example, in defense of one's country.

[7] For an argument supporting allowing elective abortion which begins by assuming (for the sake of the debate) that prenatal human beings are persons, see Thomson (1971). Thomson suggests a thought experiment, which involves imagining that a violinist is unwelcomely hooked up to one's kidneys and will die unless he remains connected. Assume the connection is necessary for some months (i.e., comparable to bringing a fetus to term or viability). Thomson argues that even though the violinist is clearly a person with a strong right to life, and even though it would be "decent" of one to stay attached for the duration, disconnecting the violinist would not violate any of his moral rights. We mention this position only to set it aside, since many people have argued that the analogy between Thomson's example and pregnancy fails. For another discussion contending that the question of personhood is irrelevant to determining the morality of elective abortion, see Lomansky (1984).

PRENATAL PERSONHOOD: DECISION VERSUS DISCOVERY

Those who oppose elective abortion often say that "human life begins at conception." But it cannot be emphasized strongly enough that this is factually wrong. Life which is unquestionably human begins long before conception. Though not complete "human beings," human spermatozoa and ova are very much alive, and they are not bovine or feline or canine — they are living human gametes. To couch the question in terms of the beginning of life is really to muddle the issue, since this language makes the question of the morality of elective abortion seem like one that can be answered by a competent biologist. But the question is not when life begins. Life begins before conception, and the human conceptus, even at the very earliest stages, is unquestionably alive. What we want to know is whether the prenatal human being should be recognized as a bearer of the same range of fundamental moral rights possessed by paradigmatic persons, among them the right not to be killed without *very* good reason. The most able biologist in the world cannot answer this for us, since the question is simply not a biological one.

But it might be objected that although some who are opposed to elective abortion and who have not thought carefully enough about the issue do make the mistake of thinking that the question is when biological life begins, it is also true that not everyone who talks in terms of the beginning of human life is making this mistake. For surely many who are opposed to elective abortion mean to contend that the life of a *unique* human being, of a distinct *person*, begins at conception and that it is because of this that measures taken to prevent birth after conception are wrong.

The problem with this response, however, is that it is not a single claim. For one can grant that the life of a unique human being *begins at* conception without granting that a distinct person *emerges at* conception, since the two claims are not equivalent unless one begs the question in favor of the personhood of the conceptus. That is, if one means by *human being* a member of the biological species *Homo sapiens*, then it is uncontroversially true that the life of a unique human being begins at conception. This is merely a scientific claim, and it can be conclusively defended by scientists as such. But the claim that a distinct person emerges at conception is not a scientific one, for to call something a "person" is already to assert that it is a bearer of moral rights. If in asserting that a human life begins at

conception or that the life of a unique human being begins at conception the opponent of elective abortion means to assert the biological claim, that can be granted immediately. But if the opponent
of elective abortion means to assert that a person emerges at conception, this is an importantly different claim. It is a moral claim
and the very moral claim that is at issue in the abortion debate.
What the opponent of elective abortion needs to tell us is *why* we
must accept that the truth of the biological claim commits us to
accepting the moral claim.

But the opponent of elective abortion might assert that those
who admit that the life of a unique human being begins at conception are indeed committed to granting that, insofar as human
conceptuses become distinct persons, the life of a distinct person
begins here as well. For where did the life of any adult person begin
but at conception?

There are, however, at least two responses to this. The first is
simply to make the logical point that one can allow that the life of a
person begins at conception without allowing that the biologically
human being present at conception is yet a person. That is, just as
one can allow that the first tiny bud in an acorn is the beginning of
the life of a future oak tree without being committed to saying that
the bud is already an oak tree, one can allow that conception marks
the beginning of the life of a potential or future person without
being committed to saying that the human conceptus is already a
person.

This logical point leads to a second, more substantive response,
namely, that we think the tiny bud in the acorn is quite clearly *not*
an oak tree. And we think this because the bud does not yet have
the characteristics of oak trees. Indeed, acorns with tiny buds are
very unlike oak trees, even though every oak tree begins as a bud in
an acorn. In just the same way, the new conceptus is very unlike
beings who have the kinds of characteristics which compel us to
recognize them as persons. What kinds of characteristics are these?
We cannot offer a full account here. But perhaps it will be enough
to point out that if we came across a being like E.T., a being that
was not biologically human but that had certain characteristics we
recognize paradigmatic persons as having (e.g., the capacity to suffer mental and physical pain, the ability to make plans, a sense of
itself as an ongoing being), we would be compelled to hold that this

being was a person and therefore must be treated in certain ways.[8] A human conceptus, however, has none of these characteristics. Indeed, like the mystery of the acorn and the oak, what is amazing is that such a radically *different* being will emerge from such a beginning.[9]

When, then, must we say of a developing human being that we must recognize it as a person? If we are talking about at what point in development we have a being with the kinds of characteristics that compel us to recognize it as a person, it seems that persons (at least human persons) are, like oak trees, emergent beings, and that deciding when to classify a developing human being as a person is like deciding when to classify a shoot as a tree. Very young trees lack many of the characteristics of grown trees (e.g., children cannot swing on them), but when a shoot begins to take on at least some of the characteristics of full-fledged trees, we think we are not confused in beginning to think of and speak of that shoot as a tree. Similarly, there is no clear distinction between where the Mississippi River ends and where the Gulf of Mexico begins. But we settle the issue by setting a *convention* that does not seem counterintuitive or unreasonable. We are faced with quite the same kind of question when it comes to the matter of human persons. Since prenatal human beings do not have the kinds of characteristics which compel us to recognize them as persons, we must, whether we like it or not, *decide* whether they are to be recognized (i.e., treated) as full-fledged persons as a matter of public policy even though they lack virtually all the morally relevant characteristics of paradigmatic persons.

---

[8] Notice that films like *E.T.* turn on just this insight. In that film, the children recognize that E.T. is a person with the moral rights that attend personhood. The adults (particularly the bureaucrats) fail to see this. The audience, of course, identifies with the children.

[9] For discussions of the kinds of characteristics which compel recognition of beings (including nonhuman beings) as persons, see, e.g., Warren (1973, 1985), English (1975), Fletcher (1979), Tooley (1972, 1983, 1984), and Feinberg (1980). For a somewhat different approach to the question of personhood, see Solomon (1983).

THE CASE FOR PRENATAL PERSONHOOD:
THE LOGICAL WEDGE

One possible convention is to set the legal recognition of person-hood at birth. Another is to set it at conception. Other conventions set the legal recognition of personhood at various stages of prenatal-ity or at various points after birth. Those who oppose elective abor-tion generally insist that we *must* decide that personhood is to be recognized by the law from conception onward.

One common argument for this position is a theological one, resting on the doctrine of immediate animation, that is, the doctrine that a soul is infused by God at the moment of conception. This soul, it is held, is constitutive of personhood. This is the current dominant theory in Roman Catholicism. Interestingly, however, this has not always been the Roman Catholic view. Indeed, early, medi-eval, and premodern theologians (including St. Jerome [347–419], St. Augustine [354–430], Peter Lombard [1095–1160], St. Bonaventure [1221–1274], St. Thomas Aquinas [1227–1274], and the Council of Trent theologians [1566]) held that the human (or "rational") soul is not infused into the conceptus until the conceptus takes on a char-acteristically human morphology, that is, a characteristically human shape with basic human organs (which occurs roughly by twelve weeks into gestation). This is the doctrine of mediate or delayed animation or hominization (see, e.g., Donceel 1970a, 1970b; Hurst 1983).

Reminiscent of the theological doctrine of delayed hominiza-tion is the secular doctrine of quickening utilized in British com-mon law from the thirteenth century to 1803 and until the second half of the nineteenth century in American common law. Prior to the acceptance of Lord Ellenborough's Act by Parliament in 1803, abortion in England was not considered morally wrong, nor was it legally prohibited before the quickening of the fetus (i.e., the first perception of fetal movement by the pregnant woman, usually around week sixteen of gestation). It was not until 1828, with the passage of New York's first statute dealing with abortion, that elec-tive termination of pregnancy prior to quickening was proscribed by any American law. The legality of elective abortion prior to quick-ening was sustained at common law in a number of jurisdictions late into the nineteenth century (Quay 1960–61; Means 1968; Mohr 1978).

The secular ground for recognizing quickening as a significant point in gestation rested on the fetus's giving evidence of its capacity (ultimately) for independent survival, a reason, as we have seen, appealed to in slightly diffferent form by the Court in *Roe*. But between 1860 and 1880, "regular" physicians stridently attacked the doctrine, arguing that gestation is a continuous process and that quickening is no more crucial to it than is any other point along the way to full development. Their moral campaign against elective abortion resulted in a burst of anti-abortion legislation which left decisions regarding when a woman could procure a legal abortion in the hands of physicians (see, e.g., Mohr 1978).[10] The argument used against the moral relevance of quickening is one version of the central philosophical argument which is given today by opponents of elective abortion—an argument known as the *logical wedge*.

The logical wedge argument holds that if we are going to recognize adult human beings as persons with fundamental rights, including the right not to be killed, then logic compels us to recognize that, from the moment of conception, the human being must have those same rights. The argument proceeds by starting with beings everyone recognizes as having the rights in question and then by pointing out that a person at twenty-five, for example, is not radically different from one at twenty-four and a half, that a person at twenty-four and a half is not radically different from one at twenty-four, and so on. The argument presses us back from twenty-four to twenty-three to twenty-two and through adolescence and childhood to infancy. From infancy, it is a short step to late-term fetuses, because (the argument goes) change in location (from the womb to the wider world) does not constitute an essential change in the being itself. After all, you do not lose your right not to be killed simply by walking from one room to another. Similarly, it is argued, mere change of place is not philosophically important enough to justify a radical difference in treatment between infants and late-term fetuses.[11] The argument then presses us back

---

[10] Regular physicians were generally the most highly educated and professionalized of nineteenth-century medical practitioners, who organized and took the political steps which led to the full professionalization of medicine as a licensed practice. See, e.g., Mohr (1978), Luker (1984), Petchesky (1984), and Hartmann (1987).

[11] Much the same is said of the various physiological changes

to embryos and finally to conception, which is the only point in development where a clear line can be drawn between radically different kinds of beings. Logic and fairness, it is argued, force us to accept that even the zygote has the same fundamental right to life as the mature human being (e.g., Wertheimer 1971).

One objection to this argument is that conception itself is not clearly a discrete event. As we have seen earlier, it takes a bit of time for the conceptus to develop even into a two-celled being. Further, as we have also seen, until the blastocyst stage, the cells of the conceptus are not yet differentiated into the separate masses that will give rise to the placenta and embryo (see Chapters 4 and 5). Thus, until the time of implantation, there is not even a very early embryo. But these biological facts are generally taken to be morally irrelevant by those who appeal to the wedge argument, since their reply is that it is still the case that after conception a being exists that is essentially and radically different in kind from the gametes which combined to issue in that new being. And this is why, it is held, conception is the only nonarbitrary point that can be used for marking the commencement of personhood and its attendant rights.

The significant objection to the wedge argument for prenatal personhood is that it turns on the assumption that we can never treat beings that are not radically different from one another in radically different ways. But if we accept this assumption, we shall be unable to justify all sorts of public policies which we believe are both necessary and fair. For example, this assumption entails that we cannot be justified in setting driving or voting ages, since withholding these privileges until a certain age unfairly discriminates against those who are close to that age (an eighteen-year-old is not radically different from a seventeen-year-old, and so on). Thus, the implication of the logical wedge argument is that setting ages for the commencement of certain important societal privileges cannot be morally justified: We must give the four-year-old the right to vote, the five-year-old the right to drink, the six-year-old the right

---

accompanying birth and closely following birth. That is, these changes are held not to transform the essential nature of the young human being and therefore not to be of moral import. Another way of arguing for the position we shall defend might include holding that such changes *are* of moral import, since once they occur, the young human being can be supported by persons other than its biological mother.

to drive. But these implications, it is rightly argued, show that this kind of argument for prenatal rights is unsound (see, e.g., Glover 1977).

The response to this criticism of the argument, however, is that the granting of societal privileges is not fundamentally arbitrary even if there is some arbitrariness in selecting ages for the commencement of such privileges. Proper use of these rights, it may be argued, requires a certain degree of maturity — a sense of responsibility, background knowledge, experience, independence, and, in the case of driving, a certain degree of developed physical dexterity. Thus, it is because certain changes normally occur as a child matures into an adult that it is appropriate to set policies that acknowledge those changes. But this, it is further argued, is not the case when it comes to recognizing the right to life. That is, the proponent of this argument insists that after conception *no* changes occur that are relevant to recognizing the personhood, and thus the right to life, of a human being.

But this takes us back to the acorn and the oak. The bud and the tree simply are significantly different kinds of beings. And an adult human being simply is significantly different from a conceptus, which has none of the characteristics that compel us to recognize it as a being with the fundamental rights accruing to persons. Prenatal human beings do, of course, possess a full human genetic code. But this characteristic is neither necessary nor sufficient for personhood, since a genetically nonhuman being (recall E.T.) might possess the kinds of characteristics that compel recognition of it as a person, while any living human cell (e.g., a living skin cell) possesses a full human genetic code but is clearly not a person. It will not do, then, simply to assume that a human genetic code is sufficient to compel recognition of personhood. And it will not do simply to deny that there are significant, morally relevant changes between the time of conception and the time when we have a being which we unquestionably must recognize as a bearer of rights. Thus, we are once again confronted with the question of *deciding* where we shall set recognition of personhood and its attendant rights.

THE INFANTICIDE OBJECTION

There is, however, yet another response open to the opponent of elective abortion, namely, that the kind of reasoning used to defeat the argument for prenatal rights cannot be correct, since it not only rules out our being committed to the rights of conceptuses, embryos, and fetuses but also entails that we are not compelled to accept that human infants are beings of a kind which must be recognized as having the full range of fundamental moral rights. Infants are, it can be argued, more like very young kittens in regard to the characteristics in question than they are like paradigmatic persons.

But this objection is not devastating. For, again, the question before us is one of deciding what convention we shall adopt. We can allow that even if infants do not yet have the characteristics that compel us to accept them as persons, there are other considerations which provide excellent reasons for taking birth as the best place to set the recognition of personhood and the full range of fundamental moral rights — despite the fact that infants are far more like very young kittens than they are like beings whose characteristics compel us to accept them as full members of the moral community.

Chief among these considerations are that persons other than an infant's biological mother are able to care for the infant and have an interest in doing so. Although there are intriguing physiological changes accompanying birth, there is no change in the morally relevant characteristics of a human being itself just before birth and just after birth; all else being equal, if it is sustained, it will develop the characteristics of paradigmatic persons. But once a viable human being emerges from the womb and others are able and willing to care for it, there are radical changes in what is involved in preserving its life. And the *crucial* change is that sustaining its life does not violate its biological mother's rights to self-direction and bodily integrity. Thus, even though birth, unlike conception, is not a point at which we have a radically new kind of being, it is *not* a morally arbitrary point for commencing recognition in our public policies of young human beings as persons.

It is important to notice here that to hold that a woman has a right to terminate a pregnancy is not to hold that she also has a right to the death of her fetus if that fetus can survive and others are interested in assuming responsibility for it. Thus, quite the same reasons that can justify a proscription on elective infanticide can justify a requirement to sustain certain fetuses that survive abortion. What we are not entitled to do is to force a woman to complete a pregnancy because others have an interest in having her fetus. But it does not follow from this that a woman may kill an infant that can be cared for by others who want it. Thus, it does not follow from the argument that the defender of a policy allowing elective abortion is committed to a policy allowing elective infanticide (see, e.g., Warren 1975). Indeed, this position is fully consistent with holding that even though infants do not yet possess the kinds of characteristics which compel recognition of them as persons, the fact that they are now biologically independent beings that can be sustained without forcing an unwilling woman to serve as a life-support system provides an excellent reason for setting recognition of personhood at viable emergence, whether that emergence be a function of natural culmination or intentional termination of a pregnancy.

This, we submit, is the moral relevance of the capacity for independent existence which the Court left unexamined in *Roe*. Unlike the Court in *Roe*, however, we suggest that birth is the morally appropriate point at which the state's interest in protecting the young human being ought to be recognized as compelling, since at this point others can assume responsibility for the young human being without overriding extremely important fundamental moral rights of women. As viability pushes back earlier into pregnancy with the development of technologies allowing us to sustain younger and younger prenatal human beings, the potential for disallowing abortion from virtually the onset of pregnancy comes closer and closer to actuality. And as technology advances to make possible increasing numbers of medical and surgical interventions held to be helpful to prenatal human beings, attempts to impose those interventions through the bodies of unwilling women will also increase (see Chapter 9). Setting conventional recognition of personhood at birth disallows attempting to justify such interferences with women on the basis of an argument from prenatal personhood and thus has the moral advantage of taking the actual, unequivocal personhood of women far more seriously than does setting conventional recognition of personhood at any earlier point.

## THE ARGUMENT FROM FETAL SENTIENCE

It is sometimes argued that abortion, particularly later abortion, is morally unacceptable because it inflicts pain on the fetus. The view we have just defended, however, can allow that even kittens have *some* moral rights. As sentient beings (beings capable of suffering pain), they have a moral right not to be treated cruelly, that is, not to

ave pain wantonly imposed on them. Insofar as fetuses are sentient, they have the same right. But it is very unlikely that fetuses,
even late in pregnancy, are highly sentient. By nine or ten weeks,
the fetus is capable of swallowing, squinting, and a variety of local
reflexes, as well as moving spontaneously. But even late stage fetuses,
for all their developing physical complexity and for all their physical resemblance to human persons, are not yet fully neurologically
functional, and this provides a good reason for believing that their
capacity for sentience is far less than the capacity for sentience in
paradigmatic persons.

Although it has been argued, most notably in *The Silent Scream*,
a videotape produced by Nathanson (1985), that fetal movement conclusively shows that fetuses experience fear and pain during surgical abortion, there are a number of reasons for rejecting this argument. Among them is the fact that one can render a normally sentient
subject insentient without eliminating the physical impulses which
the conscious brain can interpret (i.e., experience) as pain. In surgery, for example, unless sufficient local or systemic anaesthesia is
administered, an unconscious subject will still respond appropriately to stimuli by jumping, withdrawing, and so on, even though
the subject is not conscious and hence cannot interpret the physical
impulses as pain. Given the relatively rudimentary mental development of fetuses, and given that the period of fetal development, like
a period under anaesthesia, is lost to conscious memory, it is not
unreasonable to suppose that, like surgical subjects under anaesthesia,
fetuses are unable to interpret as pain the physical impulses that a
conscious, fully functioning human brain interprets as pain. Further, the gross fetal movements appealed to in Nathanson (1985) are
quite obviously a result of the physical displacement of the contents
of the amniotic sac (which includes the fetus) caused by thrusts
against the exterior wall of the sac as attempts are made to break
into the sac with a suction tube. And the single facial movement
appealed to as evidence for the claim that the fetus experiences fear
is easily explained as an instance of the spontaneous movements
fetuses are capable of at the point of gestation of the fetus in the
videotape, which is roughly twelve weeks.[12]

---

[12] For additional discussion of the problems with Nathanson's (1985)
case against abortion, see Callahan (1986c).

We do not, however, want to pass too quickly over the question of fetal sentience, since the capacity of a being to suffer is always relevant to determining morally acceptable treatment of that being. Given this, it is surprising that the question of fetal sentience has received little attention in the philosophical literature on abortion. The work of L. W. Sumner (1981) is exceptional in this regard. Sumner suggests that the onset of sentience falls somewhere in the second trimester, when the basic physiological structures of the brain which are necessary for sensation (i.e., the subcortical areas of the forebrain) are relatively complete. But even if we allow that some capacity for pain or otherwise unpleasant experience emerges during the second trimester of gestation, it seems clear that this capacity would be rudimentary, in large part because the nerves that transmit the impulses associated with pleasure and pain are routed through the cerebral cortex, which is not fully functioning in the fetus. Thus, as sentience emerges, there is not a sudden change from preconsciousness to a full-blown capacity for sensation. Further, the fetus has virtually no use for full-blown sentience, since it cannot, for the most part, either seek pleasurable experiences or avoid painful ones. If the fetus has a capacity for experiencing pain by, for example, the middle of the second trimester, it seems that that capacity, like its other mental capacities, would be primitive, that is, not a fully developed capacity like that of adult human beings (Sumner 1981; Callahan 1986c).

This much said, it must be allowed that insofar as fetuses can suffer pain, the defender of elective abortion can quite coherently hold that any pain imposed on a fetus in abortion must be justified. To say this, however, is not to be committed to holding that fetuses must be recognized as having the full range of fundamental rights that attach to persons. It is, rather, to allow fetuses at least the moral standing of any being of comparable sentience and, hence, to hold that there is always a moral obligation to not wantonly impose pain on fetuses sufficiently developed to experience pain. But given the exquisite intimacy of pregnancy and the dangers associated with any pregnancy, and given that it is reasonable to assume that fetal sentience is rudimentary, any woman who does not want to bring a pregnancy to term has strong reasons for seeking an abortion. Thus, if pain is imposed on a fetus in abortion, it is neither great nor wantonly imposed.

But it will surely still be objected that human fetuses and human infants are beings that are potentially like paradigmatic persons and that this makes them radically unlike other beings of comparable sentience. Kittens, after all, will never develop the kinds of characteristics that compel us to recognize them as full-fledged members of the moral community, and because human fetuses will—all things being equal—develop these capacities, we must recognize them as having a far more significant moral standing than other beings of comparable sentience. Sometimes opponents of elective abortion point this out, saying that from the moment of conception a developing human being is a *potential* person and must, therefore, be granted the same right to life as grown persons. But the problem here is that to say that a being is a potential person is just to say that it is a person-not-yet, which is, of course, to deny that it is now a person.[13] This gives the defender of a policy allowing elective abortion the very point that is crucial to his or her argument against the argument for prenatal personhood, and it thereby turns the focus back to the question of deciding on a convention.

ACTUAL AND POTENTIAL PERSONS

Does it follow from the disagreement over prenatal personhood that there is some serious doubt about the personhood of prenatal human beings, that is, that these beings might be persons? Sometimes those who support allowing elective abortion say things like this: The prenatal human being *might* be a person, but the evidence just is not conclusive. But if this is the position being held, the opponent of elective abortion has a strong response, namely, that we should give these beings the benefit of the doubt. After all, if a hunter hears a movement in the bushes and shoots without making sure the target is not a person, and if it turns out that the shot kills or injures a person, we charge the hunter with gross recklessness. Saying that it was possible that the target was not a person is no defense. The hunter simply should not have shot if there were even a remote possibility that some person would get injured. In just the same way, the opponent of elective abortion argues that if there is any possibility that the prenatal human being is a person, we have a duty to act as if it were a person—a duty to avoid acting recklessly

---

[13] Cf. Benn (1973): "A potential president of the u.s. is not on that account Commander-in-Chief." See also Feinberg (1980).

(see, e.g., Grisez 1970). And part of what *that* means is that another person may not kill such a being for reasons less than those that would normally justify killing a person.

This is an attractive argument, but it misses an important point. For the real doubt is not whether a prenatal human being is a person. Rather, if there is a doubt, it is about whether we should treat a being that is a potential person (in the sense that it has potentially the characteristics of paradigmatic persons) as if it were a person already. And this is not something that can be decided by going and inspecting the conceptus, embryo, or fetus as the hunter might go and look in the bushes. For on looking, we shall find that these beings lack the kinds of characteristics that compel us to accept them as persons. The question to be resolved, then, is whether we should accept that these beings which will eventually become paradigmatic persons if their lives are supported must, at this stage of their development, be treated as if they were persons already — beings with a compelling moral right to life that must be protected by the coercive power of the law.

When we are trying to resolve the real doubt, a large part of what we need to ask is what deciding to treat prenatal human beings as persons would really involve in practice and whether our shared views about morally acceptable treatment of paradigmatic persons will allow us to accept these things. Let us, then, look for a moment at just three of the implications of deciding to admit prenatal human beings into the class of full-fledged persons with full-fledged fundamental moral rights to be protected by law.

## SOME IMPLICATIONS OF ACCEPTING
## PRENATAL PERSONHOOD

If we decide to recognize prenatal human beings as full-fledged persons, it immediately follows that abortion in cases of rape or incest must be ruled out. Suppose that you were to discover that one of your neighbors is the product of rape or incest. You would not think (and none of us would think) that it followed from this that you could kill that neighbor because he is not a person. Fundamental rights are not possessed as a consequence of someone's origins. If we allow that prenatal human beings are persons, we could not, for example, with consistency allow abortion for an eighteen-year-old woman who has been raped by her father. What is more, if this woman were to perform an abortion on herself and be found out, we would be obligated to treat her as we would treat any murderer. Given existing laws pertaining to the murder of persons, in some jurisdictions this might well lead to life imprisonment or even execution.

Those who oppose elective use of abortion often try to avoid the question of what we should do with women who abort for reasons less compelling than self-defense by contending that this question should be left up to the states to decide. But the opponent of elective abortion needs to confront this question squarely and candidly. Precisely what are states to do with women who abort? Can we accept that states may decide to imprison them or execute them? If the opponent of elective abortion confronts this question earnestly and cannot comfortably hold that jurisdictions should treat these women as they typically treat murderers, then he or she needs to begin to think carefully about *why* such treatment seems morally unacceptable. Accepting prenatal human beings as full-fledged persons commits us to measures in practice that even those who are deeply opposed to elective abortion cannot fully accept, among them that the eighteen-year-old who aborts a pregnancy resulting from rape by her father is to be treated as any murderer of a helpless, innocent person. We are not, even in this pluralistic society, free to kill other persons for reasons less compelling than the immediate defense of our own lives, and if we do kill a person for less compelling reasons, we are subject to severe legal penalties, possibly including execution.

If prenatal human beings are to be recognized as full-fledged persons, it follows that those who kill them for reasons less compelling than self-defense must be recognized as full-fledged murderers and treated as such. Those who are rigorously opposed to allowing elective abortion on the ground that prenatal human beings are persons must confront this implication sincerely and sensitively, and they must be explicit about what they are willing to accept as the practical implications of their position. If they are not willing to accept that those who abort should be subject to exactly the same treatment as others who murder, then they need to recognize that they do not *really* believe that prenatal human beings have the moral status of persons. And this is true of those who hold that such matters should be left up to the individual states, since states are not, in other cases, free to allow those who murder innocent persons to be at large in the community.

What is more, those who argue against elective abortion on the ground that prenatal human beings are persons need to realize that their position is not coherent with the position on the question of prenatal personhood informing the statutes that were struck down by the *Roe* decision, since none of these statutes treated abortion as murder. Thus, arguments from prenatal personhood against allowing elective abortion entail that statutes disallowing elective abortion must be far more punitive than those in place prior to *Roe v. Wade* (1973; see, e.g., Mohr 1978).

There is yet another important implication of accepting fetuses as persons. Many who oppose elective abortion would allow abortion in cases of self-defense, that is, in cases where the woman's life is threatened by the pregnancy. But there is a problem with this position that generally goes unnoticed. For if public policy is to recognize that the prenatal human being is genuinely an innocent person, then its threat to a woman's life is an innocent threat and the state can have no good reason for preferring the life of the woman to the life of the prenatal human being. The argument from self-defense must extend to the prenatal human being as well as the woman, and a fair government simply cannot allow women to have access to safe and effective medical procedures that will systematically prefer the life of the woman to the life of the prenatal human being. If the prenatal human being has precisely the same moral status as the woman, the state must, as a matter of equal protection, do nothing that would involve it in giving the woman an unfair advantage in this battle for life between moral equals. The argument from self-defense, then, entails far greater restrictions on abortion than even the most fervent opponents of elective abortion are generally willing to support, including prohibiting access to safe medically or surgically assisted abortion for even those women whose lives are threatened by their pregnancies. If opponents of elective abortion want to allow professionally assisted abortion in cases where the woman's life is at stake, then they must realize that implicit in their position is the view that the woman and the prenatal human being are *not* of equal moral status after all (see also Benn 1973; Davis 1984).

Finally, as we have already mentioned, if prenatal human beings are to be recognized as persons from conception onward, there are important implications regarding the use contemporary birth control methods, since most of these methods have abortifacient actions. The argument from prenatal personhood entails that their use must be outlawed. If the opponent of elective abortion cannot accept that such a prohibition is morally required, then he or she does not really believe that the prenatal human being must be accepted as a person from conception onward.

ABORTIFACIENTS AND INFORMED CONSENT

Our position is that there are insurmountable obstacles to finding an even moderately strong argument for setting the convention of recognizing personhood and its attendant rights at conception, fetal viability, or any other point prior to birth. Since the personhood of the prenatal human being is the only consideration which could even conceivably justify imposing on another person the physical risks and the exquisitely intimate burden of carrying an unwanted pregnancy to term, we must conclude that legislation prohibiting women from aborting unwanted pregnancies cannot be justified, nor can legislation be justified which prohibits elective use of birth control methods with abortifacient actions simply because they have such actions.

At the same time, we are not suggesting that abortion is value-neutral. The view that we have defended is completely consistent with accepting that abortion almost always sacrifices something of value. Defenders of the pro-choice position do not hold that abortion is intrinsically good.[14] Even those who most militantly sup-

---

[14] See Whitbeck (1983) and Callahan (1986c) for a fuller discussion. However, see also Petchesky (1984) for an example of the position that a policy of elective abortion should be thought of, not as a necessary evil, but as a "positive good" analogous to education, because it is crucial in a number of respects to the well-being of women. This argument is put forward because even with effective contraceptives available, maintaining reproductive control will always make it necessary for some women to seek abortion (see Chapter 6). The position that abortion is a positive good is underpinned by a concern to establish an overriding legal right to elective abortion on the ground of a compelling moral right that will preclude prohibiting elective abortion even if safe, cheap, and highly effective contraception is universally available. But this position is entirely consistent with the position that prenatal human life is almost always of

port a policy protecting women's access to elective abortion generally hold that contraception is not only medically but also morally preferable to abortion as a method of birth control. And many women who support retaining choice in this area would not themselves opt for abortion — because of the value they place on all human life at all stages. It is inexcusably distorting, then, to attribute indifference to human life to everyone who supports a policy protecting women's freedom to elect abortion. The pro-choice position is not a pro-abortion position, and those who insist on calling it a pro-abortion position sacrifice argument for propaganda and weaken the reasonableness of their own position by attacking a position that no one holds.[15]

For those who find contraception and abortion equally acceptable methods of birth control, the abortifacient actions of many birth control technologies presents no moral problem. But for those who hold that there is a moral difference between contraception and abortion, regular use of abortifacients and induced abortion may be deeply morally troubling, even if they strongly support a policy protecting elective abortion. Because of this, physicians or other health care personnel who provide birth control methods have an obligation to be scrupulous in explaining the precise actions of the applied technology, making it clear to recipients when they are accepting a technique that routinely acts or sometimes may act as an abortifacient by intervening after conception or implantation. Failure to so inform recipients is common, and when it occurs, a practitioner has failed to obtain an adequately informed consent to medical intervention.

·    ·    ·    ·    ·

Despite the concern with informed consent that we have just expressed, our argument in support of allowing elective abortion denies that prenatal human beings must or should be recognized as persons. A different problem arises, however, when a woman elects

---

significant value and that contraception is morally preferable to abortion as a method of birth control.

[15] For discussion of women's reluctance to choose abortion and of postabortion depression, see, e.g., Denes (1977), Francke (1978), Harrison (1983), Whitbeck (1983), and Hartmann (1987).

not to abort a pregnancy but her actions or the actions of others result in damage to a prenatal human being that will eventually emerge as a person. A number of actions and omissions of pregnant women can be harmful to their conceptuses, embryos, or fetuses, and a number of environmental toxins, particularly in some workplaces, can be harmful to human gametes, resulting in the birth of damaged children. We shall take up several of the important moral and legal issues arising from these facts in Chapter 9. First, however, we need to ask whether the birth control methods discussed in Chapters 5 and 6 have potentially deleterious effects on human gametes, conceptuses, embryos, or fetuses. We turn next to this question.

# 8
# Mutagenicity, Teratogenicity, and Birth Control

## INTRODUCTION

In Chapters 5 and 6, we described the potential risks to women posed by various birth control methods. One part of the overall risk associated with contemporary birth control products that we have largely (and deliberately) ignored in our previous discussions is the risk to offspring. Reports of fetal anomalies following prenatal exposure to various synthetic sex steroids began to appear in the literature in the late 1950s (see, e.g., Keith and Berger 1980). Reports implicating oral contraceptives (OCs) in cases of prenatal harm began appearing in the literature shortly after their introduction in the 1960s. By the mid-1970s, the intrauterine device (IUD) was also said to be linked to birth defects. Most recently, charges linking vaginal spermicides to birth defects have appeared in the literature as well as in the courts. Since these methods are employed throughout the world by millions of women, even a low risk of prenatal malformation caused by their use constitutes a significant public health issue. Fortunately, as we shall see, many of the more widely publicized initial reports associating prenatal anomalies with maternal use of birth control technologies now appear to be unsubstantiated.

Prenatal anomalies may result from the actions of two kinds of reproductive toxins, namely, teratogens and mutagens. A teratogen is an exogenous agent (e.g., a drug, a chemical, a virus, radiation) that alters normal embryonic or fetal development. *Teratogenic* means causing anomalies of formation; hence, teratogens exert their effects only during pregnancy. In contrast, *mutagenic* means causing genetic change. Mutagenesis, therefore, involves a heritable change in the genetic material of germ cells. This change (or mutation) occurs through the interaction of the mutagen (i.e., the causative drug, chemical, etc.) with the DNA of the cell, and it consists of an alteration in the DNA molecule and its informational content. If affected germ cells are subsequently involved in reproduction, the germinal mutation may result in an alteration that is passed on to future generations. Alternately, a germ cell mutation may have a lethal effect at some point during development, resulting in spontaneous abortion. Exposure to a mutagen may affect only a part of the total germ cell population. Thus, mutant genes or chromosomal abnormalities can result in anomalies in offspring conceived years following exposure to the mutagen and despite intervening births of nonaffected children.

Reproductive toxicology is a nascent and complex science. As we have seen, reproduction is not a singular process but rather a complex sequence of events involving integration of specific phenomena, including gametogenesis, gamete transport, fertilization, implantation, and prenatal development. Toxic materials may affect any of these processes (and several others as well). Likewise, the biological mechanisms underlying toxicology (e.g., absorption, distribution, toxification, excretion) are similarly complex. We are only now beginning to develop a body of knowledge in this area, largely because the mechanisms involved are complex, the science is relatively new, and there are thousands of potential products which may adversely affect reproduction. As our knowledge of reproductive toxicology has evolved, however, we have also been able to see the fallacy of some earlier claims and more appropriately evaluate reproductive risks from toxins.[1]

PROBLEMS IN RISK ASSESSMENT

Reproductive impairments of various types affect both sexes and are frequent and widespread. For example, Mosher (1980) estimates that, in the United States, there are roughly three million married couples of reproductive age in which one partner is noncontraceptively sterile. Although it is impossible to accurately measure the

---

[1] It is beyond the scope of this chapter to consider the broad subject of reproductive toxicology and the involvement of all potential toxins in male and female reproductive function. For a broader discussion of the subject of reproductive toxicology, see the reviews by Berry (1976), Wilson (1977), Dixon (1980), Council on Environmental Quality (1981), and Mattison (1983).

specific extent of toxin-caused reproductive impairment in men and women, it is now well known that numerous drugs, chemicals, and other environmental factors are substantial contributors to certain types of reproductive impairment. Large-scale surveillance studies have not been conducted to identify all toxic hazards to reproduction, but many agents have been clearly identified.[2] Largely as a result of the extent of their use, cigarettes and alcohol are the two agents that have been shown to have the greatest deleterious influence on human reproduction. Other chemical agents clearly linked to reproductive impairment include certain therapeutic drugs (notably thalidomide and diethylstilbestrol [DES]) and agents to which workers may be exposed in the workplace (notably lead, anesthetic gases, and certain pesticides).

However, only a limited number of drugs and occupational exposures have been studied for potential adverse effects on reproduction. As noted in a 1980 Environmental Protection Agency (EPA) report, of the approximately 55,000 then known chemical substances and mixtures in commercial production (not including drugs, pesticides, food additives, and agents in other minor classes), few have been thoroughly tested for their effects on reproduction. Further, innumerable chemicals and complex mixtures have not been tested in food, water, and air. Indeed, the number of single chemicals and mixtures tested to date is too small to properly estimate potential hazards to reproduction posed by products to which men and women are commonly, and in some cases constantly, exposed. The cumulative effects of widespread, low-level exposure to a potential hazard are exceedingly difficult to assess, and very few studies of such effects have been reported.

The practicality and reliability of studies in the field also depend on identifying an exposed group, documenting its exposure, and examining the effects of exposure on reproduction. We have rather reliable data on the effects of prescription drugs simply because their use and quantitative exposure is generally documented. Assuming that individuals are truthful in reporting patterns of use, it is also relatively easy to examine the reproductive effects of cigarette smoking, alcohol use, and use of recreational drugs. Studies involving

---

[2] Lists of substances shown to be toxic hazards to reproduction are available in several sources, including Council on Environmental Quality (1981) and Mattison (1983).

occupational exposures are more difficult to evaluate, because the magnitude of exposure is more difficult to assess. Virtually impossible to assess are the effects of environmental chemicals, because their distributions and the magnitudes of exposure to them are extremely difficult to document. Any effects caused by general environmental pollutants are unlikely to be identified unless they are unusually conspicuous.

Compounding the difficulty of making these evaluations are the complex interactions that may exist among individual factors. For example, it is extremely difficult to evaluate toxic effects in an individual who is exposed to potential hazards in the workplace, in the home environment, and through behavioral habits. In all cases, reproductive performance is often difficult to investigate unless the affected individuals are willing to be candid with researchers and to allow objective measures (e.g., semen analysis) to be made. Other practical problems common to all epidemiologic studies must also be considered when evaluating the results presented by researchers in this area, including selection of appropriate control groups and documentation of their exposure, inherent bias in the experimental design, and the existence of confounding factors. As we shall see shortly, the lack of appropriate control data invalidates or at best severely compromises many of the reports on teratogenic risks posed by the administration of exogenous steroids and by various birth control methods.

A final factor limiting accurate risk assessment is the unavoidable incompleteness of data. Many reproductive impairments either cannot be or are not recorded. For example, reproductive failures resulting from impotence or infertility are not routinely recorded unless a physician is consulted. Early spontaneous abortions may go completely unnoticed or not be reported to a physician. These reproductive impairments and early losses are probably substantial in number. But because they generally go unreported, while later spontaneous abortions and anomalies in offspring at birth typically are reported, we tend to underestimate the extent of reproductive impairment caused by various toxins. As a result, we get a misleading picture of the processes that are impaired. Further, a complete assessment of reproductive impairment caused by chemical agents is also impossible, because the vast majority of the population of reproductive age is employing birth control measures to suspend fertility. Thus, for most of the population of reproductive age failure to conceive is generally expected and likely to be noted only when there is an attempt to conceive.

## GENDER DIFFERENCES REGARDING SUSCEPTIBILITY TO TOXINS

In the next chapter we shall examine some of the moral issues surrounding potential mutagenic and teratogenic harm posed by the workplace environment. As a prelude to that discussion, we need first to examine the relative susceptibility of male and female systems to reproductive toxins and identify where harmful exposure may occur in the reproductive process.

Both male and female gametes are at potential risk following exposure to mutagenic agents. However, as we shall see shortly, the risk to women's gametes seems to be greater than the risk to men's. In contrast to mutagens, teratogens affect only women (by definition, teratogens are a risk only after conception). Since far more chemical agents have been identified as teratogenic than have been identified as mutagenic, it follows, at least at present, that the known risks of impairment in offspring resulting from effects in women exceed the risks of such impairments resulting from effects in men.

For men, the primary manner in which reproductive function is likely to be impaired is through interference with spermatogenesis (see Chapter 3). During spermatogenesis, the developing gametes are differentially sensitive to toxic agents at various stages. However, since spermatogenesis is a continuous process in a postpubertal male, permanent damage will result only if the stem cells (spermatogonia) are damaged. In other words, damage to a man's "current crop" of spermatozoa may well leave future sperm unaffected. However, if permanent genetic damage to a large population of spermatogonia should occur, the nature of male gametogenesis makes this a very serious problem, since a lifetime of "mutant sperm" would continue to be produced through mitotic divisions of the damaged stem cells. Fortunately, the male system includes a protective barrier, the blood–testis barrier, which is composed of myoid cells in the basement membrane of the seminiferous tubules and, of even greater functional importance, tightly occluding junctions between Sertoli cells (see Chapter 3). While this barrier does not provide absolute invulnerability, it does prevent many potentially harmful toxins from reaching spermatozoa.

There is, however, no equivalent protection for the oocytes of women. Further, even if some of the millions of spermatozoa ejaculated during intercourse were damaged, there would be a low probability that a damaged sperm would be the one to achieve fertilization. In contrast, women are born with a finite supply of oocytes that have been aging from embryonic life onward (see Chapter 3). Thus, if a woman's oocytes are negatively affected by an environmental toxin, the damage to her capacity to produce healthy offspring can be permanent. Since only a single egg is normally ovulated each menstrual cycle, it will be either damaged or normal, unlike the potentially mixed population of spermatozoa in which damaged spermatozoa could exist without impairing reproductive function.

These points relate only to gametogenic differences between the sexes. In comparing relative risk factors, it is also obvious that since far more reproductive processes essential for the production of a healthy offspring occur in women (e.g., menstrual cyclicity, ovulation, sperm capacitation, gamete transport, fertilization, implantation, placental function), there are many more potential points at which reproductive toxins can intervene.

Although these facts make it clear that women are more vulnerable to reproductive toxins than are men, there is a greater awareness of the potential effects of various toxins on male reproductive function. It has sometimes been suggested that a greater awareness of the potential dangers posed to male gametes is an example of sexism, reflecting a greater concern for protecting male fertility. While this might be true in some instances, it should also be pointed out that there are two straightforward nonsexist reasons for the greater understanding of risk factors affecting men.

First, male gametes are easily, readily, cheaply, and painlessly accessed for evaluation (i.e., by masturbation). Within each ejaculate, millions of subjects are available for study. In contrast, female gametes can be obtained only through far more complicated, costly, and painful invasive surgical procedures. Even through surgical intervention, the number of oocytes that can be obtained for evaluation is meager compared to the number of sperm in a single ejaculate. Second, even assuming availability of the gametes, objective evaluation criteria (e.g., morphology, motility, swimming velocity, acrosomal integrity) can be rapidly, simply, and cheaply applied to sperm.

Applying comparable measures of viability to oocytes (e.g., capacity for in vitro protein syntheses) is much more difficult.

## PRENATAL SUSCEPTIBILITY TO TERATOGENS

We have only recently recognized that a drug harmless to a woman could impair prenatal development of her offspring and cause congenital malformations. During prenatal development, there is a continuous interplay between genetic factors, which are in essence the "program" for the production and healthy development of a fetus, and environmental factors, which provide the setting for expression of this program. Many exogenous agents, at appropriate points of sensitivity, can modify the expression of inherited genes and cause congenital malformations.

As described by Tuchmann-Duplessis (1983), the consequences of congenital malformations are increasing. At present, developmental accidents are the main cause of perinatal mortality and postnatal morbidity. More infants are permanently handicapped through developmental impairments than by any other cause. It has been estimated that 7 percent of Americans suffer from some type of congenital defect and that 700,000 infants are born defective each year (Tuchmann-Duplessis 1983). With the rising number of women employed in industry and the increasing environmental pollution resulting from industrial waste, insecticides, herbicides, defoliants, and other xenobiotics, the potential hazards for developing human offspring are ever increasing.

Depending upon the time of exposure — from gametogenesis to the fetal period and through lactation — the adverse actions on the capacity to reproduce healthy offspring are variable. Potential impairments range from infertility to embryonic death, from gross congenital malformations to more subtle impairments of biochemical functions. Some defects may not be recognized at birth. They may go unrecognized for several months after birth (like some heart anomalies) or even for several years (like some kidney and central nervous system malformations). Some anomalies are only recognized after puberty, for example, adenosis (glandular diseases), impaired reproductive function, and vaginal cancer controversially attributed to prenatal diethylstilbestrol (DES) exposure, which we shall discuss shortly.

The processes of fertilization, blastulation, gastrulation, and early erosion of the endometrium take place in the pre-implantation period (see Chapter 4). It is not widely realized that chemical insult at this stage sometimes leads to the death of the conceptus but only rarely to nonfatal teratogenic effects. According to Edwards (1980), the distinct resistance of the pre-implantation conceptus to teratogens may be due in part to the absence of major morphogenetic movements in this early stage, except for the separation into inner-cell mass and trophoblastic cells (see Chapter 4). The component cells of the cleaving conceptus appear to have similar metabolic requirements, at least in comparison with the great variations which appear later in growth, and exposure to adverse influences either causes no serious damage to any of the cells or impairs and destroys all of them, resulting in death of the conceptus.

After implantation, the embryo becomes increasingly sensitive to a wide array of teratogens that can impair or distort its growth. The formation of the germ layers and the early stages of organogenesis (see Chapter 4) are periods when great care is needed to avoid exposing embryos to various drugs, toxins, stresses, and other agents that can interfere with cellular differentiation and organ formation. Organogenesis occurs from approximately the third to the eighth week of gestation, and is characterized by the migration and association of cells and tissues into organ rudiments. This is a particularly vulnerable period for induction of structural defects. Individual organ systems are vulnerable for a relatively short span of time, and the same teratogenic agent can induce different malformations (or none at all) depending on when an embryo or fetus is exposed to the agent (Wilson 1977). Since differentiation of organ systems is characterized by a dissimilarity in the protein content and metabolic function of different cell populations, and since this differentiation results from a selective activation and inactivation of genes, this is a particularly sensitive point for modification of gene action by teratogenic agents.

The fetal period is characterized mainly by differentiation of the embryonic primordium into definitive organs (a process termed *histogenesis*), general growth, and the storage of energy substrates. Morphological maturation of organs is paralleled by an increase in functional activity, with protein content increasing more than DNA content. Increase in the rate of growth results from two phenomena, cell proliferation and increases in cell size. Growth begins with an increase in DNA followed by accelerated protein synthesis. Growth is linear and continuous, with the greatest increase in the rate of a growth occurring in the first three months of gestation. The rapid growth that is characteristic of fetal development predisposes the fetus to the damaging effects of various toxins and is the reason why fetuses are far more susceptible to damage from toxins than are adults.

Chemical insult during the fetal period can lead to a broad spectrum of effects, from growth retardation to functional disorders to transplacental induction of cancer. The latter two effects are difficult to measure, because long latency periods are often required for their expression and detection. Although the fetus is more resistant than the embryo to lethal effects, exposure to some toxic chemicals can still lead to fetal death. As placental development proceeds, the placenta becomes an increasingly effective barrier limiting fetal exposure to harmful chemicals absorbed by the woman. The placenta also protects the fetus by metabolizing chemicals, generally to less toxic forms. The efficiency with which it may perform these two functions depends on the chemical or toxin in question. And in some cases, metabolism of chemicals may actually result in an undesired effect — conversion of an innocuous product into one that is teratogenic or mutagenic. The development within the fetus itself of enzyme systems necessary to metabolize foreign chemicals is a slow process that is not completed until after birth. The liver functions in limited ways during fetal development and is incapable of the metabolic functions it performs in the adult.

Structural and functional maturation continues after birth, particularly in the nervous, immune, endocrine, reproductive, and drug detoxification systems. The neonatal period is critical, since metabolic anomalies acquired during gestation may cause a dysfunction of enzyme systems required for the autonomic life of the infant. The general metabolism is suddenly switched from an anabolic (building up) to a catabolic (breaking down) state. Before birth, the woman supplies energy to the fetus, much of which is stored as glycogen and lipids. After birth, energy is needed (and quickly) for thermogenesis, respiration, and motility. A fault occurring during the late intrauterine stages may only be expressed when postnatal demands are placed on the newborn. For example, the baby may die because surfactant cannot be produced by the lungs to prevent them from collapsing or because the metabolic pathways needed for energy utilization may malfunction—both faults can result from intrauterine teratogenic effects.

After birth, the neonate remains susceptible to chemical insult, especially through exposure to toxic agents in breast milk. The types of damage most extensively studied are alterations of the nervous system reflected in neurobehavioral deficiencies and childhood cancer (Council on Environmental Quality 1981).

Another difficulty in assessing teratogenic action is our inability to measure many subtle traits which may have been elicited by exposure to a teratogenic agent during pregnancy (or, on the other hand, which may be due to innumerable other causes). For example, it is difficult to imagine how subtle effects on the nervous system (possibly manifested as a speech defect, reading disability, or behavioral disorder) could ever conclusively be linked to a teratogenic agent, even though, in theory, such an agent may have been the cause of the defect. Even more difficult to know is whether prenatal exposure to the subtle effects of teratogens has reduced an intellect of potential genius to one in the average range or has reduced the motor skills of a potential star athlete to those of a benchwarmer. Could teratogens be the cause of some people's lifetime predispositions to various illnesses and ailments? It is unlikely that all such questions will ever be conclusively answered.

GENERAL PRINCIPLES OF TERATOGENESIS

Six general principles have been established to characterize the action of a teratogenic agent on the conceptus (Berry 1976; Wilson 1977; and Edwards 1980). The first principle is that the susceptibility of an animal to teratogenesis (termed *Mendelian susceptibility*) depends on its genotype and how it interacts with the environment. Although, as a general rule, a particular compound will exert similar effects over a wide range of animals, there are numerous and significant variations in responses across species and individuals. When reviewing animal data for potential extrapolation to humans, it must be kept in mind that factors such as hormonal control, anatomy, pharmacokinetics, metabolism, effective dosage or exposure, and so on, may differ dramatically among species. If an inappropriate animal model is employed for testing, results derived from the animal studies may have no relevance for predicting human response. There are many examples of reproductive toxins which have pronounced effects in one species but no effect in another. A classic and tragically instructive example is the tranquilizer thalidomide. Although harmless to the women who took it, use of thalidomide resulted in the birth of several thousand children with limb deformities ranging from shortening and torsions of the upper and lower extremities (termed *phocomelia*) to complete absence of arms and legs (termed *amelia*). A virtual epidemic of deformed babies occurred in 1961. The first reports of these defects were given by Lenz in West Germany and McBride in Australia (see Tuchmann-Duplessis 1983). In addition to limb deformities, thalidomide was subsequently also linked with anomalies of the heart, kidney, and gastrointestinal tract (Tuchmann-Duplessis 1983). Prior to its use in humans, thalidomide had been tested in rats and mice. Only in retrospect was it discovered that although rats and mice apparently are insensitive to it, developing humans are highly sensitive. On the other hand, other assorted toxins have been shown to elicit effects in test animals while eliciting no apparent effect in humans. Testing of drugs for human teratogenic potential became mandatory after the thalidomide incident.

As described by Tuchmann-Duplessis (1983), not only are there differences in response to drugs among different species, there are also differences in response among strains of animals within a species and even between individuals of the same strain. These findings have led researchers to two basic conclusions about teratogenic susceptibility: (1) susceptibility is not general but is dependent on organ-specific gene action and (2) tendency to malformation of one organ may depend on several genes, each being affected by various teratogens. A strain susceptible to one agent may be resistant to another.

A biochemical explanation for strain differences in teratogenic susceptibility has been described by Tuchmann-Duplessis (1983). For example, it has been known for years that certain strains of mice are more susceptible to teratogenic effects from glucocorticoids than are others (Fraser 1978). When mice of the A/J strain are treated with cortisone between day 11 and day 14 of pregnancy, their offspring exhibit a 100 percent incidence of cleft palate. In contrast, the same treatment administered to strain C57BL/6J produces only a 20–25 percent incidence of cleft palate. Salomon and Pratt (1976) and Goldmann et al. (1977) have shown that these differences in susceptibility are related to cytoplasmic receptors for glucocorticoids.

Comparing the facial mesenchyme cells of the two strains, the authors found that the embryonic facial mesenchymal cells of cortisone-sensitive strains have a much greater ability to bind glucocorticoids than do those of cortisone-resistant strains. Thus, in this example, susceptibility to cleft palate is closely related to the affinity of embryonic mesenchymal cells to bind glucocorticoids. There are relative susceptibilities regarding other anomalies, both across strains and across species (e.g., maternal ingestion of cortisone has no effect on cleft palate in humans).

A final point on the complex interrelationship between pharmacological properties and teratogenic action is illustrated by research that followed in the wake of the thalidomide tragedy. Two compounds (Aturban and Doriden) that are structurally and biochemically closely related to thalidomide and are used for similar purposes became suspect and were tested extensively. However, exposure to these drugs induced no malformations in a variety of test animals (even using very high doses, including those toxic to the mother), and no malformations have ever been reported in humans (Tuchmann-Duplessis 1983). Thus, agents which are structurally, physiologically, and pharmacologically quite similar to one another may yield widely differing effects.

The second principle of teratogenesis — that the susceptibility of a prenatal being varies with the stage of development at the time of exposure — has already been discussed.

The third principle of teratogenesis is that teratogens act in specific ways to initiate abnormal embryogenesis. Growth of a fetus, for example, may be impaired by gene mutation, chromosomal or meiotic damage, restriction or limitation of precursors or energy sources, and interference with enzymes, osmotic pressure, or membranes. A single teratogen can invoke multiple types of damage.

The fourth principle is that the manifestations of abnormal growth are death, malformation, growth retardation, and functional disorders.

The fifth principle is that access of teratogenic agents to the conceptus, embryo, or fetus varies according to the nature of the agent. For example, irradiation passes directly through a woman's body to the fetus. Chemicals gain access to the woman's blood and, depending on the nature of the chemical, may cross the placenta, gaining access to the fetus. As our knowledge of placental properties and placental functions has grown, we have come to realize that the placenta is not, as originally thought, an impenetrable protective barrier. Numerous physiological and pathological attributes of a woman can affect the action of a teratogen on a fetus. Physiological factors include a woman's age, diet, hormone balance, and uterine environment. Examples of pathological factors which may increase the action of potential teratogenic agents include metabolic diseases, diabetes, and obesity (Tuchmann-Duplessis 1983).

The sixth principle of teratogenesis is that abnormal development is related to the dose of the teratogen. Below certain levels, many teratogens have no effect. This nil effect may be due to the ability of tissues to be repaired or recolonized from neighboring cells; thus, the level of damage would have to reach a certain plateau before the developing being can no longer repair it and disorder is expressed in the tissues. Once levels of the teratogen rise above the nil-effect level, dose-response relationships may intervene and result in a steep increase in damage, including death (Edwards 1980). Thus, as we have already pointed out, a toxin may have no effect or a devastating effect on a prenatal human being.

Little is known about drug interactions that might cause teratogenic effects (i.e., cases in which two drugs, neither of which is teratogenic alone, interact to produce adverse effects). Further, teratogenic effects may be elicited only under unique predisposing conditions. For example, a normally nonteratogenic agent might be teratogenic if there is a deficiency of a particular vitamin or mineral. It is virtually impossible to test for all of these possibilities.

With this overview of the principles of teratogenesis and with an appreciation of the complexity of this area of study, let's now turn our attention to the literature suggesting a link between prenatal risks and contraceptive methods.

## TERATOGENICITY AND ORAL CONTRACEPTIVES

Simply stated, and despite initial claims to the contrary, we have no good reasons for believing that the OCs in use today pose substantial teratogenetic risks. Early reports ascribing deleterious teratogenic effects to OCs have been refuted by more numerous and better-designed studies that indicate contraceptive steroids (i.e., OCs, implants, and injectables) are not teratogenic (e.g., the reports of Keith and Berger 1980; World Health Organization 1981; Wilson and Brent 1981; Gray 1983; Simpson 1984, 1985a, 1985b). We shall consider the initial studies upon which claims of teratogenicity were based, and we shall argue that flaws in or limitations of these studies justify dismissing their conclusions. It is, of course, a principle of logic that a bad argument may have a true conclusion. The same principle applies to scientific studies — a flawed or unacceptably limited study may draw a true conclusion. However, the combination of methodological problems in the early studies linking ocs to prenatal anomalies and the conclusions of better-designed recent studies suggesting that there are no such links strongly support the conclusion that contemporary ocs do not pose teratogenic risks. As we proceed through the chapter, we shall see that much the same is true of the purported links between ocs and mutagenesis and also the purported links between some other birth control methods and teratogenic and mutagenic harms.

*Fetal Masculinization*   Perhaps the first report on the adverse effects of administering synthetic analogues of sex steroids during pregnancy was given by Hayles and Nolan (1957). They reported that a masculinized female fetus was born to a woman who received methyltestosterone during pregnancy. Reilly et al. (1958) reported similar occurrences in two women, one treated with testosterone and the other treated with 17α-ethinyl testosterone (ethisterone). In addition to the logical potential of these androgenic agents to cause virilization of female fetuses, certain 19-nor-testosterone progestins (i.e., norethindrone and probably norgestrel) can also virilize female fetuses when administered at susceptible periods of pregnancy (Carson and Simpson 1983; Simpson 1985a, 1985b). However, the doses required for virilization (e.g., 20–40 mg per day of norethindrone) are considerably higher than the levels present today in ocs (e.g., 0.2–1.0 mg per day). Thus, virilization of female fetuses should not be of concern for women using contemporary ocs.

Questionable reports linking exposure of progestational agents to cases of masculinized female fetuses include those of Wilkins et al. (1958), Grumbach, Ducharme, and Moloshok (1959), and Breibart, Bongiovanni, and Eberlein (1963). Exogenous steroids cited by these researchers included ethisterone (most frequently cited), diethylstilbestrol (DES), conjugated equine estrogens, ethinyl estradiol, and "pure progesterone."

These and many other studies which purport to establish a link between exogenous sex steroids and fetal anomalies are seriously flawed in several ways. There is often a lack of knowledge concerning the population at risk and the existence of other risk factors and often a failure to calculate incidence rates as well. The studies also generally fail to state clearly why the hormones were prescribed, and they contain frequent errors in chemical terminology. Dose levels and duration and timing of administration are often omitted. Of greatest importance, virtually all of these early studies were devoid of appropriate control groups for comparison. Because of these serious methodological errors, we cannot reasonably conclude from these studies that the OCs in common use today pose a risk of masculinization of female fetuses in women who become pregnant while on OCs.

*Cardiac Anomalies*   The somatic anomaly most often attributed to the use of exogenous progestins involves the heart. That progestins were cardiac teratogens was first claimed in a 1973 report by Levy et al. Given the flaws and vagueness of this report, it is surprising that it was viewed as having any credibility. It was reported that six of seventy-six mothers who received "sex hormones" in the first trimester of pregnancy delivered infants with transposition of the great vessels. The report did not specify or identify which sex hormones were administered, nor did it specify the dose or duration of treatment.

Nora and Nora (1973) claimed similar findings based on a retrospective study. They reported that 20 of 224 mothers giving birth to infants with cardiac defects recalled receiving an estrogen or progestin compound. Reliance on the subjects' recall, as well as generalizations concerning the compounds used, time of treatment, and reason for treatment, invalidates the study's findings.

A later report by these same investigators (Nora and Nora 1975) concerned nineteen patients with various congenital anomalies. They concluded (again in retrospect) that exposure to hormonal contraceptives during pregnancy was a factor in these anomalies. In light of the small number of subjects involved, the lack of appropriate controls, the lack of specifics regarding the hormones used, and the retrospective nature of the study, it is difficult to understand why the conclusions of this report received widespread publicity and credence.

Janerich et al. (1977) identified infants with cardiac defects through birth certificates. Of 104 mothers of affected infants interviewed, 18 had received hormones (16 for pregnancy diagnosis, 2 through inadvertent use of OCs). Again, recall bias in this study is a possibility. Further, the report left it unclear whether exposure occurred during the period of embryogenesis when the developing heart is susceptible to damage.

According to Simpson (1985b), the major impetus for claims of teratogenicity was the outcome of a U.S. Collaborative Perinatal Project, published by Heinonen et al. (1976) and Heinonen, Slone, and Shapiro (1977). Of 1,042 offspring said to have been exposed to "sex hormones" during their gestation, 19 had cardiac defects (1.82 percent; 385 of 49,240 (0.78 percent) unexposed offspring were affected (relative risk = 2.3, $p < 0.05$).

The conclusion of this study — that exposure to progestins increased risk of prenatal cardiac anomalies — has been invalidated. Wiseman and Dodds-Smith (1984) re-evaluated the same data from the U.S. Collaborative Perinatal Project and found that of the 19 progestin-associated cardiac defects, 2 involved coding errors (no progestagen exposure occurred). Two other infants with cardiac defects had trisomy 21, and the aneuploidy, not the progestins, likely caused the problems. Two more were found to be exposed only during the first two weeks of pregnancy, when anomalies cannot ordinarily be induced. Five other infants were not exposed until after cardiac embryogenesis was complete (i.e., after day 42 of gestation). Thus, only 8 of the 19 cardiac defects originally attributed to progestagen teratogenicity could not more logically be attributed to other causes. But this incidence in infants of progestin-exposed women (8 of 1,042 offspring, or 0.77 percent) is virtually identical to the incidence of cardiac defects in the nonexposed control population. Thus, the most reasonable conclusion is that OCs do not cause prenatal cardiac anomalies.

Numerous other studies have reported no evidence that progestins are cardiac teratogens. These are summarized in the reviews of Keith and Berger (1980), World Health Organization (1981), Wilson and Brent (1981), Gray (1983), and Simpson (1984, 1985a, 1985b). We shall mention just a few of the larger studies which support the conclusion that steroidal contraceptives are not cardiac teratogens.

Simpson (1985b) cites a 1972 study in which Spira and coworkers evaluated 20,000 French women throughout pregnancy. Nearly one-half (9,566) received progestins (most for pregnancy diagnosis or pregnancy maintenance). The anomaly rate did not differ between progestin-exposed and nonexposed groups.

In Sweden, Kullander and Kallen (1976) followed 6,379 pregnant women; of these, 194 had abnormal infants. Of the 194, only 5 (2.5 percent) were exposed to progestagens; 2.0 percent of controls (normal infants) were exposed. A British report (Royal College of General Practitioners 1976) cited anomaly rates of 1.5 percent among 136 infants exposed to OCs, 1.6 percent among 11,009 infants of women who never used OCs, and 1.6 percent among 5,530 infants of women who discontinued OCs prior to pregnancy.

Nishimura, Uwabe, and Semba (1974) microdissected 108 embryos that had been exposed to hormones and detected no cardiac anomalies. Several controls had anomalies. Katz et al. (1985) examined women who reported vaginal bleeding during pregnancy. Of note is that both the group treated with progestagens and the untreated control group experienced comparable vaginal bleeding. Anomalies were not increased in the embryos of the women exposed to progestagens.

In summary, the evidence overwhelmingly suggests that progestins are not cardiac teratogens. The relatively few older studies suggesting a teratogenic involvement in cardiac anomalies are riddled with flaws. As we pointed out earlier, methodological shortcomings combined with the contrary conclusions of valid studies justify dismissing the conclusions of studies purporting to show a positive link between progestins and cardiac defects. Specifically, retrospective studies based on recall are inherently biased. Prior pregnancy outcome was rarely taken into account in these studies, despite a known genetic association between the birth of one child with a cardiac defect and the increased risk in subsequent pregnancies. One crucial problem is that the reasons for administering progestins were often not discussed, despite the logical assumption that the very factors threatening pregnancy maintenance may have been the cause of the cardiac defects rather than the progestins used to maintain pregnancy. Finally, few studies restricted analysis only to the interval of embryogenesis during which exposure can produce cardiac defects.

*Penile Anomalies* Penile or neoscrotal hypospadias (a developmental anomaly in males in which the urethra opens on the underside of the penis) were linked to progestins (especially medroxy-progesterone) by the report of Aarskog (1971). Reports of Czeizel, Toth, and Erodi (1979) in Hungary and Monteleone, Castilla, and Paz (1981) in Latin America also showed an enhanced statistical risk of hypospadias in male infants exposed to progestins during pregnancy. However, Aarskog's study was uncontrolled, and the Hungarian study overlooked a high prevalence of hypospadias in the male relatives of many affected infants (Simpson 1985b). The Latin American study did not include crucial information on time and extent of exposure.

In contrast, the better-designed studies of Sweet et al. (1974), Avellan (1977), and Bracken et al. (1978) failed to show a link between hypospadias and progestins. According to a review by Simpson (1985b), not a single prospective study has shown such a relationship. Thus, the combination of flaws in the studies suggesting a link between progestins and penile anomalies and the lack of evidence of any such link in better-designed studies suggests that the most reasonable conclusion is that there is no such link.

*Limb Anomalies*  Janerich, Piper, and Glebatis (1974) reported that 15 of 108 women (13.9 percent) who gave birth to infants with some type of limb reduction deformities (e.g., shortening or absence of a limb, finger, or toe) ingested "progestational steroids." Once again, the hormones involved were not specifically identified. A similar number of "controls" were selected, but selection was based only on approximate date of birth and county of residence. Four of 108 controls (3.7 percent) had been exposed to progestins. Using these figures, the authors alleged that progestin exposure increased the risk of limb deformities some fourfold. But several flaws in this study are obvious. The control group differed significantly from the treatment group, since those in this group did not have problems in early pregnancy that indicated hormonal treatment (again no consideration was given to the conditions leading to progestin treatment). Thus, the purported control group was not really a proper control group at all. Also, some exposures may have occurred during the early all-or-none period (i.e., the period when there is either death or no teratogenic effect).

Greenberg et al. (1977) and McCredie et al. (1983) also claimed an increase in limb reduction deformities following progestin exposure. However, both reports invite criticism and invalidation because of their reliance on memory recall.

The purported link of limb reduction deformities to progestins has also been undermined in a large number of studies. Oakley, Flynt, and Falek (1973) conducted an especially well designed study of malformed infants in metropolitan Atlanta and reported no link between maternal hormonal exposure and limb reduction deformities. Bracken et al. (1978) reached the same conclusion. Lammer and Cordero (1986) reported on a large case-control study involving 1,091 malformed infants and found no association between any of eleven malformation categories and ocs. Only 1 of 98 mothers of infants with limb reduction defects reported a hormone exposure from failed ocs. Interviews were conducted with the mothers as soon as possible after birth of the infant, most within six months and all within one year. While this report is also limited by its dependence upon memory recall, in this case the women needed only to recall whether they were taking ocs at the time of pregnancy.

The conclusion that limb reduction teratogenicity is not associated with progestin exposure is strengthened by the fact that, unlike the more subtle defects, limb shortening is obvious to even the casual observer; thus its occurrence would not be overlooked and its incidence would not likely be underestimated. The 1974 report of Janerich et al. was the primary evidence offered to support the initial claim of a link. Later, Janerich himself (Janerich and Polednak 1983) modified his initial opinion. He apparently now shares the view that current-dosage ocs do not pose a substantial risk for limb deformities.

*Neural Tube Anomalies* Neural tube defects (e.g., spina bifida, anencephaly, encephalocele) were also once claimed to be associated with progestin exposure. The claim was largely based on two reports (Gal, Kirman, and Stern [1967] and Greenberg et al. [1977]) that are invalid for the kinds of reasons previously given. Numerous case-control studies (e.g., Laurence et al. 1971; Bracken et al. 1978; Lammer and Cordero 1986) show no link between neural tube defects and progestins, and earlier claims of a link have now been rejected.

In summary, early reports purporting to link progestins or ocs in general to teratogenic effects have subsequently been countered by a much greater and more convincing body of evidence. A review of the valid scientific evidence leads us to conclude that there are no substantial teratogenic risks associated with use of current-dosage OCs.

## MUTAGENICITY AND ORAL CONTRACEPTIVES

OCs have also been said to be mutagenic. Induction of both gene-mutations and chromosomal abnormalities have been claimed to be the result of OC use, but, as we shall see, these claims have been convincingly discredited.

*Gene Mutations*   Ideally, since mutability varies among genes, possible mutations responsible for Mendelian or polygenic disorders resulting from exposure to exogenous steroids should be assessed locus by locus. However, this is mathematically impossible, given baseline mutation rates of $10^{-5}$ to $10^{-6}$ per locus per gamete per generation (Simpson 1987). Therefore, investigators are reduced to comparing overall anomaly rates in gametes exposed and not exposed to exogenous steroids. This approach is obviously less than ideal, since it results in a pooling of anomalies of Mendelian, polygenic, chromosomal, and environmental etiologies.

Simpson (1985b) reviewed the results from seven independent investigations involving a total of over 20,000 offspring from women who used OCs prior to conception. He concluded that there was no evidence of any increased anomaly rates. Similarly, he reported that various national surveillance reports indicate no increase in any genetically related disorder after the introduction of OCs in the 1960s. Importantly, the report also shows that there has been no change in the sex ratio since OCs have been in wide use. A constant sex ratio is quite significant, since induction of lethal X-linked recessive mutations would decrease the proportion of liveborn males. Mutations at any of the many X-linked loci associated with genes essential for life would obviously contribute to an altered sex ratio favoring females. Further, agents inducing X-linked mutations would also likely have induced autosomal mutations which would be observed. Once again, the bottom line is that there is overwhelming evidence from numerous sources to contradict the few small-sample studies that initially were believed to suggest OC mutagenicity, and there is virtually unanimous agreement within the scientific community that ocs pose no threat of mutagenicity. Moreover, as Simpson (1985b) points out, the fact that progestins clearly seem not to induce mutations in germ cells also offers some reassurance that they are unlikely to have mutagenic effects in somatic cells which may cause cancer later in life. However, as we previously pointed out, since the potential effects of exogenous agents always occur in the future and are therefore not completely measurable, there is a theoretical possibility that ocs may subtly affect oocytes. And since the potential effects of exogenous agents on different kinds of cells may vary, absence of mutagenic effects on germ cells does not entail that the same agent will not have mutagenic effects on other cells. However, given the current evidence, which suggests that contemporary ocs (and other steroidal birth control products) do not cause cancer in women (see Chapter 5), the absence of evidence of mutagenic effects of these products on gametes supports the more general view that they do not function as mutagens.

*Chromosomal Abnormalities* Given the nature of the process of oogenesis (see Chapter 3), it is not unreasonable to assume that prior hormonal exposure may induce chromosomal abnormalities. In theory, the oocytes which "hibernate" in the first meiotic division from embryogenesis until ovulation many years later might complete meiosis inefficiently as a result of hormonal exposure, resulting in chromosomal abnormalities.

The report of Carr (1970) prompted initial concern about possible chromosomal abnormalities resulting from mutagenic actions of ocs. In this study, 48 percent of abortuses of women who previously used ocs were found to have some chromosomal abnormality compared with a 22 percent abnormality rate in controls (women who had not used ocs). Most of the excess was due to polyploidy (having more than two full sets of chromosomes). However, as with initial well-publicized reports in other areas, Carr's observations were not confirmed in several later studies.

Boué and Boué (1973) reported 66 percent abnormal complements (16 percent polyploidy) among abortuses of 243 previous oc users compared with 63 percent (18 percent polyploidy) among 604 controls. Lauritsen (1975) found 61 percent abnormalities in previous oc users and 49 percent in controls. However, this numerical but statistically nonsignificant increase was due to monosomy X and structural abnormalities, not polyploidy, as reported by Carr (1970). Alberman et al. (1976) observed 32 percent abnormalities in 524 prior OC users and a similar rate of 26 percent in 428 controls.

As emphasized by Simpson (1985b), failure to confirm the initial findings of Carr (1970) is especially noteworthy, because either of two biases might spuriously yield increased abnormality rates in exposed groups. First, unrecognized induced abortuses are more likely to be included inadvertently among controls than among women going off the pill in order to conceive. Surreptitious illicit abortions are a likely explanation for the unusually low frequency of chromosomally abnormal abortuses in Carr's control group. Second, as indicated in our discussion in Chapter 5, ovulation may be delayed during the cycle immediately following discontinuation of OC use. This delay will result in pregnancies of less advanced gestation than those of controls, who are more likely to have normal cycles. Because the frequency of chromosomal abnormalities is inversely related to gestational age, unrecognized younger gestation ages would lead to an inflated abnormality rate in prior OC users.

As further evidence that OCs cause neither numerical nor structural chromosomal abnormalities, Simpson (1985b) suggests that one should also note the conditions not shown to occur. For example, if OCs do have deleterious effects, the frequency of spontaneous abortions should increase after hormonal discontinuation, because 50–60 percent of first-trimester abortuses show cytogenetic abnormalities. But, to the contrary, pooled data from numerous large studies show no increase in frequency of spontaneous abortions. Also, an increased frequency of liveborns with Down's syndrome (trisomy 21) should be evident in prior OC users, because trisomy in both abortuses and live births is presumably caused by the same cytological nondisjunction. No such increase is known to occur. Finally, an increase in liveborns with cytogenetic abnormalities would be reflected by a generalized increase in anomalies following cessation of use of OCs. Again, the evidence suggests that this does not occur. Thus, the clear consensus of scientific opinion is that use of OCs does not predispose women to oocyte chromosomal abnormalities which lead to anomalies in children.

MUTAGENICITY, TERATOGENICITY, AND
INJECTABLE AND IMPLANT PROGESTINS

Few studies have specifically concentrated on the potential teratogenic and mutagenic effects of implant and injectable progestins.
As we saw in Chapter 5, the development of such progestins is
more recent and their use is less widespread than that of OCs. However, we have already considered data concerning the two progestins
most commonly used in these preparations (medroxyprogesterone
and norethindrone). As we saw in Chapter 5, maternal serum progestin levels with implants and injectables are considerably lower
than serum levels of hormones in OC users. This is one of their major
advantages. Thus, it is logical to assume that if certain adverse effects
do not occur in users of the higher-dose OCs, injectable and implant
preparations are even less likely to cause such problems. Given the
large numbers of women worldwide who have participated in various studies of these two progestin delivery systems, it seems likely
that teratogenic and mutagenic effects would have been noted and
reported if indeed there were adverse effects. But no direct claims of
teratogenicity or mutagenicity have been made. Since use of implants
and injectables is fairly recent, however, and since there is some
concern about the reliability of some investigators in certain countries (see Chapter 9), we should not too hastily take lack of reports
of adverse effects to show that implants and injectables are defi-
nitely not teratogenic or mutagenic.

MUTAGENICITY, TERATOGENICITY,
AND DIETHYLSTILBESTROL

Diethylstilbestrol (DES) is a nonsteroidal, synthetic estrogen that is
effective as a postcoital interceptive (i.e., a morning-after pill) following unprotected intercourse (see Chapter 6). DES was widely
prescribed for women, especially in the United States, in the late
1940s and early 1950s as a treatment for threatened spontaneous abortion and premature labor. Numerous reports that began appearing
in the mid-1970s suggest that daughters of women treated with DES
may have suffered teratogenic effects, including susceptibility to a
rare type of vaginal and cervical carcinoma. Other more controversial effects of exposure to DES in utero have also been suggested. In
reviewing the literature on the potential teratogenicity of DES, a

sharp distinction must be made. On the one hand, DES probably does not have teratogenic effects if used properly as a postcoital interceptive (i.e., as recommended by the FDA). On the other hand, DES may well have caused teratogenic effects in the daughters of women who received it therapeutically decades ago based on the mistaken belief that it would prevent miscarriage. It is currently used only as a postcoital interceptive, and, as we saw in Chapter 6, there are now other products that are more efficacious for that purpose.

Although the consensus is that daughters of women who received DES during pregnancy have a risk of vaginal, cervical, or endometrial cancer that may be up to four times greater than in the general population, there is not unanimous agreement on this point (Ziel and Finkle 1975; Smith et al. 1975; Mack, Pike, and Henderson 1976; Kaufman et al. 1977; Lipsett 1977; Bibbo et al. 1978; Sloane 1980; Henzl 1986). Likewise, there are studies which conclude that DES exposure resulted in menstrual cycle irregularities (e.g., Bibbo et al. 1977), while other studies refute that claim (e.g., Barnes 1979). Even more controversial is the uncorroborated report of Ehrhardt et al. (cited by Schumacher et al. 1987), which suggests that daughters of DES-treated mothers show an increased adult incidence of homosexuality and bisexuality when compared with the general population. There are at least two other studies that refute these claims (see Meyer-Bahlburg 1984). There are no reports that suggest mutagenic effects of DES exposure.

Earlier in this chapter we outlined some of the more significant variables affecting the action of a potential teratogenic agent. No doubt the inconsistencies among the reports mentioned above regarding the effects of in utero exposure to DES are due to the interplay of several of these variables. Perhaps the single most important factor affecting response is time of exposure. As we saw earlier, there are finite periods in prenatal development during which developing systems are vulnerable to damage. Once a system has passed through its critical periods of development, it is relatively immune to damage. On the other hand, exposure of developing cells to DES during the organogenesis of a woman's reproductive tract may adversely affect her development and predispose her to subsequent aberrant growth under certain conditions. But this implies an additional variable, namely, adult exposure to a set of conditions that can trigger malignant growth of prenatally altered cells. Other obvious variables include the duration of exposure to DES, the effective dosage reaching the fetus, and interactions with other drugs and predisposing conditions. Since all reports concerning the potential teratogenicity of DES are, by necessity, retrospective clinical studies, it is impossible to know the specific set of variables associated with each case.

## TERATOGENICITY AND INTRAUTERINE DEVICES

Barrie (1976) first proposed that IUDs could cause congenital malformations. This suggestion was based upon the birth of two infants with limb reduction defects whose mothers had IUDs in place at conception and throughout pregnancy (one a Graefenberg ring, the other a Dalkon Shield). Stevens and Fraser (1974) and Leighton, Evans, and Wallis (1976) each reported single cases of anomalies (cleft palate and limb reduction respectively) in users of copper IUDs.

As use of medicated IUDs containing copper became more widespread in the 1970s, the safety of IUDs became of increasing concern. The toxicity of copper was studied by several investigators, especially in regard to the effects of systemic absorption of copper and its potential teratogenicity in cases of accidental pregnancy.

Although it has been shown in rats that dissolved copper may enter the systemic circulation and be distributed in many body parts, there is no evidence that the small quantities of copper (10–50 $\mu$g per 24 hours) lost from the Copper-T IUD result in any toxic manifestations in women (Tatum 1977). As Tatum (1977) point out, the adult minimum daily requirement for copper is 2,000–5,000 $\mu$g.

Detailed studies by Chang and Tatum (1973) in rats, hamsters, and rabbits indicated that copper wire did not produce any teratogenic effects on developing fetuses. Not only did the copper not affect gestation, parturition, and lactation, but subsequent development and fertility of the $F_1$ and $F_2$ generations were also normal. Reviews by Furst and Haro (1969) and Gilman (1962) provide extensive evidence that neither metallic copper nor copper salts have carcinogenic properties.

Guilleband (1976) reported that of 20,684 insertions of the Copper-7 IUD, 714 pregnancies occurred with the device in place. Of these pregnancies, 167 continued full-term and 5 dissimilar anomalies occurred. This rate of anomalies in infants approximates that in the normal population.

Tatum, Schmidt, and Jain (1976) reviewed 918 pregnancies that commenced while a Copper-T device was in use. Of the total, 465 women elected abortion. For the remainder, the spontaneous abortion rate was 20.3 percent (24 of 118) with the device removed or expelled and 54.1 percent (85 of 157) with the device left in place. The stillbirth rate was 0.9 percent with and 1.9 percent without IUD removal. However, only 1 anomaly (vocal cord fibroma) was detected among 157 births and 9 abortions late in pregnancy.

In the United Kingdom, Snowden (1976) reported no anomalies in 317 pregnancies of women with an IUD in situ. Albert (1983) likewise failed to observe anomalies in pregnancies of women conceiving with copper devices in place.

In a case-control study of limb reduction defects and the IUD, Layde et al. (1979) compared 96 infants with limb defects with appropriately selected controls and found no significant increase in limb defects in the IUD group. In a large study (involving 2,191 anomalous infants), Bracken and Vita (1983) assessed contraceptive usage of all types. Again, no significant increase in congenital malformations were linked to IUDs.

As with copper IUDs, no studies have shown any teratogenic effects of IUDs impregnated with progesterone or progestagens.

As we saw in Chapter 6, pregnancies with an IUD in place are associated with increased frequencies of ectopic pregnancy, spontaneous (often septic) abortions, and other risks to women. Given that one of the IUD's primary actions is to create a uterine environment which is extremely inhospitable to a conceptus (see Chapter 6), it is reasonable to assume that a being developing in such an environment would be adversely affected. But reasonable assumptions often turn out to be mistaken, and this seems to be one of those cases. In fact, studies of tissues obtained from 394 women who spontaneously aborted showed that there was a lower incidence of embryonic abnormalities in women using IUDs (21 percent) than in women using no contraceptive technology (44 percent) (Poland 1970). Tatum (1977) reported that in more than 200 accidental pregnancies allowed to progress with an IUD in place and resulting in live births, there was no evidence of an unusual incidence of congenital abnormalities. As discussed by Simcock (1985), although there is no evidence of a teratogenic effect exerted by any IUD, many physicians still persist in advising pregnant women using IUDs to abort their pregnancies. Simcock (1985) reports from his personal experience that despite reassurance of the apparent normality of the fetuses, many of his patients who conceive with an IUD in place request abortion because of their fears of teratogenic effects of the IUD. As we described in Chapter 6, the standard practice is to remove a pregnant woman's IUD at the earliest opportunity if she elects to continue with the pregnancy (the purpose of removal is to minimize the risk of a septic abortion). Finally, because IUDs act locally rather than systemically (see Chapter 6), it is not possible for an IUD to affect a woman's gametes. And while IUDs increase the mortality rate of spermatozoa, no effect of an IUD on the genetic content of sperm cells has ever been shown or, to our knowledge, alleged.

MUTAGENICITY, TERATOGENICITY, AND
VAGINAL SPERMICIDES

The active ingredient of most spermicidal creams, jellies, foams, suppositories, and sponges is nonyl-phenoxy polyoxyethylene-ethanol (nonoxynol-9). The mode of action of nonoxynol-9 is straightforward; as implied by the term *spermicide*, it immobilizes and kills spermatozoa. Spermicides may be used alone or, far more effectively, in conjunction with barrier methods (see Chapter 1). Some three million women in the United States employ birth control methods utilizing spermicides (Wilbur 1986).

A recent and highly publicized lawsuit alleging that the Ortho spermicidal product a woman was using at the time of conception caused her daughter's birth defects has produced considerable consternation among pharmaceutical companies and within the medical community in the United States (*Wells v. Ortho Pharmaceutical Corporation* 1986). A federal appeals court upheld a $4.7 million award and the Supreme Court has declined to review the case. Of particular concern is the court's contention in *Wells* that "legal decisions may be based on evidence unacceptable by today's scientific standards" (see Mills and Alexander 1986). As we shall see shortly, there is a clear scientific consensus that vaginal spermicides are not associated with increased prenatal malformations. However, despite strong scientific evidence invalidating the claims of litigants, in the wake of such court decisions pharmaceutical companies must now consider removing spermicides from the market for economic reasons (cf. Searle's decision to remove its copper IUDs from the market, discussed in Chapters 1 and 6).

Before examining specific reports on the possible mutagenic and teratogenic effects of vaginal spermicides, we need to consider the theoretical plausibility of these claims. For a number of reasons, teratogenicity resulting from the use of vaginal spermicides is not likely. If a woman knows that she is pregnant and elects to continue the pregnancy, there is no reason for her to use spermicides or any other birth control method. If she is early in her pregnancy (i.e., prior to her first missed period), she is in the all-or-none phase during which teratogenicity is unlikely. Thus, only when there is an unknown pregnancy of greater than two weeks duration is there even a theoretical risk of teratogenic harm from a spermicide. Even then, that nonoxynol-9 is embryotoxic and that it migrates from the vagina to the uterus in a quantity sufficient to affect the developing embryo must be shown if claims of its teratogenicity are to be credible. Although it is not known to what extent nonoxynol-9 (or other spermicidal agents) may be stored or transferred within a woman's body, to our knowledge no one has established the presence of the spermicide at the site of embryonic development nor demonstrated it to be embryotoxic. Since migration to the site of embryonic development seems unlikely, if conception of a malformed offspring results from a failure of the spermicide, it seems that the cause would be mutagenic, not teratogenic. The only way this could occur is through chromosomal damage to the spermatozoon participating in fertilization. Although it has been hypothesized that spermicides may cause chromosomal abnormalities by damaging spermatozoa, this has yet to be established as more than a theoretic possibility.

The well-publicized report of Jick et al. (1981) was the first to claim an association between spermicides and birth defects. The investigators studied the incidence of birth defects in 790 Seattle women who had filled prescriptions for spermicides within 600 days of miscarrying or delivering a baby. They compared the miscarriage rate and the incidence of birth defects in infants of women in this group with that observed in a much larger population of women (approximately 4,000) who had not purchased spermicides. They reported a 3.5 percent miscarriage rate and a 2.2 percent birth defect rate for the spermicide purchasers, compared with rates of 2.0 percent and 1.0 percent respectively for the control group.

Despite the glaring errors in the experimental design of the Jick study on which they were based, reports that spermicide usage "more than doubled a woman's chances of producing an infant with birth defects" received considerable attention in the news media. Most striking among the deficiencies of experimental design in the study is the lack of verification that women in the group under study actually used the spermicide purchased or that they used it at the time of conception or early in their pregnancies.

Adding to the controversy, Silberner (1986) reported that two of Jick's coauthors on the original report are now disassociating themselves from its conclusions. One coauthor, Richard N. Watkins, is quoted by Silberner (1986) as saying that the original conclusion "was based on an inaccurate presumption of exposure to spermicide near the time of conception." Watkins re-examined the medical records of eight women who produced deformed infants and found that four of them indicated that their pregnancies were planned and that they were not using spermicides at the time of conception. A second coauthor, Louis B. Holmes, has noted that no subsequent investigations have suggested a link between spermicides and birth defects and that reservations expressed in the original article tended to be ignored in courts of law (Silberner 1986). Holmes is quoted by Silberner as saying, "In retrospect, I believe our article should never have been published." However, Jick stands by the original report. He believes that the 1981 report "addressed plausible hypotheses" and that while an association of spermicides with limb defects "remains in substantial doubt," he feels the literature on possible chromosomal abnormalities "is more supportive [of the link than not] . . . but it is far from definitive" (Silberner 1986).

The only report subsequent to that of Jick et al. (1981) claiming any relationship between spermicides and birth defects is that of Rothman (1982). In this report, an increased exposure to spermicides in Down's syndrome infants having cardiac defects was claimed. However, spermicide use was not associated with infants who had cardiac defects but not Down's syndrome. Rothman's conclusions, limited as they are, are probably invalidated by recall bias.

In contrast to the reports associating use of spermicides with birth defects, numerous well-designed, large-scale studies clearly suggest that there is no causal connection (e.g., Huggins, Vessey, and Flavil 1982; Mills et al. 1982, 1985; Polednak, Janerich, and Glebatis 1982; Shapiro et al. 1982; Bracken and Vita 1983; Cordero and Layde 1983). Shapiro et al. (1982) reported on 462 women who used spermicides during the first four months of pregnancy (438 of these also reported use during the month preceding the last menstrual period). In theory, therefore, both teratogenic and mutagenic effects were possible. The 462 exposed women delivered 23 infants with birth defects (5 percent), compared with 2,254 infants with birth defects among 49,825 controls not exposed to spermicides (4.5 percent).

Polednak, Janerich, and Glebatis (1982) used a case-control experimental design to assess the specific anomalies reported by Jick et al. (1981). They found no significant difference between spermicide users and nonusers for any of the defects assessed, namely, limb reduction defects, hypospadias, Down's syndrome, neural tube defects, and cardiovascular defects.

Mills et al. (1985) conducted a case-control study involving 34,660 women. Included were 3,146 women who had used spermicides before but not after their last menstrual period and 2,282 who had used spermicides only after their last menstrual period. The investigators documented use of other contraceptives and other possible confounding variables and analyzed by time of exposure for 157 types of anomalies. No significant differences between controls and users of spermicides were found for any anomaly. Likewise, no change in sex ratio occurred following spermicidal exposure, which, as we have already seen, offers reassurance concerning lethal X-linked recessive mutations and lethal mutations in general.

Recently, Louik et al. (1987) and Warburton et al. (1987) reported results from two large studies examining maternal exposure to spermicides in relation to birth defects. Louik et al. (1987) concluded that the risks of five specific birth defects — Down's syndrome, hypospadias, limb reduction defects, neoplasms, and neural tube defects — are not increased by exposure to spermicide contraceptives in the first four months of pregnancy, at the time of conception, or at any time before conception. Warburton et al. (1987) specifically examined whether the risk of fetal trisomy was increased with use of spermicides. They found no evidence of an association, either when all types of trisomy were combined or when trisomy 21 alone was considered. These conclusions were based on an examination of 13,279 women who were undergoing prenatal fetal chromosome studies at seventeen different medical centers but who were not as yet aware of the results of their screening studies. All responses were coded in order to eliminate any opportunity for differential recall of spermicide exposure.

The extremely thorough, well-designed, and carefully controlled studies of Mills et al. (1985) should be accepted as sufficient to finally lay to rest concerns about teratogenicity and mutagenicity of vaginal spermicides.

After the *Wells* decision, a decision which apparently was not based on the scientific evidence regarding spermicides and birth defects, Mills and Alexander (1987) expressed the concern of many scientists in a letter to the editor published in the *New England Journal of Medicine* on April 23, 1987. They said, "Our point is that justice is best served by determining whether or not the alleged cause of a malformation is the true cause. Applying uncritical standards does not promote justice, nor is unscientific thinking in society's best interest."

Despite public perception to the contrary, then, virtually all earlier, often highly publicized studies claiming teratogenic and mutagenic effects of birth control methods do seem to have been refuted by more numerous and better-designed studies showing no such effects. We are completely unwilling to minimize concerns about any potential adverse effects of birth control methods. But, in all candor, we were genuinely surprised by the dearth of evidence supporting the general misconception that various birth control methods carry a high risk of teratogenicity and mutagenicity. Such a misconception is likely to lead a number of women who do not presently want a child to use less effective methods (e.g., unmedicated barriers) or to avoid using birth control technologies altogether, resulting in increased numbers of unwanted pregnancies and more unwanted children or more abortions. We believe it is important, then, for women to realize that, in general, fear of teratogenic and mutagenic harm should not lead them to avoid using most contemporary birth control devices or agents or to seek an abortion in cases where the conceptus, embryo, or fetus has been exposed to one of these devices or agents. Such fears are undoubtedly in great part perpetuated by the materials commonly provided to women by manufacturers of birth control products (e.g., the package inserts which accompany ocs). Given our examination of the reports linking these products to teratogenesis and mutagenesis and of the studies undermining those reports, we must conclude that either manufacturers have not themselves carefully reviewed the literature or (more likely) that the purpose of the warnings is to allow manufacturers to claim that women and their prescribing physicians have been warned in the event that mutagenic or teratogenic damage is alleged to have resulted from product use (see also the discussion of harm to women in Chapter 5). If a woman wants to avoid pregnancy but is fearful of the purported teratogenic and mutagenic effects of available technologies, she would do best to find a physician or other professional who will be able to give her a competent assessment of the grounds for believing that her fears are warranted.

.   .   .   .   .   .

There are significant concerns today surrounding the issue of preventing harm to human beings before their birth. The most pressing of these concerns arise with certain behaviors on the part of some pregnant women and exposure of pregnant women and fertile men and women to toxins in the workplace. These potential sources of harm to human gametes and prenatal human beings have raised questions of increasing moral urgency, particularly about restricting the life-style choices of women, about holding women legally liable for causing prenatal harm, about prohibiting fertile or pregnant women from taking certain positions in the workforce, and about requiring some women to choose sterilization if they want to work in certain positions. We turn next to these issues.

# 9
## Mutagenesis, Teratogenesis, and Informed Consent: Some Moral Issues

INTRODUCTION

As we saw in Chapter 6, a number of contemporary birth control methods are potentially injurious to women using them. Fears that these methods are also teratogenically injurious (i.e., harmful to conceptuses, embryos, or fetuses) and mutagenically injurious (i.e., harmful to women's gametes) persist, and they are encouraged in a number of ways, for example, by the warnings that are commonly included in package inserts accompanying various oral contraceptives. But we argued in Chapter 8 that the initial reports linking teratogenic and mutagenic harms to birth control technologies have been invalidated by more recent and better-designed studies. As indicated at the end of that chapter, the most pressing contemporary concerns about harm to prenatal human beings and oocytes arise with certain behaviors on the part of some pregnant women (e.g., use of tobacco, alcohol, and other drugs), with lack of good prenatal nutrition, with maternal refusals of medical and surgical interventions that are believed to prevent prenatal harm, and with exposure to toxins in the workplace.

The issues of mutagenesis and teratogenesis and harm to women from the use of birth control technologies have raised a number of questions of increasing moral urgency. The two we shall focus on in this chapter are the question of prevention of and liability for mutagenic and teratogenic harms and the question of producing, testing, and distributing birth control products in populations where securing a genuinely informed consent to acceptance of birth control methods is problematic. Within the issue of prenatal harm, we shall be most concerned with evaluating suggestions for policies that attempt to protect prenatal human beings from potentially harmful maternal actions or decisions, since such suggestions are becoming more and more common and such policies are daily becoming more hotly debated (see, e.g., Johnsen 1987). We shall also take up the question of so-called fetal protection policies which exclude pregnant or fertile women from certain positions in the workplace, since this issue is receiving growing attention in the courts. In concluding the chapter, we shall focus on the problem of procuring an adequately informed consent to the acceptance of birth control technologies by individuals in certain populations.

## POTENTIAL AND FUTURE PERSONS

We argued in Chapter 7 that prenatal human beings should not, at any stage, be considered persons with the full range of fundamental rights attaching to persons. Such a position is consistent with the U.S. Supreme Court's decision in *Roe v. Wade* (1973) for, as emphasized by Glantz (1983), the Court in *Roe* did *not* argue that a fetus becomes a person at viability (see Chapter 7). On the other hand, the Court did not say that the state has no interest in protecting even previable fetuses, embryos, or conceptuses from injury. That is, although the *Roe* decision guarantees women the legal right to elective abortion through the end of the second trimester of pregnancy, a very different issue regarding protection of the prenatal human being arises when a woman elects not to abort a pregnancy and either her actions or the actions of another result in the birth of a damaged child (e.g., Mathieu 1985; Robertson and Schulman 1987). Indeed, the decision in *Roe* has been used with increasing frequency in legal decisions and by legal commentators to shore up other arguments for expanding liability for prenatal harm, for restricting the behaviors of pregnant women, and for imposing medical and surgical interventions on women to protect prenatal human beings expected to reach term.[1]

In order to see how it may be held both that elective abortion is acceptable and that people should be held liable for or forced not to contribute to prenatal harm, a distinction needs to be made between potential persons and future persons. In Chapter 7, we distinguished

---

[1] See, e.g., *Jefferson v. Griffin Spalding County Hospital Authority* (1981), Bowes and Selgestad (1981), Parness and Pritchard (1982), Robertson (1982, 1985, 1986), Lenow (1983), Dougherty (1986), Mathieu (1985), Parness (1985, 1986, 1987), Green and Brill (1987).

between (1) the time when a human being has developed the kinds of characteristics which compel us to recognize beings as persons (metaphysical or actual persons) and (2) the time set by convention when a being which does not yet have these characteristics is accepted into the community of persons (conventional persons). We argued that the conventional recognition of personhood should be set at birth. We now need to make some further distinctions in order to address the questions at hand.

A prenatal human being is a potential person when it is the case that (1) if that being were supported, it would eventually develop into a being that has the kinds of characteristics which would compel us to recognize it as a person, and (2) if that being were supported, it would be born and gain conventional entry into the class of persons. Notice that not every prenatal human being is a potential person (in either the metaphysical or conventional sense), since many conceptions terminate in spontaneous abortion (see Chapter 6), and often this is because the conceptus, embryo, or fetus has an anomaly that is incompatible with life or that prevents it from ever developing the kinds of characteristics which would compel us to recognize it as a person.

A prenatal human being is a future person (1) if it has the capacity to develop the morally relevant characteristics, and (2) it *will* gain conventional entry into the class of persons through birth. All future persons are potential persons; but since not all potential persons will endure to reach either actual (metaphysical) or conventional personhood (they may die because of abortion, accidents, etc.), not all potential persons are future persons (cf. Langerak 1979). The complex moral and legal issues which concern us involve prenatal human beings as both potential and future persons. Our focus, however, will be on prenatal harm to future persons.

## LEGAL ACTIONS FOR PRENATAL INJURY

*Wrongful Death Actions*   A prenatal human being which is a potential person may be fatally injured as a result of someone's action(s) or someone's omission(s).[2] Were it not for the injury (it is assumed),

---

[2] Whether omissions are properly understood as causes is a question beyond the scope of this book, and we shall ignore it here. For discussions of this question, see, e.g., Fitzgerald (1967), Foot (1967), Harris (1974),

the developing human being would have endured and been born undamaged. In cases like this, the agent causing the damage can be held liable for the death of a viable or previable prenatal human being. Such cases are known as *wrongful death cases*. Traditionally, wrongful death suits have been brought under statutes designed to compensate beneficiaries for losses which result from the death of a family member. Initially, nearly every U.S. jurisdiction required that an infant be born alive and then die as a result of injuries sustained prenatally for there to be a cause for legal action under a wrongful death statute. Damages for the death of a prenatal human being were not recoverable, because the prenatal human being was not considered separate from its biological mother (*Dietrich v. Inhabitants of Northampton* 1884).

Such thinking has carried forward in some decisions.[3] But the livebirth requirement has been attacked, primarily on the ground that, since no suit can be brought if a death occurs before birth, if someone has caused prenatal injury, ensuring or allowing prenatal death is more attractive to that person than allowing a potentially damaged being to come to birth. Thus, the livebirth requirement, at worst, encourages lethal violence from those who have reason to believe they have caused prenatal injury; at best, the requirement creates an incentive for such persons to withhold any efforts to save the lives of prenatal human beings they might have injured, for example, by bringing the pregnant woman to the hospital (Lenow 1983). Such reasons led the Minnesota Supreme Court to become the first court to allow recovery for the death of a fetus under a wrongful death statute (*Verkennes v. Corniea* 1949).[4] In *Rainey v. Horn* (1954), the court accepted the inseparability thesis but allowed recovery anyway, on the ground that since, if born, the offspring could have brought suit for injury, the parents had a rightful action for wrongful death. Although wrongful death suits involving prenatal harm have generally been limited to cases involving prenatal death after the point of viability, the trend has increasingly been toward allowing actions for prenatal death at any stage, on the ground that,

---

Rachels (1975), Mack (1976, 1980), Benjamin (1979), Green (1980), Husak (1980), Feinberg (1984a), Callahan (1988a).

[3] See, e.g., *Libbee v. Permanente Clinic* (1974), *Salazar v. St. Vincent Hospital* (1980), *Vaillancourt v. Medical Center Hospital of Vermont* (1980).

[4] See also, e.g., *Chrisafogeorgis v. Brandenberg* (1973).

but for the wrongful action(s) or omission(s), the offspring would have reached viability (Lenow 1983).[5]

Very different from wrongful death actions are wrongful birth, wrongful pregnancy, and wrongful life actions, which also differ from one another.

*Wrongful Birth Actions*   Wrongful birth actions are brought by parents against physicians, genetic counselors, laboratories, pharmacists, contraceptive manufacturers, and so on. Claims are for recovery of the costs parents incur in taking care of a disabled child and sometimes for their pain and suffering in being burdened with such a child. Usually, these cases involve a negligent failure to warn potential parents that their children are likely to inherit a disabling condition, failure to diagnose or warn parents about the presence of such a condition in a fetus, incompetent sterilizations and unsuccessful abortions, laboratory diagnostic errors, faulty contraceptives, pharmacist errors in filling prescriptions for oral contraceptives, and so on. The central claim in such cases is that the wrongful error of the defendant resulted in a "harmful birth" which the woman, if properly informed, could have prevented by aborting (Feinberg 1985a).

*Wrongful Pregnancy Actions*   Wrongful pregnancy actions involve unplanned pregnancies that occurred because of the error of some third party (an error leading to sterilization failure, failure of an abortion procedure, etc.). Such actions can be brought irrespective of whether a healthy infant is born. Wrongful birth and wrongful pregnancy can, in principle, be charged in the same suit (Feinberg 1985a).

*Wrongful Life Actions*   Actions for wrongful life are, as Feinberg (1985a) points out, far more controversial than are the previous kinds of actions, and they have been far less successful. What distinguishes these actions from others is that they are brought, not by parents,

---

[5] From a scientific perspective, suits for wrongful death are problematic, especially when they involve previable human beings. Given the figures on spontaneous abortion (see Chapter 6), it is *extremely* difficult to establish a causal connection between some external event and prenatal death, particularly when the death is early in a pregnancy.

but by the damaged child. The action for damages is not brought because the defendant caused the injuries defeating hope for a reasonably high quality of life. Rather, the claim is that the defendant wrongly allowed the child to come into existence at all, given his or her afflictions. Suits for wrongful life can be brought against physicians or genetic counselors for failure to provide information to the parents which might have motivated the parents to avoid conceiving or to abort a pregnancy. But they can also be brought against parents for allegedly wrongfully conceiving or not aborting. The main reason that wrongful life suits have not been widely successful is that courts have great difficulty evaluating the claim made by damaged plaintiffs that being born is itself an injury — that is, that this individual would have been better off never having been brought into existence at all (Feinberg 1985a; see, e.g., *Speck v. Finegold* 1979; *Phillips v. United States* 1980).

*Actions for Nonfatal Prenatal Injuries*   The case law involving recovery for nonfatal prenatal injuries closely parallels the case law involving recovery for wrongful death, moving from the early view that the physical inseparability of the prenatal being from its mother precluded actions being brought in its behalf to the later view that an infant born alive which was injured as a viable fetus could recover damages. The first such decision, *Bonbrest v. Kotz* (1946), opened the door to wide acceptance of recovery by damaged plaintiffs for prenatal harms occurring after the point of viability (Lenow 1985).

But a number of courts (as happened with the development of wrongful death cases) have gone further and allowed recovery for injuries sustained prior to viability (e.g., *Hornbuckle v. Plantation Pipe Line* 1956; *Bennett v. Hymers* 1958; *Smith v. Brennan* 1960). In fact, over the last decade we have begun to see cases in which a plaintiff has recovered for injuries resulting from the actions of others prior to the plaintiff's conception. *Renslow v. Mennonite Hospital* (1977), for example, concerned a child who was born suffering from hyperbilirubinemia (an excess of bilirubin in the blood, which, when sufficiently high, produces visible jaundice and may cause severe neurological damage; it often occurs in fetuses as a result of blood group incompatibility). The child recovered for permanent brain and nervous system damage alleged to have resulted from the hospital's twice negligently transfusing her mother with blood from the wrong blood group nine years prior to the child's birth. By allowing recovery for preconceptive harm, such decisions have helped to pave the way for controversial restrictions that prevent fertile women from working in environments which might have deleterious effects on their gametes, a topic we shall touch on below.

Today, most courts hold that the time of prenatal injury is irrelevant if a causal connection can be "shown" between the harm suffered and someone's actions or omissions (Glantz 1983).

## PROTECTING FUTURE PERSONS

Central to the reasoning in decisions granting recovery for prenatal injuries is a concern to protect the interests of liveborn persons, or, under our distinction, future persons (Glantz 1983).[6] This concern

---

[6] Traditionally, the class of liveborn persons includes all infants, even those with an anomaly (e.g., anencephaly, an invariably fatal condition involving absence of the cerebral hemispheres of the brain) that precludes their ever developing the kinds of characteristics that compel recognition of a being as a person (see Chapter 7). Thus, as traditionally understood, all liveborn persons will not qualify as future persons under our distinction, since the class of future persons does not include beings incapable of developing the kinds of characteristics that compel recognizing the moral rights that attend personhood. We shall not pursue this distinction here, since the position we shall defend will turn out not to depend on it. We should mention, however, that the distinction between the traditional class of liveborn persons and the class of future persons is important and useful for dealing with other questions, particularly with questions about when infanticide might be morally permissible. For example, in 1987, Brenda and Michael Winners of Arcadia, California, decided not to abort their anencephalic fetus but to attempt to bring her to term and then keep her on a life-support system long enough to arrange for transplanting her organs to infants in vital need of replacement organs. It is customary not to place such infants on life-support systems, and the decision drew criticism from a number of groups and individuals, including some ethicists, who contended that going forward with the plan violated a first principle of medical ethics, namely, that the treatment of one patient must not be modified for the purpose of treating another patient. Other objections included the contention that treatment of the infant (i.e., sustaining her on a life-support system) solely for the sake of "harvesting" her organs showed lack of respect for her as a human being (e.g., Clark et al. 1987). We believe that the distinction between the traditional class of liveborn persons and the class of future persons (especially when combined with other distinctions we have made in this chapter and in Chapter 7) can be effectively used to show why the

was captured in a Canadian decision, quoted by the court in *Bonbrest* (1946):

> If a right action be denied to the child it will be compelled without any fault on its own part to go through life carrying the seal of another's fault and bearing a very heavy burden of infirmity and inconvenience without any compensation therefore. To my mind, it is but natural justice that a child, if born alive and viable, should be allowed to maintain an action in the courts for injuries wrongfully committed upon its person while in the womb of its mother (*Montreal Tramways v. Leveille* 1933).

This same concern is captured more succinctly and forcefully in the court's judgment in *Smith v. Brennan* (1960) that a child has a legal right to begin life with a sound mind and body (reiterated in, e.g., *Womack v. Buckhorn* 1976; *Berger v. Weber* 1978; *In re Baby X* 1980).

Such reasoning can be used to justify recovery for both nonfatal prenatal injury and wrongful life. As we pointed out previously, wrongful life actions have enjoyed little success in the courts to date. But a California appellate court decision suggests that courts may change that trend, not only in allowing more recoveries for wrongful life in general but in allowing recovery from parents as well as third parties. The case involved the failure of a laboratory (which had previously been alerted to failures in its testing) to diagnose a couple as carriers of Tay-Sachs disease (a recessive disorder characterized by progressive retardation in development, paralysis, dementia, blindness, and death by age three or four). The child's claim was recognized, and the court added this comment:

> If a case arose where, despite due care by the medical profession in transmitting the necessary warnings, parents made a conscious choice to proceed with a pregnancy, with full knowledge that a seriously impaired infant would be born, that conscious choice would provide an intervening act of proximate cause to preclude liability insofar as defendants other than the parents were concerned. Under such circumstances, we see no sound public policy which would protect those parents from being answerable for the pain, suffering, and misery which they have wrought upon their offspring (*Curlender v. Bio-Science Laboratories* 1980, *in dictum*).

---

Winners fetus was not a person, a future person, or even a potential person, and why decisions like the Winnerses' are justifiable and ought to be carried out. (As it turned out, the infant could not be sustained long enough to arrange any organ transplants.)

In cases where the potential for a severe genetic defect is discovered prior to conception, such reasoning entails that unless the
would-be parents practice contraception or seek abortion if they do
conceive, they may well find themselves legally liable for producing a wrongful life. In cases where a severe genetic defect is discovered after conception or a severe prenatal harm is suspected, such
reasoning would clearly place parents in the position of choosing
abortion or potentially facing legal liability for bringing a pregnancy to term. And since biological fathers (at least at present) have
no legal right to interfere with a woman's right to abort or not
abort a pregnancy,[7] any such liability for wrongful life must fall on

---

[7] But see *Taft v. Taft* (1983), in which the husband of a woman in her
fourth month of pregnancy sought a court order giving him authority to
require that she submit to surgery involving suturing her cervix to
minimize her risk of miscarriage (a cerclage or "purse string" operation),
surgery the woman had refused on religious grounds. The lower court
appointed a guardian *ad litem* for the fetus and granted the husband
authority to consent to the surgery. Although the Massachusetts Supreme
Court reversed the decision, it did so only because no legal precedent
ordering such a submission to protect a previable fetus was cited by the
husband or found by the court and because no facts had been presented to
show that the surgery would be a genuinely lifesaving one as opposed to a
merely precautionary one. The reasons for the reversal leave it open that
the original decision might have been upheld in another case. The court
makes this explicit in saying, "We do not decide whether, in some
circumstances there would be justification for ordering a wife to submit to
medical treatment in order to assist in carrying a child to term." Even more
recently, in the well-publicized Baby M Case, which involved a custody
battle for a child conceived by Mary Beth Whitehead via artificial
insemination with the sperm of William Stern, the court's reasoning
implies that biological fathers have what seem to be property rights over
offspring containing their genetic material. Whitehead argued that the
arrangement she had agreed to, which included her being paid $10,000
when she turned the child over to Stern, involved selling a baby. In reply,
Judge Harvey Sorkow of the New Jersey Superior Court claimed:

> The fact is, however, that the money to be paid to the surrogate is not
> being paid for the surrender of the child to the father.... The
> biological father pays the surrogate for her willingness to be impreg-
> nated and carry his child to term. At birth, the father does not purchase
> the child. It is his own biological genetically related child. He cannot
> purchase what is already his (*New York Times* 1987).

Notice that such an arrangement cannot coherently be construed as a widow women who do not abort.[8]

As regards prenatal injury more generally, there is also a rising trend toward holding women legally liable for causing prenatal harm and toward imposing invasive procedures on pregnant women in order to prevent prenatal harm.[9] The reasoning in many of the relevant post-*Roe* cases and commentaries turns on the belief that (1) if a woman has decided to carry a pregnancy to term, then *ceteris paribus* she carries a future person, and (2) that future person has a compelling moral right not to begin its independent life disadvantaged by avoidable harms resulting from the actions or omissions of others, including its mother. This reasoning has led to using child protection statutes to impose transfusions and cesarean sections on women to save their fetuses and it has also given rise to arguments for holding women criminally liable for acting in ways thought to cause prenatal harm during pregnancies expected to be brought to term.[10]

In one recent California action, a woman, Pamela Stewart, was criminally prosecuted when her failure to follow medical instructions (including instructions not to take amphetamines, to stay off her feet, to refrain from having intercourse, and to seek immediate

---

contract for a service rather than as a contract for a product, since the arrangement makes payment contingent on the delivery of a product, i.e., "the surrender of the child to the father." Notice, too, how the label "surrogate" misrepresents the role of the woman in such cases and presumes the biological father's authority over the offspring. Whitehead is not a surrogate mother at all—she is the child's biological mother.

[8] Wrongful life cases and the growing emphasis on prenatal testing raise a number of concerns. Pregnant women are increasingly pressured to undergo such testing and increasingly face the expectation that they will abort a pregnancy if there is any potential of its issuing in a disabled child. Such pressures foster an already worrisome societal attitude which disenfranchises the disabled (see, e.g., Blatt 1987; Henifin 1987; Saxton 1987; Henifin, Hubbard, and Norsigan 1989).

[9] See, e.g., *Application of President and Directors of Georgetown College* (1964), *Raleigh Fitkin-Paul Morgan Memorial Hospital v. Anderson* (1964), *People v. Estergard* (1969), Leiberman et al. (1979), *Jefferson v. Griffin Spalding County Memorial Hospital Authority* (1981), Bowes and Selgestad (1981), Parness and Pritchard (1982), Robertson (1982, 1985, 1986), *Taft v. Taft* (1983; see note 7 above), Shaw (1983), Mathieu (1985), Parness (1985, 1986, 1987), Mackenzie and Nagel (1986), Johnsen (1987).

[10] See, e.g., Leiberman et al. (1979), Bowes and Selgestad (1981), Annas (1982, 1986), Parness (1983, 1985), Johnsen (1987).

medical treatment if she began bleeding) led to her fetus being born severely brain-damaged. The child died five weeks later and Stewart was arrested for causing the death of her son. Annas (1986) reports that police officials wanted her charged with murder, but the district attorney decided instead to prosecute under a California child support statute. Stewart was charged with a misdemeanor which carried a possible sentence of a year in prison or a fine of $2,000. The case was dismissed only because the defendant was able to convince the court that the 1872 law (California Penal Code, Section 270) under which she was being prosecuted was intended to ensure that fathers provide child support, including (following a 1925 amendment to the statute) financial support for women pregnant by them (e.g., Annas 1986; Brown et al. 1987; Johnsen 1987; *People v. Stewart* 1987).[11]

The situation becomes even more complex as prenatal therapies, including fetal surgical techniques, are developed. As these procedures pass from experimental status to being recognized as safe and effective treatments, we are likely to see increasing support for requiring women to submit to them for the good of their offspring (see, e.g., Robertson 1982, 1985, 1986). It is not uncommon for those supportive of physically intrusive prenatal protection policies to suggest that recent advances in medicine which have made prenatal human beings potential patients somehow change their moral status, endowing them with the right to treatment we recognize other human beings as having (e.g., Bowes and Selgestad 1981). But nothing about the moral status of a being follows from the bare fact that it can be effectively treated medically or surgically. Veterinarians, after all, are able to provide remarkable treatment to a great variety of animals, and some treatment of nonhuman animal fetuses is also now possible. But we do not think that this fact endows these beings with personhood and an attendant right to treatment (cf. Ruddick and Wilcox 1982). On the contrary, the question of the moral status of a being is prior to the question of entitlements, and those who argue from the fact that a prenatal human being can now

---

[11] Cases like this raise some additional puzzles. For example, if physicians in such cases fail to so advise women, should *they* be subject to prosecution? What medical advice must be explicitly stated and what may be left up to "common sense"? Must a woman be told about *all* the drugs and other potential toxins that could cause prenatal harm and be advised to avoid them? Must she be advised not to sky-dive, etc.?

be treated as a patient to the moral claim that prenatal humans (but not prenatal pigs, prenatal cattle, etc.) have a right to treatment fail to understand that they are simply begging the question in favor of prenatal personhood for human beings.

Again, however, arguments for requiring women to submit to therapies for the good of prenatal human beings need not be based on any claim that these beings are persons. All that needs to be claimed is that insofar as a prenatal being is a *future* person, it has a right not to be injured in a way that will importantly set back the interests it will have as a person (see, e.g., Mathieu 1985). We need, then, to ask whether the fact that a woman intends to bring a pregnancy to term justifies imposing medical and surgical procedures on her or otherwise legally restricting her behavior for the sake of the future person she carries.

### DIRECT INTERFERENCE WITH PREGNANT WOMEN

Much of the case for such impositions rests on the argument that in deciding to bring a pregnancy to term, a woman both waives her right to abortion and takes on a set of special duties of care toward the prenatal human being as the current embodiment of a future person. But, in fact, a woman never waives her right to abortion (Smith 1983; Annas 1987). She may decide not to exercise that right, but this does not count as a waiver of the right itself any more than the decision not to buy a certain kind of car amounts to a waiver of the right to buy that kind of car. As we saw in Chapter 7, a woman (at least in the United States) retains a legal right to elect abortion for any reason at all through the end of the second trimester of pregnancy, and even after the second trimester if the pregnancy is sufficiently threatening to her health.

Further, those who argue for the view in question assume that in making the decision not to abort, a pregnant woman waives her right to bodily integrity in favor of the future person she carries (see, e.g., Mathieu 1985; Green and Brill 1987). But waiving a right involves voluntarily relinquishing it, and in just the kinds of cases that concern us (i.e., cases in which a woman refuses a procedure or engages in a certain behavior that is believed to cause prenatal harm) we find women who clearly have *not* relinquished their right to bodily integrity. As Smith (1983) has rightly pointed out, the concept working here is not one of waiver at all. It is, rather, the concept of forfeiture. For example, a felon forfeits, but does not waive, his or her right to be at liberty in the community. The argument, then, is one from forfeiture of rights, and once this is understood, the picture becomes far less benign than the picture of a woman voluntarily relinquishing bodily integrity to protect the welfare of a future person. The pregnant woman becomes analogous to the criminal who can no longer demand that he or she not be interfered with by the state. Indeed, in arguing for the position that impingements on a pregnant woman's bodily integrity to protect a future person are justified, legal commentators often point out that bodily seizures and bodily intrusions without a person's consent are not unknown to the law (e.g., Bowes and Selgestad 1981; Mathieu 1985). The examples given include imposing prison sentences, execution, forcible medical and surgical treatment, and forcible feeding for the sake of prison discipline and imposing surgery to retrieve evidence of a crime (e.g., Robertson 1982, 1985, 1986; Robertson and Schulman 1987). The analogy is chilling. Pregnant women are not felons, nor are they, to use another example in the literature, incompetents who may be ordered by courts to submit to bodily invasions to aid others because they are not capable of making such judgments for themselves.[12]

The argument for these policies to protect prenatal future persons also often includes (explicitly or implicitly) analogizing the prenatal cases to ordinary pediatric cases. It is widely accepted that in pediatric cases the state may interfere with parents to provide treatment for a child or to provide for other fundamental needs of a child (see, e.g., Robertson and Schulman 1987). And though it is generally recognized that there is an important difference between prenatal and pediatric cases (since prenatal cases involve providing treatment through the woman's body or otherwise directly interfering with a woman's behavior and pediatric cases do not), recommendations for when women might justifiably be imposed upon tend to be discussed in terms of comparing the risks of harm to the woman attendant to the bodily invasion (or other imposition) and

---

[12]See, e.g., *Strunk v. Strunk* (1969) and *Hart v. Brown* (1972), where kidney transplants from incompetents were ordered to save the life of a sibling. See also the argument from these examples in Bowes and Selgestad (1981) and the discussion of court-ordered bodily invasions in Mathieu (1985).

the risks of harm to the future person if there is no intervention (see, e.g., Robertson 1982, 1985, 1986). The quick movement to the pediatric model seems again to rest on the assumption that a woman who intends to bring a pregnancy to term waives her right to bodily integrity in favor of the right of a future person not to be harmed. In this way, bodily integrity and individual autonomy tend to drop out as considerations, and justifiable impositions are taken to be decidable by weighing the potential risks of intervention to the woman and the potential costs of nonintervention to the future person. But we have already seen that this model really involves forfeiture rather than waiver of rights; thus, the leap to deciding whether to forcibly intervene on the basis of comparing relative potential harms has not been justified.[13]

The very serious problem with all the arguments for imposing prenatal treatment through a woman or forcibly limiting a woman's behaviors for the sake of a future person is the failure of proponents of these arguments to address the issue from the point of view of the pregnant woman (cf. Whitbeck 1983; Johnsen 1987; Levi 1987). The comparison of prenatal to pediatric cases fails precisely because prevention of harm in the pediatric cases does not involve the violations of autonomy or bodily integrity involved in the prenatal cases. The obligation not to harm proposed for the prenatal cases involves much more than what is involved in ordinary cases of avoiding harming other persons, even one's own children. The duty to avoid harming others is generally dischargeable by simply refraining from running them over with cars, dropping things on them, and so on. But if pregnant women have a duty to avoid prenatal harm, this requires actually nurturing a future person (Bolton 1979). Although this makes the prenatal cases unlike most cases of not harming others, it does make them somewhat like the pediatric cases, because we do recognize that parents have special positive duties of

---

[13] In saying this, we certainly do not mean to approve all the kinds of impingements on individual autonomy and bodily integrity that have been allowed against prisoners. There are, for example, serious moral questions raised by force-feeding prisoners, and serious moral and constitutional questions raised by forcible surgical interventions on prisoners to gain evidence in criminal cases. And it goes without saying that capital punishment is extremely difficult to justify in a society which has the resources to effectively protect innocent persons from those who have murdered.

nurturing and aiding their children. But to avoid speciousness, proponents of the analogy must be willing to hold that morality requires court-ordered invasions of the bodily integrity of parents for their children's welfare as well as severe restrictions on parental behaviors when those behaviors are believed to be damaging to children. Once the movement is made to comparing the potential harms to parents resulting from intervention with the potential harms to children resulting from nonintervention, it follows from the analogy that parents could be forcibly taken to medical centers to donate blood, bone marrow, or even transplantable organs, such as eyes or kidneys. And since it is well known that substance abuse in parents is severely psychologically harmful to children, the position requires that the state must attempt to ensure that no such abuse goes on in families.

Rather than so dramatically interfere with individual lives, however, we have not allowed such forcible interventions. Where parents grossly fail to nurture their children or where their behaviors otherwise seriously harm their children, the acceptable intervention is physical removal of the children from the family. In the prenatal cases, however, protecting conceptuses, embryos, and previable fetuses would require taking custody of pregnant women, and removal of the offspring would involve forcible induction of labor or forcible surgical retrieval of viable fetuses, a draconian measure not even the most strident supporters of fetal protection have explicitly endorsed, although the cases involving forced cesarean sections are extremely close to this.[14]

The implications of making the prenatal and pediatric cases analogous are, we submit, simply too morally costly. On the one hand,

---

[14] See also Parness's (1983) discussion of taking custody of prospective parents, with examples of several attempts by states to take custody of fetuses by taking custody of pregnant women. See, as well, Robertson and Schulman (1987), who seem to be in favor of accepting the implications of the analogy with the pediatric cases. Although there is some slippage, Robertson and Schulman also attempt to keep the protection of women's liberty and bodily integrity as the considerations to be balanced against the prevention of prenatal harm. However, this raises another pair of problems: (1) deciding when a potential harm to a future person outweighs the rights to noninterference and bodily integrity of an actual person, and (2) deciding who should be charged with making such decisions.

upholding the analogy would require applying to the pediatric cases the doctrine of forfeiture of rights to bodily integrity and giving to the state a right to extreme and constant interference with parental behavior. On the other hand, it would involve giving the state the right to take a pregnant woman into custody, disable her, induce labor or cut her open against her will to rescue the viable fetus. We describe the implications of the analogical argument this way, not as an exercise in inflammatory rhetoric, but to make as evident as possible the very harsh realities that accepting the view in question entails for pregnant women and parents. And we submit that confronting these realities lucidly should make it evident that the moral costs of giving such intrusive powers to the state are just too high. Thus, overriding a woman's right to control what will be done to or through her body for the sake of a future person cannot be justified on the basis of an argument from the analogy between prenatal and pediatric cases, which is the only argument that holds out any real hope of justifying the kinds of impositions on pregnant women that are currently being proposed. As Rothman (1986) argues, pregnant women may not be treated as mere maternal environments; as Annas (1986) argues, neither may they be treated as mere fetal containers that may be opened and shut or otherwise forcibly manipulated for the protection of future persons.

## LEGAL SANCTIONS FOR WOMEN WHO CAUSE PRENATAL HARM?

*Criminal Sanctions*   One alternative to allowing direct interference with pregnant women is to apply sanctions in cases of prenatal injury, relying on the deterrent value of the criminal law (e.g., Parness 1985, 1986). The analogy with pediatric cases fails to justify direct intervention, but it has been argued that child protection statutes might be interpreted in such a way that women causing prenatal harm could be charged with crimes. For example, Leiberman et al. (1979) contend that since pregnant women are the natural guardians of prenatal offspring, it is logical to construe rejection of a potentially lifesaving prenatal intervention (which does not put the woman's life at comparable risk) as a felony, and they suggest that physicians should be able to warn refusing patients that they are committing a felony. Parness (1983) suggests that a woman who risks addicting to heroin a fetus she intends to bring to term could be deemed to have undertaken both tortious and criminal conduct toward her child. And we have seen that an attempt to interpret an existing statute as criminalizing a woman's causing prenatal harm was recently made in the Pamela Stewart case. Although some of these cases cannot appeal to any argument from the rights of future persons, and although we believe that the arguments against the justifiability of direct intervention tell as well against using criminal sanctions to prevent prenatal harm to future persons (since such sanctions would coerce women into "accepting" intrusive interventions), there are other noteworthy issues raised by the suggestion of using the criminal law against women for causing prenatal harm.

The first point to realize is that the movement to criminality by interpreting existing statutes to include prenatal harm caused by pregnant women is too quick. If we are to make women who act (or refuse to act) in the ways at issue into criminals, this requires that we enact new statutes or revise existing statutes to expressly and unambiguously make criminal the particular behavior and refusals of medical or surgical intervention in question. In the United States, crimes (unlike torts) do not emerge through case law. Common law crimes were abolished many years ago (see e.g., *In re Greene* 1892), and it is now a well-established principle in our law that crimes must clearly be identified as such so that people are provided with advance notice that engaging in certain behaviors will mark them as enemies of the community and may justify the state's removing them from the community. Thus, unless criminal codes are revised to amply warn pregnant women who intend to continue their pregnancies to term that potentially damaging behaviors and refusals of prenatal medical or surgical intervention are now crimes, criminal prosecution of women under existing statutes (be they child protection statutes or more general criminal neglect or battery statutes) cannot be justified.

Rewriting criminal codes to expressly protect prenatal future persons has been suggested (e.g., Parness 1985). And if we take Leiberman et al. (1979) seriously, at least some intervention refusals ought to be felonious. But felonies are crimes punishable by death or imprisonment. What would be an appropriate punishment for felonious refusals of prenatal medical and surgical interventions? Laying the possibility of execution aside, imprisonment of nonconsenting women is neither morally nor legally justifiable, since such women cannot reasonably be construed as societal menaces.

In cases where a woman's behavior leads to prenatal injury, criminal sanctions are equally unjustifiable. Prenatal harm resulting from a pregnant woman's behavior nearly always involves low birthweight, often accompanied by fetal drug addiction. Low birthweight is a major cause of infant mortality and has been identified as the single greatest hazard for surviving infants, for it results in a heightened vulnerability to various developmental problems and in a substantially increased risk of death from common childhood diseases (e.g., National Academy of Sciences 1985; Hartmann 1987). Low birthweights are associated with poor prenatal nutrition, pregnancy in the very young, smoking tobacco and drinking alcohol during pregnancy, and other kinds of drug use, including use of crack, the extremely potent form of cocaine, which is thought to account for a 20 percent rise in infant deaths in at least one American community in 1986 (Monmaney et al. 1987). That community is the impoverished black community in Harlem (in New York City), which has a high rate of teenage pregnancy and in which, like many similar communities, prenatal education and prenatal care have not been readily available.

The Harlem example is a telling one, and proponents of holding women criminally responsible for prenatal harm need to realize that the harms they seek to prevent are neither justifiably nor effectively dealt with by bringing the massive powers of the state to bear against women to coerce medical or surgical intervention or by treating women as criminals after the fact. The often-interrelated problems of pregnancy in the very young, chemical abuse, poor nutrition, ignorance, and poverty are social problems, appropriately and most effectively dealt with by positive measures that enhance the social, economic, and intellectual position of the least well-off members of society and of women generally. Treating women as mere uterine environments that can be invaded or punished involves the kind of blaming the victim that can only seem correct when one flatly ignores the complex social conditions that typically give rise to the evil that is to be avoided (in this case, the evil of harm done to future persons by their mothers). As Annas (1986) argues, the best chance the state has for protecting prenatal future persons is through positive actions that enhance the status of women rather than by cutting funds for maternal education, health care, and nutrition and then assailing often resourceless women for not doing the best that can be done for their future children (cf. Henifin, Hubbard, and Norsigan 1987; Johnsen 1987).

*Civil Sanctions*  The use of civil sanctions against women who cause prenatal harm is equally unacceptable, although holding a woman financially responsible for the costs associated with caring for a child who is handicapped as a result of her actions or decisions seems in principle to involve no violation of a woman's basic moral or civil rights. But one problem here is that such sanctions seem pointless, since parents with the resources to support their children are already commonly required to support them; thus adding specific sanctions for women who cause prenatal harm is redundant. And requiring full support from parents without the necessary resources is as futile in these cases as it is in other cases where children of impoverished parents require special care.

Another problem is that such sanctions seem gratuitously hostile to women, since the case for such sanctions ignores the fact that prenatal human beings are begotten by fathers and that fathers often encourage precisely the kinds of behaviors that may lead to prenatal harm (e.g., drug use). Recall that part of the case against Pamela Stewart was that she had intercourse with her husband after being advised to refrain from doing so. Yet her husband was not prosecuted (Annas 1986).

Other problems with such sanctions include worries about abuse by fathers and prosecutors as well as concern that fear of lawsuits will surely motivate unnecessary interventions, as has been the case with cesarean deliveries. That physicians tend to overestimate the need for intrusive interventions to prevent prenatal harm is demonstrated by a number of cases involving atttempts to force cesarean deliveries on women who subsequently successfully delivered vaginally (see, e.g., *Jefferson v. Griffin Spalding County Hospital Authority* 1981; *North Central Bronx Hospital v. Headley* 1986; Rhoden 1986).

Finally, introducing any of these forms of interference with women will surely lead a number of the pregnant women most likely to cause prenatal harm (e.g., those using teratogenic drugs) to avoid the medical establishment as completely as they are able, thus making such policies patently counterproductive (see also Johnsen 1987).

Our conclusion, then, is that a woman's bodily integrity must never be impinged upon for the sake of a prenatal future person, even if it is clear that an intervention is not seriously risky for her and will prevent substantial damage to a future person. Nor should a woman whose behavior causes prenatal harm be a candidate for forcible interference or criminal prosecution. The proper policy is to find the political will to take positive action to reduce both the ignorance that may underpin some maternal refusals of prenatal medical and surgical intervention (Shriner 1979; cf. Leiberman et al. 1979) and the ignorance that so often leads to poor prenatal nutrition. The task is to introduce policies that will increase, rather than decrease, the welfare of pregnant women (e.g., Annas 1986, 1987) and to encourage the avoidance of pregnancy among those who are not prepared to be committed to the welfare of prenatal future persons. This cannot be accomplished without including frank and detailed sex and family education in schools, beginning at the elementary level. Finally, it should also be realized that a significant number of teens will be sexually active despite their parents' hopes to the contrary and that we need to make birth control aids, particularly barrier aids (condoms most of all), readily available to them. Not only are such measures desirable to help curb the tide of teenage pregnancies and to protect prenatal future persons from harm without violating the moral rights of their mothers, they are also potentially lifesaving measures given the increasing number of deaths caused by AIDS in both the homosexual and heterosexual communities.

## MUTAGENIC AND TERATOGENIC HARM
## IN THE WORKPLACE

Harm to future persons resulting from the actions or omissions of third parties does not raise the same sorts of problems that are raised by the harmful acts and omissions of pregnant women. Because the intimate physical relationship that exists in pregnancy does not exist between third parties and prenatal future persons, use of the law to prevent prenatal harm does not involve the intrusions which the maternal cases involve. One of the main moral problems arising here, however, pertains to how potential third party perpetrators of preconceptive and postconceptive prenatal injury may respond to being liable for mutagenic and teratogenic harms. In particular, there are serious problems that have arisen with the exclusionary treatment of fertile women from many positions in the workforce.

As we have already seen, most courts today will allow recovery for injury at any prenatal stage if a causal connection can be "shown" between an agent's act(s) or negligent omission(s) and the injury (Glantz 1983). This includes recovery for both preconceptive and postconceptive prenatal injuries. The response by some employers in industries where certain jobs involve exposure to environmental conditions thought to be teratogenic or mutagenic with respect to female germ cells has been to exclude fertile women (and sometimes all women) from these positions. Such exclusionary policies have been adopted by a number of the largest U.S. corporations (e.g., General Motors, Gulf Oil, B. F. Goodrich, Firestone, Dow, DuPont, Eastman Kodak, Union Carbide, and Monsanto) and the Lead Industries Association has opposed employing fertile women in its industry for over a decade—all with the result that hundreds of thousands of lucrative jobs are not open to women of childbearing capacity (Bertin 1989). It has been argued that allowing such policies not only disenfranchises women by disallowing them access to a substantial number of employment opportunities but also suggests that it is appropriate to force a woman's interest in employment to yield to her capacity for reproduction (Bertin 1989). This perpetuates the view that women are, first and foremost, "mother machines" (Corea 1985), potential "fetal containers" (Annas 1986), or potential "maternal environments" (Rothman 1986) and that, as a result, they may be disallowed important choices on what positions they will take in society.

That such exclusionary policies are blatantly discriminatory in nature has recently been argued by Bertin (1989), who contends that they often rest on the unexamined assumption that women's germ cells and prenatal human beings are uniquely susceptible to ill-effects from workplace environments. That is, fertile women are often excluded from certain jobs absent any demonstration that their oocytes or their conceptuses, embryos, or fetuses are likely to be harmed by employment environments. If there is suspicion of mutagenic or teratogenic effects, the assumption is that the environment is harmful unless proven otherwise, and fertile or pregnant women are quickly excluded. On the other hand, says Bertin, when an environmental component might be mutagenic to men's germ cells, the assumption is the opposite: The environment is presumed safe unless proven otherwise. In cases where it is demonstrated that an environmental component is mutagenic to sperm, the toxin is banned. Bertin suggests that "these patterns . . . reinforce the notion that the workplace must accommodate the needs of men, but not of women, and that society requires and benefits from the paid labor of men, but not that of women."

There is much to be said for Bertin's argument. But, as we have seen in Chapter 8, important differences between female and male gametogenesis, differences in the physiological capacity of women and men to protect gametes from toxins, and the characteristics of prenatal offspring support the presumption of hypersusceptibility of oocytes and prenatal offspring to workplace toxins. A number of regulatory agency restrictions reflect these differences in susceptibility to toxins. Allowances for radiation exposure, for example, are higher for men than for women and higher for nonpregnant women than for pregnant women. And handling certain materials which are easily inhaled (e.g., prostaglandins) can lead to spontaneous abortion but present no threat to either male or female gametes or adult human beings.

These facts show that the presumption that oocytes and prenatal humans are more susceptible to harm from environmental toxins than are spermatozoa or human adults is, in general, justifiable. But it is also true that these replies do not address questions regarding men's continuing capacity to produce healthy sperm. One reason for more studies on the male reproductive system is increased understanding of potential environmental hazards to male gametogenesis. Also, since the criteria used for evaluating sperm (see Chapter 8) cannot identify genetic changes, the replies we have just offered to the previous argument do not disallow that a sperm affected by an environmental toxin might be fully motile yet have suffered damage to its genetic material.

Further, despite the justifiability of a general presumption in favor of the higher susceptibility of oocytes and prenatal offspring, relying too heavily on that presumption may prove costly to industry in two ways. First, it may well turn out that making the presumption in favor of harmlessness when potential harm to male gametogenesis and spermatozoa is involved will lead to increasing numbers of negligence cases involving mutagenic effects on sperm and deleterious effects on men's capacity to produce adequate numbers of healthy sperm. Second, as Bertin (1989) notes, the three federal appeals courts which have examined the legality of exclusionary policies have found them to be discriminatory, even if the proposed justification is protection of health (*Wright v. Olin Corporation* 1982; *Zuniga v. Kleberg County Hospital* 1982; *Hayes v. Shelby Memorial Hospital* 1984). Bertin points out that although two courts allow that a defense should be available for defendants, a heavy burden of justification is placed on companies that have such policies, which includes showing that the environmental condition poses a known significant or unreasonable risk, not simply a speculative or hypothetical one; showing that the male reproductive system is not similarly at risk; and showing that no alternative with a less discriminatory effect is available. These requirements suggest that companies with exclusionary policies may soon find themselves more frequently in court for unjustified discrimination against fertile women as a result of leaning too heavily on even justifiable presumptions.

As we said in commencing this section, protecting prenatal future persons from the harmful actions and negligence of third parties does not raise the kinds of moral problems raised by attempting to protect them from the potentially harmful actions or decisions of pregnant women. Thus, use of the law to ensure the protection of oocytes and prenatal offspring from hazards in the workplace is morally appropriate. But the blanket exclusion of fertile or pregnant women from large segments of the workplace is seriously problematic, raising, as it does, critical questions of fairness. Systematic exclusion of any group from any societal position always raises serious concerns about justice, and societal institutions, including businesses, need to strive to avoid any such exclusions. Where that effort is not made voluntarily, use of the law to ensure the effort is justifiable. Although some conditions potentially harmful to oocytes and prenatal offspring cannot be completely eliminated from the workplace, Bertin (1989) suggests a solution that should be approximated as far as possible, namely, that industries and individual employers should try to make their workplaces safe for *all* persons, present and future, and if a company cannot achieve safety, then whatever is preventing it should be eliminated rather than excluding certain people.

But again, not all risks can be eliminated. Taking this into account, our own view is this: If the maximal safety levels that can be reached have been reached but there is still a known, serious, ineliminable risk to prenatal offspring or oocytes, it would not be unjust to exclude pregnant women (temporarily if the risk is teratogenic) or fertile women (if the risk is mutagenic) from positions where exposure to the risk is *demonstrably* unavoidable. The problems that will arise under such policies, of course, are problems of evidence, which make blanket exclusion of women from certain workplace environments the easier course for employers. How will an employer *know* that a woman is not pregnant or that she is not fertile? It seems that employers cannot know, and asking women to prove that they do not fall into an excluded group raises worries about intrusion. The reasonable solution is to put the responsibility into the hands of women themselves, releasing employers from liability should teratogenic or mutagenic harms result from an ineliminable hazard. Approaching the question of these exclusionary policies this way has the virtue that it (1) requires employers to make and keep the workplace as safe as reasonably possible for all, since any remaining hazards must be genuinely ineliminable; (2) protects conscientious employers; and (3) respects the privacy, autonomy, and moral agency of women.

BIRTH CONTROL RISKS AND INFORMED CONSENT

Among the most serious moral problems arising from the risks associated with birth control technologies is the problem of acquiring a subject's genuinely informed consent to assuming such risks. The problem cuts across all populations insofar as the long-term risks of some of these methods are unknown even to those who develop, produce, test, and distribute them. But even when risks are well known, the problem of informed consent to risks remains a serious one in developing nations where population control has been accepted as a high priority.

Population control is one of the several values which have led to selecting areas for trying out new birth control technologies when long-term risks are unknown and to continuing use of products known to be especially dangerous. In the late 1950s, for example, clinical trials of the pill, which was being developed by Searle, were conducted on poor women in Puerto Rico expressly because of the population pressure there. Hartmann (1987) reports that at least one woman in the study is known to have died from congestive heart failure, and Corea (1985) reports that of 1,250 women in the study, 5 died, 3 with symptoms suggesting blood clots. Although research-ers conducting the study denied that such effects were associated with the pill (Hartmann 1987), no autopsies were performed either to support or to challenge their claim (Corea 1985); we now know that exogenous steroids, particularly at the high levels included in the early hormonal contraceptives for women, are indeed clearly associated with circulatory disorders (see Chapter 5). It can, of course, be legitimately asserted that the relatively small number of deaths just mentioned does not of itself suggest (let alone prove) that there was any link between the preparation and circulatory disorders. Indeed, the incidence of death resulting from circulatory disorders falls within the expected range of occurrence in the general popu-lation. But the problem lies with the researchers' a priori dismissal of a possible link, particularly in so early a trial. As we have seen in Chapter 5, extrapolating from animal studies to predicting effects in human beings is a tricky business at best, and all early product trials involving human subjects necessarily hold out unknown risks. Women participating in the early pill trials could not have known the risks they were assuming, because the researchers themselves could not have known. When there is great pressure to control pop-ulation, the acceptance of previously untried birth control methods by poor, uneducated women raises especially troubling questions regarding whether genuinely informed consent to necessarily unknown risks can be secured.

Irregularities in clinical trials also raise worries about informed consent. Currently, worldwide trials of the subdermally implant-able contraceptive Norplant (see Chapter 5) are being conducted. Norplant trials commenced in Brazil in August 1984; they were halted in January 1986. The moratorium was the result of the efforts of the Special Commission on Reproductive Rights of the state of Rio de Janeiro and the Reproductive Rights Commission within the Min-istry of Health. Although the World Medical Association's Decla-ration of Helsinki (1964, revised 1975) lays out clear principles for biomedical research involving human subjects, including strong informed consent requirements, and although the guidelines for con-ducting the Norplant trials clearly met these and other requirements, a number of troubling irregularities were found in the trials, for example, failure to inform women that the drug had not been licensed or recommended by the government; failure to inform women that the drug's effectiveness was uncertain; failure to inform women that the drug could induce certain anticipated (and unantic-ipated) side effects; failure of physicians to report adverse or toxic effects; failure to adequately examine women prior to implantation; failure to implant on the fifth day of women's menstrual cycle to ensure that subjects were not pregnant (at least one center implanted three pregnant women); participation of unapproved centers; and implantation of an even newer version of Norplant (Norplant 2), which was not authorized for the trials. As pointed out by Lucia Arruda, president of the Rio commission, all the women in the study were extremely poor, poorly educated, and "desperate in their search for contraceptive methods" (Women's Global Network on Repro-ductive Rights 1986d). The Puerto Rican and Brazilian examples are just two which point out how serious the problem of informed con-sent can be in clinical trials of new birth control products in the third world.

At the same time, products known to be especially dangerous are sometimes "dumped" on developing nations; A. H. Robins' Dalkon Shield is a prime example (see Chapters 1 and 6). A few months after this device was on the market, the company was aware of reports of adverse effects. Hundreds of potentially incriminating documents apparently were burned, including documents relating to the wicking action of the device's tail. Realizing that sales on the U.S. market would drop, Robins moved quickly, and it successfully sold large quantities of the Dalkon Shield at a huge discount to the Office of Population at the United States Agency for International Development for distribution in the third world (see, e.g., the dis-cussion and sources in Hartmann 1987).

As the term implies, informed consent involves a cognitive or knowledge component and a volitional or will component. A person's right to give an informed consent to a medical or surgical intervention can be violated, then, if that person is not given infor-mation relevant to making a reasonable judgment on an interven-tion or is coerced into accepting an intervention. Coercive anti-natalist practices in developing nations, therefore, also critically raise the problem of informed consent to accepting birth control tech-nologies. China's antinatalist policy and the practices adopted to implement it provide one example (see Chapter 2). Other recent and current examples have occurred in the following countries: India, where the early 1970s saw mass vasectomy camps, and where the middle 1970s saw emergency rule and sterilization quotas, with the threat of fines and imprisonment for couples who failed to be sterilized after their third child and the withholding of food and government services from the unsterilized; Indonesia, where "Smiling Family Safaris" have been used to bring thousands of women together in a picniclike atmosphere to become *apsari* (angels) by accepting intrauterine devices; Thailand, where women have been required to accept Depo-Provera before being allowed to marry; and black South Africa, where adolescent girls are being injected with Depo-Provera without their consent and where many black women must document their use of birth control in order to apply for jobs (e.g., Hartmann 1987; see Chapter 5 for a description of Depo-Provera).

Particularly worrisome are societies which include quotas as part of their population control policies and in which those who find "acceptors" are given attractive incentives for meeting or exceeding quotas (see, e.g., Jacobsen 1983). Such practices give those who are charged with securing informed consent a strong motivation (1) for leaving out information which might dissuade members of the "target population" from accepting birth control technologies and (2) for using coercive measures to ensure acceptance. In some societies, penalties for reproducing have been replaced by incentives for accepting contraceptives. But where target populations are extremely poor and these "incentives" include desperately needed food and money, people often have no reasonable alternative but to accept the offers extended by their governments. Where reasonable alternatives are precluded, voluntariness is substantially diminished and genuinely informed consent is precluded. To have no reasonable choice but to acquiesce is really to have no choice at all (Callahan 1986b).[15]

As we pointed out in Chapter 2, although the need to limit population growth is often quite real, excessive concentration on pop-

---

[15] It might be asked just how these programs differ morally from "incentives" to procreate that we readily accept (e.g., tax exemptions or direct payments for additional children through welfare). In certain cases, such practices clearly do raise serious moral worries. For example, if a woman has no reasonable alternative to having children (or more children) as a way of "making a living," the same problem exists. The point is that where no reasonable alternative to accepting birth control or to having children is available, an acceptably voluntary choice is not possible. See Callahan (1986b) for a more complete discussion of this aspect of voluntariness.

ulation control too often overlooks the fact that the social conditions and economic arrangements in societies where population is
taken to be the cause of poverty tend to be the kinds of conditions
and arrangements which breed destitution for large segments of the
citzenry.

Excessive concentration on population control can also lead to
exploitation in testing new birth control technologies and to moral
assault in antinatalist practices. Further, when these wrongs are committed, they are committed against those who are already the least
powerful and least well-off members of their societies. Certainly
not all testing programs or all programs that encourage reduction
in population raise these concerns to the same degree, but insofar as
birth control testing programs and antinatalist policies fail to respect
the moral right of persons to give an adequately informed, uncoerced
consent to any surgical or medical intervention involving their own
bodies, they cannot bear moral scrutiny. What is more, programs
which ignore the informed consent requirement are counterproductive in the long run, since people become discouraged with using
birth control technologies when they suffer unanticipated side
effects; as a result, use can quickly decline, frustrating population
control efforts (e.g., Warwick 1982; World Bank 1984; Hartmann
1987). Thus, we come back again to a point made in Chapter 2,
namely, that moral and pragmatic reasons call for moving away
from an excessive emphasis on population control efforts in developing nations to encouraging social and economic changes that make
genuine reproductive choice and therefore genuinely informed consent to birth control methods possible.

.    .    .    .    .    .

Our focus has been on existing and developing birth control
methods for women. Before closing, we need to look at the prospects for new birth control methods, including new contraceptive
alternatives for men. We turn now to a consideration of these possibilities.

# 10
## Male Contraception and Future Prospects

INTRODUCTION

While birth control options for women are more limited than many would like, options for men are even more limited. Currently there are only three methods for limitation of fertility available to men: coitus interruptus, condoms, and vasectomy. Of these three methods, coitus interruptus is neither very effective (see Chapter 1) nor emotionally fulfilling to either party. Though highly effective, vasectomy is acceptable only to men who are comfortable with the idea of permanent infertility. Therefore, the use of condoms, a less effective method than the better female methods (e.g., the pill and IUD), is really the only suitable option for most men. From the woman's perspective, even if her partner is totally willing to assume contraceptive responsibility and use condoms, it is still she who must bear the greater burden if she chooses not to employ one of the available and more effective female birth control options instead of or in addition to condoms and becomes pregnant as a result. As we have seen in Chapter 1, this is one of the primary reasons for concentrating on developing safe and effective birth control methodologies for women.

As we have also seen in Chapter 1, since fertilization and conceptus development occurs within women, there are a greater number of reproductive processes to manipulate in order to prevent a successful pregnancy. As described in some detail in Chapter 4, the two centers of neuroendocrine control in women (i.e., cyclic and tonic) allow oral contraceptives to suppress cyclic function without affecting tonic control. In men, the presence of just one center (the tonic) makes this approach less feasible. And, as we have seen in Chapters 3 and 4, the fundamental difference in gametogenesis between the sexes makes achieving temporary infertility without risk of permanent sterility far more promising for women than for

*285*

men. Finally, it is difficult to argue with the logic of attempting to prevent pregnancy by controlling the fate of a single ovum produced once a month compared with the overwhelmingly more difficult task of interrupting the continuous process of sperm production, which yields some twenty to thirty million spermatozoa per day every day throughout a man's long reproductive life.

Despite the inherently greater difficulty of the task, a number of approaches to fertility control in men have been examined. We now turn to a discussion of these research efforts and an examination of the current status of male contraceptive research.

## APPROACHES TO FERTILITY CONTROL IN MEN

### Interference with Sperm Transport: Vasectomy

As mentioned earlier, the only general approach to male fertility control that has proved to be universally successful and acceptable to users is the blockage of sperm transport. In essence, the condom (see Chapter 1) blocks sperm at the conclusion of their journey through the male reproductive tract by interposing a physical barrier that prevents their deposition into the female reproductive tract. A vasectomy is the simplest, safest, and most effective way to permanently interfere with sperm transport.

A vasectomy is a simple surgical procedure; it involves making an incision into the scrotum, severing the vas deferens (the tube that carries sperm), tying off the two ends of the vas deferens, and closing the small scrotal incision. The procedure is usually performed under local anesthesia in a doctor's office or clinic and requires only about fifteen to twenty minutes to complete. Before otherwise unprotected intercourse, enough time should be allowed for the elimination of sperm already present in the vas deferens at the time of the surgery. Minor variations in the cutting and ligating steps have been used, but these are of consequence only in regard to potential reversibility. Generally, about a 1–5 cm segment of the vas deferens is removed. If a longer portion is excised, the probability of successfully reattaching the severed ends at some future time is reduced (Silber 1980).

Compared with female sterilization (see Chapter 5), a vasectomy is simpler, safer, cheaper, and similar in effectiveness. Despite these advantages, in virtually all countries which report figures on sterilizations, the number of female contraceptive sterilizations performed each year exceed the number of male sterilizations (Goldsmith, Edelman, and Zatuchni 1985). No doubt one factor contributing to the relatively low reliance on vasectomy for family planning is a lack of understanding regarding what the procedure involves. In many cultures, and no doubt by some men in all cultures, any surgery in the scrotal area is automatically equated with castration.

Vasectomy does not affect sperm production. Sperm continue to be produced and transported to the epididymis for storage. However, since the sperm can no longer be removed by ejaculation because of the occlusion of the vas deferens, they are engulfed by phagocytes and reabsorbed by the body. Over time, this may lead to the production of circulating antibodies specific to sperm. In reality, the immunological infertility which may result from this occurrence poses no problem unless the man is interested in attempting to re-establish fertility through a vasectomy reversal.

Vasectomy has no effect on hormone production (Whitby, Gordon, and Blair 1979); therefore, it has no physiological effect on libido, erection, or ejaculation. Since spermatozoa represent less than 5 percent of the total ejaculate, no decrease in ejaculate volume is likely to be noticed. Men who do report diminished sexual interest, impotence, and other sexual dysfunctions following vasectomy are no doubt experiencing psychological side effects arising from their concern about being demasculinized by the procedure. As with several female birth control methods, including sterilization, some men report a heightened sex drive following vasectomy. But this effect, undoubtedly, is because of the new freedom to enjoy spontaneous intercourse without fear of causing pregnancy or the need to employ contraceptives (e.g., condoms, diaphragms) which may fail as well as interfere with spontaneity.

As an alternative to traditional surgical vasectomy, transcutaneous methods which employ either injection of chemical agents or electrocoagulation to block the lumen of the vas deferens have been investigated (Goldsmith, Edelman, and Zatuchni 1985). These approaches have been poorly received and, except for alleviating the fear of scrotal surgery, have no major advantages.

As with female sterilization, although considerable advances have occurred over the last few years in surgically reversing a vasectomy, it should still be considered a permanent procedure and employed only by men who are willing to accept permanent infertility. Depending on the degree of damage and method of vasectomy, reversal may be achieved through a procedure called *vasovasostomy*. This is a microsurgical technique in which the segments of the vas deferens are reattached (Silber 1980). Various types of valves, plugs, and clips have been examined over the years as a means of mechanically establishing and then reversing a vasectomy (Brueschke et al. 1979, 1980; Davis 1980; Djerassi 1981; Fawcett 1982; Harper 1983). Rather than occlude the ends of the severed vas deferens, each end is attached to a plug or valve which initially is closed to prevent passage of sperm. If fertility is desired at a later date, the valve may be opened to allow passage of sperm. There are numerous problems with the procedure, however, including difficulty in anchoring these devices satisfactorily in the vas deferens, erosion of the vas tissue, inflammatory reactions, and undesired passage of sperm through the valves over long periods of implantation.

## Interference with Spermatogenesis

Causing an azoospermic state would undoubtedly be the most effective means of male contraception. However, several principles must be understood in order to appreciate the difficulty in developing antifertility drugs that act upon the seminiferous tubules of the testes to suppress sperm production. (1) Spermatogenesis is a rather long process that takes approximately ten weeks for completion (Heller and Clermont 1964). Once spermatogonia begin this process, they are destined to either complete it or degenerate (see Chapter 3). Thus, agents interfering with the continuous process of spermatogenesis cannot be expected to produce an infertile state immediately or to allow immediate return to fertility following discontinuation of use. (2) The process of spermatogenesis requires continual replacement of spermatogonial stem cells by their mitotic division in the basal compartment of the germinal epithelium (see Chapter 3). Any drug that would destroy these stem cells would result in irreversible infertility. (3) Once meiotic division of spermatocytes begins, the chromosomes are especially vulnerable to potential mutagenic damage, for this process involves DNA replication and the interchange of genetic material between paired chromosomes. Naturally, researchers are reluctant to develop and clinically

test drugs which may damage spermatocytes. Excluding spermatogonia (stem cells) and spermatocytes as targets for attack leaves only
the later stages of spermatogenesis, when spermatids are developing into spermatozoa. To date, no drug has proved to be selective
for only the late stages of spermatogenesis (Fawcett 1982). (4) The
postmeiotic germ cells are highly dependent on the so-called blood-
testis barrier to isolate them from the "normal" fluid environment
of blood and lymph. While this protects the developing germ cells
from the potentially mutagenic effects of numerous chemicals and
toxins, the tightly occluding junctions of neighboring Sertoli cells
also limits the access of many substances which may successfully
interfere with spermatogenesis. (5) Finally, since testosterone is
required for (among other things) libido, potency, and various male
secondary sex effects, any approach directed toward inhibiting the
production or action of testosterone is very likely to be associated
with undesirable side effects. Although loss of libido and the inability to attain an erection would obviously constitute an effective birth
control measure, it is not likely to be accepted by very many men or
women.

*Early Antispermatogenic Agents*  Research on antispermatogenic
agents was stimulated by observations dating from the 1940s that
certain cytotoxic agents (e.g., nitrogen mustards, ethylene amine
derivatives, and monoesters and diesters of methanesulphonic acid,
arrest spermatogenesis at dose levels below those having systemic
toxicity (Landing, Goldin, and Noe 1949; Jackson 1970). Although
these compounds could not be considered as potential contraceptives, because they possessed alkylating, carcinogenic (e.g., toxic to
bone marrow), and potentially mutagenic properties, they did
encourage speculation that other agents capable of inhibiting
spermatogenesis but devoid of such undesirable characteristics might
be developed (Steinberger 1980).

Nitrofurans (heterocyclic compounds used to treat urinary tract
infections) were the first chemical compounds tested specifically
for their potential use as contraceptives (Steinberger 1980). Although
studies in rats showed that nitrofurans inhibit spermatogenesis at a
dose level free of systemic effects (Nelson and Steinberger 1952), at
dose levels required to suppress spermatogenesis in man, undesirable toxic side effects resulted (Nelson and Bunge 1957). Similarly,
thiophens, bis-dichloroacetyl diamines, and dinitropyroles showed

initial promise relative to suppression of spermatogenesis in trials involving rats, dogs, and monkeys. But they subsequently proved to have toxic effects, either in continued animal trials or initial clinical studies in humans (Heller, Flagsolle, and Matron 1964; Patanelli and Nelson 1964; Steinberger 1980; Fawcett 1982).

Perhaps the most interesting of all these compounds were the bis-dichloroacetyl diamines. Tests on prison volunteers in the early 1960s showed that sperm counts dropped to insignificant levels within two to three months of continuous administration of the drug, yet returned to normal concentrations upon discontinuance of use (Heller, Flagsolle, and Matron 1964). However, in the presence of alcohol, the compounds were found to have various seriously unpleasant side effects, including severe nausea and vomiting. Their alcohol incompatibility, plus concerns over possible liver damage with long-term use, resulted in their abandonment as a potential male oral contraceptive.

The indazol carboxylic acids are another group of antispermatogenic compounds that have been tested in animals. Studies in monkeys have shown them to arrest spermatogenesis and to maintain infertility with a single weekly dose (Sylvestrini et al. 1975). Potential effects of long-term use have not been established and clinical trials in humans have not been conducted (Fawcett 1982).

*Gossypol*  Approximately a decade ago, Chinese researchers found that gossypol, a phenolic compound occurring primarily in cotton seed, functions as an antifertility agent in men (National Coordinating Group on Male Antifertility Agents 1978). This initial discovery was serendipitous and based on epidemiologic investigations in the People's Republic of China motivated by the finding that Chinese men whose diets consisted mostly of foods cooked in cottonseed oil became infertile. Subsequent controlled studies in a variety of animals and human models, both in China and the United States, have confirmed that the antifertility was the result of gossypol ingestion. Specifically, it has now been established that in the first few weeks of treatment, gossypol attaches to maturing sperm stored in the epididymis and renders them immotile through interference with mitochondrial enzymes. Over the course of longer treatment, the drug also acts directly in the testes to check sperm production. Although all aspects of its action are still not fully understood, that it acts directly on the motility of mature sperm and on the growth of immature cells sets gossypol apart from other potential fertility-regulating agents. Of major significance is that gossypol acts without interfering with hormone production. Secretion of LH (luteinizing hormone) and testosterone and maintenance of libido appear to be unaffected in most trials (Segal 1985).

Despite these encouraging results, there are several problems and unanswered questions associated with gossypol that are of serious concern. Perhaps the greatest worry is in regard to possible long-term toxic effects on the heart and liver following prolonged use. Minimal effective dosage and potential residual levels are still unestablished. A recurring problem in most clinical studies is the suppression of blood potassium levels, which may diminish normal muscle function, among other effects (Steinberger 1980; Segal 1985; Edwards 1988). It has been known for a number of years that in high levels, gossypol is toxic to nonruminants; it reduces the oxygen-carrying capacity of the blood, irritates the gastrointestinal tract, produces pulmonary edema and shortness of breath, and may even cause respiratory paralysis. Prolonged exposure to high levels may also result in permanent sterility, as happened to a number of the Chinese men whose cases initially led to the discovery of gossypol's antifertility effects. While these serious side effects are greatly reduced in trials in which gossypol is administered at subtoxic levels, the potentially toxic nature of gossypol merits caution and remains an issue of concern.

Liu et al. (1981) reported results of a large clinical trial in China involving 8,806 volunteers. Three preparations were used: gossypol, gossypol-acetic acid, and gossypol-formic acid. Optimal doses were established to be 20 mg per day for sixty to seventy-five days, followed by a maintenance dose of 50 mg per week. Efficacy, based on sperm examinations, was reported to be 99 percent. Sperm counts below 4 million per ml appears after two to three months of treatment, and counts associated with fertility took at least three to four months to return after cessation of treatment. Of major concern is that 10 percent of the men remained azoospermic and an additional 16 percent continued to have subnormal sperm numbers. Longer lengths of treatment were associated with a lower rate of recovery. This finding raises serious concerns regarding the reversibility of gossypol-induced infertility.

Numerous studies on the efficacy and safety of gossypol are currently in progress. It is possible that analogs of gossypol can be developed that allow a greater separation between the toxic and antifertility effects of gossypol and allow a more efficient return to fertility following cessation of treatment.

*Steroidal Suppression of Spermatogenesis*   The idea of using steroidal compounds to suppress spermatogenesis is three decades old, dating from the studies of Heller et al. (1958). Since that time, many synthetic steroids have been examined as potential agents to interfere with spermatogenesis (see reviews by Frick et al. 1981; Fawcett 1982; Bajaj and Madan 1983; Harper 1983; Neumann 1985). Appropriate doses of all three major classes of gonadal steroids (i.e., progestins, androgens, and estrogens) can block the hypothalamo-hypophyseal–gonadal axis, resulting in an availability of testosterone in the tubular compartment of the testis that is inadequate to support spermatogenesis.

*Androgens.*   Since we have established that testosterone is essential for spermatogenesis (see Chapter 3), it may appear contradictory to state that testosterone can be used to inhibit spermatogenesis. However, the administration of high doses of testosterone does inhibit spermatogenesis, because the circulating exogenous testosterone inhibits the secretion of LH, which in turn suppresses production of testosterone within the testes. It is this locally produced and locally active endogenous testosterone that is needed for spermatogenesis. In theory, the exogenously administered circulating testosterone is adequate to maintain libido and secondary sex characteristics.

Reedy and Rao (1972) administered testosterone propionate by daily intramuscular injection for sixty days to seven men. In all subjects, azoospermia occurred, with no reported adverse side effects. Normal or near normal sperm counts followed cessation of treatment.

Bajaj and Madan (1983) summarized four studies involving weekly or biweekly administration of testosterone enanthate. Azoospermia was achieved in only about 50 percent of the treated subjects, although oligospermia occurred in at least 90 percent of the men. Although these studies demonstrate that it is possible to lower sperm counts through exogenous administration of androgens, the dosages required to do so are so high that there are serious questions about whether such high levels given for long periods of time would cause major side effects, including prostatic cancer and various cardiovascular and metabolic disorders. It must also be kept in mind that merely lowering a man's sperm count is no guarantee of infertility (Djerassi 1981).

*Estrogens.* Estrogens are highly effective and potent inhibitors of testicular function. Their ability to induce azoospermia in men has been well established for thirty years (Heller et al. 1958). However, it is equally well established that they are not suitable for fertility control in men. Major problems include their inhibition of all androgen–dependent organs and functions, including libido. Impotence, severe gynecomastia (breast development), and severe cardiovascular side effects result from their application. Finally, nonreversible changes in testicular function are likely to result from long-term administration (Frick et al. 1981; Bajaj and Madan 1983; Neumann 1985).

*Progestins.* The antispermatogenic effects of numerous progestins are also well established, and specific details concerning various synthetic products are available in the reviews previously listed. In general, administration of progestins alone in doses sufficient to induce azoospermia or severe oligospermia also results in loss of libido and potency, gynecomastia, and loss of the secretory activity of accessory sex glands.

*Progestin-androgen Combinations.* Trials have been conducted, the largest involving twenty-five major dosage regimens, with combined administration of progestins and androgens (Schearer et al 1978; World Health Organization 1978, 1979). The idea behind this approach is to avoid or minimize the adverse effects of long-term use of progestins described above. Additionally, because of the synergistic action of the two drugs, the doses of both progestins and androgens can be less than when either is used alone.

None of the twenty-five dosage regimens reported by Schearer et al. (1978) was fully effective in causing azoospermia. Some regimens were associated with decreased libido, gynecomastia, and weight gain. A major disadvantage of this approach is that, even when spermatogenesis is suppressed, a delay of six to eight weeks is required following initiation of treatment. Return to fertility is also delayed following termination of treatment (Schearer 1978).

Of the various combinations tested, the combination of depot medroxyprogesterone acetate (DMPA, 200 mg per month) plus testosterone enanthate (200 mg per month) or testosterone cypionate (250 mg per month) seems to be the most effective (World Health

Organization 1979). Oligiospermia was achieved in almost all subjects on this regimen, although azoospermia was manifested by only 50–60 percent of the men. Although more effective than either steroid alone, the combination approach, because of side effects and the failure to induce azoospermia, does not appear very promising.

*Gn-RH Antagonists and Agonists*   The potential application of Gn-RH (gonadtropin releasing hormones) antagonists and agonists as a female contraceptive method was discussed in Chapter 5. Theoretically, both kinds of substance could also be used for male fertility regulation. The antagonist would act at the level of the anterior pituitary to interfere with the synthesis and release of both LH and FSH (follicle-stimulating hormone). While this approach is likely to interfere with spermatogenesis, a reduction in circulating LH would also lower circulating testosterone, thereby affecting libido and secondary sex characteristics. With a reduction in the negative feedback of testosterone, enhanced endogenous synthesis and release of Gn-RH from the hypothalamus would result, which would necessitate an increase in the dosage of the antagonist to maintain its therapeutic effectiveness; thus a vicious cycle would be created (see Chapter 4). At present, Gn-RH antagonists of sufficient biological potency and of proven safety are not available for use in men.

As we saw in Chapter 5, Gn-RH agonists apparently work by overstimulating the receptors of the anterior pituitary, leading to refractoriness, diminished gonadotropin secretion, and subsequent effects on gonadal steroidogenesis. Reductions in spermatogenic activity have generally been accompanied by the unwanted side effects of reduced serum testosterone and consequent reduced libido and potency (Labrie et al. 1980; Belenger et al. 1980; Linde et al. 1981; Rabin et al. 1981).

Although trials are continuing in this area, the prospects of using Gn-RH agonists or antagonists for male contraception are not very promising. It would appear that the only way to restore libido and potency decreased by treatment is through exogenous testosterone supplements — an inconvenient solution not likely to be accepted by most men.

*Inhibin*   McCullagh (1932) first postulated the existence of a water soluble substance of testicular origin which was capable of regulating FSH production via negative feedback. This hypothetical substance, which McCullagh designated *inhibin*, remained more fiction than fact until several laboratories independently presented evidence to firmly establish its existence in the late 1970s (see the review by Steinberger and Ward 1988). Purification and amino acid sequencing of inhibin was not achieved until 1985.

There is evidence that incubation of pituitary halves or cultures of pituitary cells with inhibin in vitro and injection of inhibin in vivo does lower FSH production (Steinberger and Ward 1988). What is not clearly established is whether inhibin performs that function under normal physiological conditions. Likewise, the role of FSH in spermatogenesis is unclear. Thus, the consequences of over- or undersecretion of FSH in the mature male remain speculative (Steinberger and Ward 1988). There is at least one study involving monkeys that suggests suppression of FSH by antibodies impairs spermatogenesis and leads to infertility (Moudgal 1981).

The theoretical approach to the use of inhibin as a male contraceptive, therefore, is based on the observed inverse relationship between inhibin and FSH and on the assumption that lowering FSH will inhibit spermatogenesis. Theoretically, the advantage of inhibin would be its selective inhibition of spermatogenesis without interfering with LH and hence testosterone production (which would lead to decreased libido and related problems).

Although several laboratories continue to pursue this line of research, it should be viewed with cautious optimism, at best. To date, no inhibin preparation is available which is known to reduce the level of circulating FSH to zero or to result in azoospermia. Also, most inhibin preparations tested to date also show some suppressive effect on LH (Bajaj and Madan 1983; Steinberger and Ward 1988), although this may be nonspecific suppression due to impurities. Our knowledge of several complex forms of inhibin-related proteins in only now evolving. Thus, even if inhibin should prove successful in suppressing spermatogenesis without affecting testosterone production, the testing that would be required to determine appropriate dosage regimens, delivery systems, assess potential side effects, determine reversibility, and so on, would put its availability as a male contraceptive well into the next century.

## Interference with Sperm Maturation and Epididymal Function

Spermatozoa are not capable of fertilizing an ovum when they leave the testis. Since spermatozoa must undergo further physiological maturation in the epididymis in order to attain fertilizability (Fawcett 1982), this suggests that the epididymis is a potential target for anti-fertility drugs. This approach is attractive for two major reasons: Since all cellular divisions have occurred by the time that spermatozoa reach the epididymis, the potential for adverse genetic effects is minimal. At this point, the genetic material in the condensed sperm head is metabolically inert and highly resistant to chemical alteration. Also, the latency period before an antiepididymal agent becomes effective would be relatively short (i.e., seven to fourteen days).

Changes associated with epididymal maturation of spermatozoa include the development of progressive motility, modification of metabolic capabilities, changes in nuclear chromatin, surface modification of the plasma membrane and acrosome, and movement of the cytoplasmic droplet (Bedford 1975). Unfortunately, the chemical mediators of most aspects of sperm maturation are still largely unknown. Several epididymal secretory proteins have been identified, but their functions have not been established (Orgebin-Crist, Danzo, and Davies 1975; Lea, Petrus, and French 1978; Fawcett 1982). As indicated in the review by Robaire and Hermo (1988), once more is known about the specific controlling factors in the maturation process, a variety of approaches involving the development of inhibitory drugs may appear worthy of investigation. Basic approaches include modifying the action of hormonal factors known to regulate epididymal function, altering the microenvironment of spermatozoa as they acquire their fertilizing ability, and directly altering the spermatozoa themselves (e.g., preventing the addition of or altering the glycoproteins that are normally added to the cell coat of the surface of the sperm during storage in the epididymis).

*α-chlorohydrin*   Several compounds have been tested in an attempt to alter epididymal function. Beginning in the late 1960s, a series of studies appeared on the ability of the drug α-chlorohydrin to reversibly inhibit fertility in several species (see the reviews by Jackson and Robinson 1976; Jones 1978; and Lobl 1980). Brown-Woodman et al. (1978) and Ford and Harrison (1983) reported that, at low doses, α-chlorohydrin (a monochloric derivative of glycerol) inhibits the enzyme glyceraldehyde-3-phosphate dehydrogenase that is essential for the energy metabolism of sperm while in the epididymis. However, at higher doses α-chlorohydrin was found to result in the formation of spermatoceles (cystic distentions of the epididymis containing spermatozoa). These spermatoceles resulted in the blockage of sperm transport through the tissue and in the consequent atrophy of the seminiferous tubules, which was caused by increases in back pressure (Reijonen, Kormano, and Ericsson 1975; Jones 1978; and Ford and Waites 1982). Wong, Yeung, and Ngai (1977) and Wong, Au, and Ngai (1980) demonstrated that α-chlorohydrin blocked resorption of sodium and water from the cauda epididymis in rats. This compound has also been shown to have severe toxic effects (bone marrow depression) when tested in primates (Kirton et al. 1970); therefore its investigation as a potential male contraceptive has been abandoned. Future efforts utilizing structural analogs of α-chlorohydrin devoid of these undesirable side effects and targeted at the epididymis is a possibility (Robaire and Hermo 1988).

*Antiandrogens* The androgen dihydrotestosterone (DHT) is required for sperm maturation and the acquisition of fertilizing capacity in the epididymis (Robaire and Hermo 1988). Therefore, an obvious approach to inhibiting sperm maturation is to use an antiandrogen, such as cyproterone acetate or flutamide, to block the epididymal DHT receptors and thereby block epididymal function. However, as might be expected given our previous discussion of the use of anti-androgens, results of several studies indicate that the action of androgens in other target tissues is also blocked, and therefore these compounds have undesirable side effects.

*Inhibitors of 5α-reductase* An alternate approach to blocking the action of DHT in the epididymis is to prevent its synthesis by the enzyme 5α-reductase, which is responsible for converting testosterone to DHT (see Chapter 3). A vast array of compounds have been reported to block 5α-reductase in a variety of tissues. However, reports on only three families of drugs have appeared on the ability to block epididymal 5α-reductase (Robaire and Hermo 1988).

Robaire et al. (1977) demonstrated the in vitro inhibition of epididymal 5α-reductase by a family of 5,10-secosteroids. These compounds have not been tested for their effect on fertility in vivo.

The compound diethyl-4-methyl-3-oxo-4-aza-5α-androstane-17β-carboxamide (4-MA) is one of the more extensively tested inhibitors of 5α-reductase in a number of tissues, and it has also been found to be a competitive inhibitor of the epididymal enzyme (Cooke and Robaire 1986). Brooks et al. (1982) reported that 4-MA did not alter the fertility of male rats. However, these investigators did not establish that the dose used was sufficient to inhibit epididymal 5α-reductase. Since 4-MA at concentrations sufficient to inhibit epididymal 5α-reductase also inhibits other enzyme systems (Robaire and Hermo 1988), it is an unlikely candidate as a selective blocker of epididymal function.

The third group of potential inhibitors of 5α-reductase are the 17-chloroformate analogs of testosterone (Robaire, Duron, and Lobl 1986). No trials testing their efficacy as in vivo blockers of epididymal function have been conducted.

*Gossypol*  As we saw in the section on compounds that interfere with spermatogenesis, gossypol has an initial effect on sperm maturation and suppresses spermatogenesis over the longer term. Given current information, early speculations that gossypol selectively inhibits epididymal functions no longer appear warranted. The blood-epididymis barrier and epididymal functions remain intact in the presence of this drug (Segal 1985).

### Immunological Approaches to Male Fertility Control

As we have seen in our discussion of birth control methods for women, the basis of the immunological approach to fertility control is to administer or stimulate the development of antibodies that are capable of inactivating a hormone or a reproductive tract protein necessary for successful reproduction. In the male reproductive tract, there are a wide variety of antigens whose neutralization may theoretically result in infertility.

*Hormone Antibodies*  Given our knowledge of the hormonal regulation of male reproductive function (see Chapter 3), there would appear to be several potential sites of immunological intervention. However, as we have noted on several occasions, although hormones produced at each level of the hypothalamo–pituitary–testicular axis can be neutralized by antibodies, this approach is not feasible because of its many adverse side effects, most notably depressed libido and impotence. The only hormonally directed immunological approach that offers any real promise is the neutralization of FSH. More information is still needed about the mode of action of FSH on spermatogenesis and about the stage at which spermatogenesis is interrupted by the blockage of FSH (Wickings and Nieschlag 1983). In addition, long-term studies are required to evaluate possible side effects of active immunization, including possible irreversible tissue damage.

*Antisperm Antibodies* Spermatogenesis can take place only because the rigorously controlled environment of the germinal epithelium sequesters it from the general body circulation by means of the blood-testis barrier (see Chapters 3 and 8). Unlike the differentiation products of other systems, the specialized proteins required for the construction and function of spermatozoa are not produced until puberty — well after the point at which the immune system is fully functional. Without a functional blood-testis barrier, new protein synthesis associated with the cell surface, acrosome, nucleus, cytoplasm, and mitochondria of the spermatozoa would be recognized as "foreign" and an autoimmune response would result. Disruption of the blood-testis barrier and immunization against sperm-specific proteins is, therefore, a logical approach to male contraception.

As indicated by Menge (1986), the observation that sperm cells are antigenic and capable of eliciting antibodies can be traced back to the turn of the century. As early as the 1920s, speculation arose regarding the possible role of sperm antigenicity as a cause of human infertility. Katsh (1959) summarized early attempts in experimental animals to induce infertility by immunization with semen. The reports stimulated several attempts to immunize women by multiple injections of human semen. During the 1950s and 1960s, several groups of clinical investigators working with infertile couples reported evidence of an association between human infertility and antibodies to sperm (see Menge 1986). A summary of numerous reports indicates a rather clear and significant negative association between serum titers of sperm antibodies of either partner and the capacity to reproduce (Menge 1980). Likewise, there is a negative association between fertility and the presence of titers of local antibodies to sperm in the cervical secretions of infertile women (Menge et al. 1982).

Studies in experimental animals have demonstrated the potential of immunizing women with sperm to induce infertility. However, trials reporting successful immunization of men have also generally reported azoospermia and aspermatogenesis caused by induction of immune orchitis (inflammation of the testis) — a pain-ful and unacceptable side effect (Menge 1986). In contrast, the nat-ural occurrence of sperm autoantibodies resulting from unknown causes following vasectomy or infection appears to involve little or no testicular effect, and the antifertility effect is exerted through the binding of the antibodies to sperm cells in the ejaculate (Menge 1986). Although the role of the secretory immune system in the female reproductive tract is well established, it is less well under-stood in the male tract. Specific antisperm antibodies of both the IgA and IgG classes have been identified in secretions of the lower reproductive tract of women and in the semen of men. Although the exact source or point of entry of the antibodies in the male reproductive tract has yet to be carefully evaluated, evidence from men who have undergone vasovasostomy suggests entry on the testicular side of the former occlusion or lesion, since in most cases antisperm antibodies appear in the ejaculate after reconnection with the vas deferens (Linnet, Hjort, and Fogh-Anderson 1981; Menge 1986). Regardless of the source, it appears that antibodies against sperm of either the IgA or IgG class are capable of interrupting normal fertility (Menge 1986).

One problem which hinders the study of sperm antigenicity is that seminal plasma is also antigenic. In many cases, seminal plasma antigens may be adsorbed to the surface of ejaculated spermatozoa, making it extremely difficult to distinguish between the two. Since there are distinct sperm-specific and seminal plasma-specific anti-gens, antiserums against each may be developed to test for antigens that are essential for fertilization. The antigenic complexity of spermatozoa and the difficulty of discerning which antigens play a role in fertilization are additional obstacles to success in this area of male contraceptive research.

Perhaps the greatest progress has been made in understanding the structure, localization, and antigenic properties of the testis-specific sperm enzyme lactate dehydrogenase $C_4$ (referred to as either LDH-$C_4$ or LDH-X). This enzyme is involved with sperm carbohy-drate metabolism. Although lactate dehydrogenase is a widely dis-tributed enzyme, LDH-X appears in the seminiferous tubules at the time that pachytene spermatocytes are first formed (Setchell 1978). The unique developmental and biochemical properties of LDH-X have been reviewed by Wheat and Goldberg (1983).

Most studies involving LDH-X have focused on immunizing females with the enzyme, and it is currently being treated as a female rather than male contraceptive; hence it does not merit extensive examination in this section. Studies in this area are summarized in the reviews by O'Rand (1980), Goldberg (1983), and Wheat and Goldberg (1983). While immunization does result in up to 67 percent reduction in fertility in female laboratory animals and nonhuman primates, it does not induce complete sterility.

Various proteolytic and mucolytic enzymes essential for fertilization are packaged in the acrosome of the sperm head. Of particular note are the enzymes hyaluronidase (important for disruption of the cumulus cells) and acrosin (essential for penetration of the zona pellucida at fertilization). Similar to the results indicated for LDH-X, immunization of females of various species with hyaluronidase and acrosin has partially inhibited fertility but has not produced sterility (O'Rand 1980).

More recently, hybridoma technology has been utilized to produce monoclonal antibodies (highly specific immunoglobulins) against sperm cell surface antigens (Alexander 1985). Although application of this technology should enhance the advancement of immunocontraceptive research, given the number of practical problems yet to be resolved it does not appear that acceptable antisperm vaccines are likely to be developed in the near future.

### Physical Approaches to Male Fertility Control

*Thermal Methods* As pointed out in Chapter 3, in humans (and most other mammals) an intratesticular temperature that is several degrees lower than body temperature (approximately 2.2°C lower in men) is essential for continuous production of fertile spermatozoa. Although several other factors are involved in testicular thermoregulation (see Setchell 1978), the presence of the testes in a pendulous scrotum contributes to the process. Studies in several species clearly indicate that replacement of the testes in the abdominal cavity or elevation of the temperature of the scrotum by insulation or by externally applied heat results in cessation of spermatogenesis (Setchell 1978; Fawcett 1982). Fawcett (1982) reported that human volunteers who immersed their scrotums in a heated water bath daily for short periods gradually decreased their sperm counts to infertile levels. Based upon these findings, several devices designed for regular application of heat to the scrotum for the purpose of inducing infertility have been suggested. These include hot water baths, infrared spot heating, and microwave diathermy (Fawcett 1982). To date, none has been proven effective as a routine contraceptive practice.

The basic problem with thermal approaches is their unpredictability — a serious limitation for a potential contraceptive. Since it is the process of spermatogenesis, not the individual spermatozoon, that is sensitive to elevated temperature, a man using a thermal method would remain fertile for many days or weeks after commencing use of the technique. If infertility were achieved, the period of infertility would be highly variable among individuals. Finally, even if treatment were conscientiously continued, achievement and maintenance of infertility would be difficult to monitor without frequent sperm counts, a procedure that most men would be unqualified or unwilling to perform. These practical limitations make thermal methods unlikely candidates for wide use or success as male contraceptive methods.

*Ultrasound*   Ultrasound is widely used diagnostically (e.g., for monitoring fetal development) as well as for treating various musculoskeletal disorders. It has been reported for several animal species that brief exposure of the testes to ultrasound induces reversible infertility without loss of libido (see, e.g., Dumontier et al. 1977). The effects apparently involve some mechanical damage produced by high-frequency acoustic vibration. Histological examination reveals extensive destruction of germinal elements, but the fact that fertility can be regained suggests that Sertoli cells and spermatogonia are more resistant to ultrasound than are other germ cells. Safety and efficacy in humans have yet to be demonstrated (Fawcett 1982).

## Summary of Status and Future Prospects of Male Contraception

Several points emerge from the material presented so far in this chapter. First, recent research explains why it is the case that, other than the condom, there is at present no safe, effective, readily reversible method of male contraception that is acceptable to large numbers of men. Second, the reasons for this fact pertain to the complex nature of and our relative lack of understanding of the controlling mechanisms of male reproduction. Spermatogenesis is a far more complex process than is oogenesis. Third, despite the relative lack of promise in developing a safe and effective nonbarrier male contraceptive, significant and extensive research has been done and continues to be done on male fertility control. Indeed, all the known theoretical approaches to male fertility regulation have been explored and a number of approaches remain under study. Finally, despite the research efforts that have been and are being made in the attempt to develop fertility regulation methods for men analogous to those developed for women, no "new" male contraceptive is likely to appear soon or even for some time to come. While there is still reason to believe that male–directed fertility control is an attainable objective, we should not expect to see that objective realized in the foreseeable future.

On the positive side, a tremendous amount of basic information relative to male reproductive function has been gained from studies aimed at male fertility regulation. Given the complexity of the processes associated with sperm production, maturation, and metabolism, this knowledge is an essential first step in the continuing search for safe, effective, and user–acceptable male contraceptives. We have come to realize that the controlling mechanisms are even more complex then previously thought. We now have a better understanding of the complex role of the Sertoli cells in spermatogenesis. For example, we now know that they possess specific FSH receptors; they respond to testosterone; they produce and utilize androgen–binding protein to maintain high intratubular androgen concentrations; they produce inhibin to regulate release of FSH from the anterior pituitary; they are responsible for movement of the clones of germ cells toward the lumen of the tubule; they facilitate spermatozoa release and degradation of residual bodies formed during spermatogenesis; they form the key component of the blood–testis barrier to regulate the internal environment of the tubule; and they create in the adluminal compartment of the tubule a unique microenvironment favorable for germ cell differentiation (see Fawcett 1979). All of these functions are essential for spermatogenesis and make the Sertoli cell the prime candidate for research regarding male contraception. We are now much closer to being able to selectively and reversibly suppress one or more of these functions and effect a control of spermatogenesis.

We should also add that both male sterilization and the male barrier approach have been improved. As noted earlier, although a vasectomy should still be sought only if a man is willing to accept the possibility of permanent infertility, considerable progress has been made in perfecting microsurgical techniques of vasovasostomy, which has tremendously increased the reversibility of vasectomies. As the field of microsurgery continues to progress, it is reasonable to assume that vasovasostomy is likely to become an even more successful procedure and, hence, vasectomy an even more viable birth control option. Condoms have also been improved in recent years in regard to their reliability, durability, and allowance of penile sensitivity. Because of their dual effectiveness in preventing pregnancy and disease, their lack of side effects, and their ready availability, condoms are likely to remain a popular birth control option even if new methods are developed.

A question often raised is whether men will accept complete responsibility for fertility control if and when effective male approaches are more readily available. Naturally, the answer to that question will vary not only from culture to culture but from individual to individual. However, at least within the United States, there does appear to be a growing interest on the part of men in sharing responsibility for family planning and a growing desire among men to achieve control over their own fertility. Given that more than 25 percent of the couples employing contraception in the United States rely upon the condom and that over half a million vasectomies are performed each year, it seems that a large segment of the male population is willing to share or assume the responsibility for fertility control.

FUTURE PROSPECTS OF BIRTH CONTROL TECHNOLOGIES

Before recapping the prospects for the future availability of specific birth control options, it will be helpful to reflect on the characteristics of the "ideal contraceptive" and examine how the conflicting desires, needs, and interests of consumers, pharmaceutical companies, and government regulatory agencies clash to limit present and future choices.

The World Health Organization defines the ideal contraceptive as one that (1) is highly efficient; (2) is easy to apply; (3) is reversible (i.e., there is normal fertility after withdrawal of the method); (4) involves no severe side effects or serious risks; (5) is inexpensive; (6) can be distributed easily; and (7) is acceptable in the light of the religious, ethical, and cultural background of the users (Rabe, Kiesel, and Runnebaum 1985). Obviously no single product or procedure exists that meets all these criteria for all persons. And given the important differences among individuals and cultures, it is unlikely that any such product or procedure ever will exist. Thus, since no product or procedure perfectly meets all criteria, each person must decide the relative importance of each criterion as it applies to his or her individual situation, values, and needs.

Obviously, high efficiency in preventing birth is the primary criterion to be met by all potential birth control methods. Even here, however, the relative worth of a method's efficacy must be subject to individual standards of acceptance. It is inevitable that some failures will occur in any population of users of methods other than total abstinence. It is important to keep in mind that the quoted failure rates of various methods are of two types: (1) lowest observed failure rate and (2) failure rate in typical users. For user-dependent methods of birth control (such as oral contraceptives, diaphragms, and condoms), the technique should not mistakenly be blamed for the failure of individuals to apply it properly. The extent to which one is willing to trade lesser efficiency for fewer side effects, easier reversibility, and so on, is once again an individual matter.

Ease of application involves a trade-off with user control and other characteristics. Methods which have a long period of effectiveness following a single administration (e.g., IUDs, Norplants) are relatively easy to apply, but they also take fertility control from their users during their long duration of effectiveness. This raises the kinds of concerns discussed in Chapter 5.

While ready reversibility is also desirable, the more efficient birth control methods will generally also be the ones of lesser immediate reversibility. High efficiency is generally achieved by a multilevel suppression or interference with key reproductive phenomena. As a rule, some period of readjustment will be needed following cessation of application of the method before the physiological or endocrinological events or mechanisms suppressed return to normal.

Severe side effects and serious health risks make any potential birth control method unacceptable. Indeed, the fact that numerous products which are highly effective also pose serious health risks is the most common reason for not pursuing further testing. However, some degree of health risk and some side effects will probably always have to be tolerated in order to achieve effective birth control. As Djerassi (1981) points out, there is no such thing as a wholly safe contraceptive. As with virtually every other type of drug, some side effects in some individuals are simply inevitable. Naturally, the consumer has a right to expect that only basically safe products are marketed. The pharmaceutical industry has a moral as well as a legal responsibility to adequately test all products to assess their potential risks and assure their basic safety. Government agencies have the mandate to assure the compliance of pharmaceutical companies with the requisite testing procedures. While we shall point out some of the current problems brought about by overregulation shortly, it must also be kept in mind that stringent FDA regulations help to ensure that the dangerous studies of the early 1960s using extremely high dose oral contraceptives will not be repeated and that unsuspecting women will not have another equivalent of the Dalkon Shield thrust upon them in the future.

Are new contraceptive options available which have a well-established record of high reliability? Yes. Included in this group are various long-acting steroidal systems (especially Norplants), RU-486, new design IUDs (especially the Progestasert and Copper T380A), and possibly Gn-RH agonists. Are these birth control methods safe? Yes. Are they totally free from side effects and can it be guaranteed that they pose no health risks? No. Are they universally acceptable in light of the religious, cultural, and moral perspectives of all potential users? Clearly, no.

Technological feasibility is not what is limiting the availability of new and expanded birth control options; it is the approval process. Given the time required for testing and approval of new products in the United States, it is inconceivable that any product not currently under investigation could be approved and available before the next century. The exceptionally long period of development and testing of new contraceptive methods entails that if work on a new product began today and proved successful, children born today would likely be sexually active well before that product was available for their use. No new birth control method (in the United States or elsewhere) can be made available to the public without the full participation of the pharmaceutical industry. But pharmaceutical companies are no longer willing to devote the resources to the development of birth control products that they once were. Simply stated, providing products for other health-related applications is more lucrative, and, in the free enterprise system, potential profits determine the selection of products for development. Clearly, more cooperation and collaboration between the industry and drug regulatory agencies is needed to ensure the fastest possible testing and approval of new products within the constraints of public health and safety.

The current status of RU-486 in the United States is illustrative of the costs of delay. Although RU-486 has been used in clinical trials by over four thousand women in twenty countries since 1982 and is now approved for use in five countries (France, Sweden, the Netherlands, Britain, and China), substantial additional testing would still be required before the FDA would even take it under consideration as a product to be marketed here (Fraser 1988). Requirements to repeat studies already well conducted in other countries is redundant, costly, and wasteful. Yet, such requirements continue to be enforced by the FDA. Further, political pressure from those opposed to the use of any abortifacient, directed toward both pharmaceutical companies and federal agencies, make approval for use of products such as RU-486 in the United States highly unlikely in the foreseeable future.

In the 1970s there were at least thirteen major pharmaceutical companies actively involved in contraceptive research. Of those companies, only one (Ortho Pharmaceutical) is still active in the field (Fraser 1988). This attrition is attributable to two causes: the costs incurred during long product development time (up to seventeen years) and the inflation of liability insurance caused by consumer litigation. Fraser (1988) estimates the current costs incurred in research, clinical trials, and FDA approval of a new contraceptive to be in the range of $30 to $70 million. And that figure does not even include the need to set aside additional funds as protection against liability claims. Fraser (1988) suggests that the future of new contraceptive marketing may lie with small companies specializing only in contraceptive products, since such companies would not risk losing enormous assets from other product divisions in a liability case. Needless to say, the long-term goal of any pharmaceutical company that wishes to stay in business must be to recover development costs and make a profit. Hence, pricing a contraceptive at a low cost, while ideal for the consumer, is not in the best interest of the pharmaceutical company. For example, contemporary birth control pills cost only pennies to produce but sell for fourteen to fifteen dollars per pack. It would be an unsound business decision to switch to production of a less profitable product (especially if speculative research costs must be incurred) or to encourage consumers to utilize a less profitable item.

Because of the exorbitant cost of developing a new contraceptive technology, most research is now dependent on direct or indirect government funding. In 1988, 60 percent of all funding for contraceptive research in the United States came from the federal government, compared with 25 percent in 1970 (Fraser 1988). When birth control research is dependent on that high a percentage of governmental support, when such research is not a top governmental priority, and when the government requires extensive testing and retesting of products before approving them for use, the difficulty of bringing new alternatives to the market is obviously substantial.

In the case of research on birth control technologies, the difficulty is compounded by a prohibition on use of public funds for research in a significant area of the technology. For example, federal funds have been expressly withheld from research on any product which may be abortifacient in action. Despite the impressive amount of research on RU-486, which has led to its acceptance and availability in other countries, federal dollars may not be used to fund research on the product. But this is morally unacceptable. As we argued in Chapter 7, the only secular argument that could possibly be compelling against the moral acceptability of using potentially abortifacient birth control technologies is unsound and hence cannot justify withholding funding for scientifically worthy and socially useful research. With no secular argument available to justify withholding public funds for research on abortifacient technologies, it becomes apparent that religious convictions motivate the prohibition. But in a pluralistic society like our own, such reasons are not morally acceptable ones for instituting public policies that interfere with individual liberty or that negatively affect the welfare of citizens who do not share those religious convictions (Callahan 1986a). The unjustifiability of this restriction is even more glaring when one considers the potentially beneficial uses of RU-486 in addition to its use as a birth control technology (see Chapter 6).

One possible solution to the problem of decreased interest in new birth control product development by pharmaceutical companies is for the government to subsidize their involvement in new product research and development (either directly or through tax incentives) and to provide them with indemnity against litigation for product failure when a product has been responsibly tested. The primary reason for the tremendous costs and long delays associated with the development and testing of a potential new birth control product is the extent of toxicity testing which is rightly required by the government to ensure that the product will present minimal health risks to the population. While long-term health risks to the user are always a legitimate concern, testing for such risks is extremely costly. Since the public wants and the government demands this type of extensive testing, it seems more than appropriate that public tax dollars be used to pay part of the costs. Djerassi (1981) suggests several ways in which this might be accomplished.

After reviewing the research that has been done on birth control methods in recent years and attempting to predict the likelihood of particular products becoming available to the American consumer in the near future, we have both an optimistic and a pessimistic conclusion. On the positive side, several products either have proven or should in the near future prove their feasibility as birth control options. On the negative side, the extensive and expensive product testing required by FDA regulation, coupled with the fact that several of the more viable birth control options raise politically volatile issues, serves to make approval and availability of new options in the near future highly doubtful.

Our assessment of potential new birth control options for women is based on the evidence regarding their efficacy and safety presented in earlier chapters. Because the selection of a birth control method must be highly individualized, and because no product is appropriate for all women under all conditions, the options available to women desiring birth control should be maximized. Paternalistic preclusion of viable birth control options is not in the best interest of women. And religious reasons for making viable birth control options inaccessible to women are not acceptable in a society where those reasons are not universally accepted.

Perhaps the most promising and exciting new birth control option — and the one least likely to gain approval in the United States in the near future — is RU-486. Because of its multiple modes of effecting pregnancy prevention, it is clearly the most versatile birth control product yet developed (see Chapter 6). Not only is it highly effective under a variety of conditions, evidence to date also suggests that because of its short biological half-life (less than forty-eight hours), its side effects are short-lived. Safe and legal use of RU-486 could make the termination of an unwanted pregnancy a more personal and private matter than at present, substantially enhancing reproductive choice. Perhaps an organized political demand by those committed to maximizing reproductive choice could lead to its approval by the FDA and overcome the fear of boycott by religious groups that is likely to make pharmaceutical companies reluctant to market it.

Several of the new long-acting steroidal products also show considerable merit. These include the Norplant subdermal implants, injectables, vaginal rings, intracervical devices, and biodegradable systems (see Chapter 5). Because they are effective for up to five years, the Norplant systems are the most attractive of the long-term options. One of their major advantages, freeing the user of the need for conscious control of her contraceptive protection, does raise the kinds of moral concerns discussed in Chapter 5. But compared with RU-486, the Norplant systems are less politically volatile, because they are primarily contraceptive in their mode of action and because they are likely to be viewed as a longer-lasting version of an already accepted contraceptive — the pill. Especially for young women who desire a long period of contraceptive protection and who would otherwise probably use the pill, one of the Norplant systems would seem to be the ideal contraceptive choice. Continued success of Norplant systems in countries where they are currently available could also heighten the pressure for their approval in the United States.

Although far less widely tested than either RU-486 or long-acting steroidal systems, Gn-RH agonists may actually have a better chance at future approval. This is because they are truly contraceptive in nature, user controlled, readily reversible, and nonsteroidal. However, potential side effects may ultimately prevent their availability (see Chapter 5).

The introduction of a new and improved IUD (Copper T380A, GynoPharma) to the market is also a welcome development. As discussed at length in Chapter 6, the IUD, while clearly inappropriate for many women, is an appropriate and a relatively safe choice for many others.

We should also add that improvements continue to be made in existing birth control options. As we saw in Chapter 5, the pill is far safer and more effective today than at any other time in its thirty-year history. Improvements also continue to be made in two major over-the-counter products: condoms and vaginal spermicides.

Continued refinement and improvement of microsurgical techniques for reversing sterilization procedures for both men and women could conceivably make planned reversible sterilizations (admittedly a misnomer) a highly popular option in the near future.

And finally, as we project into the future, it is also conceivable that couples may one day be able to employ the safe and effective contraceptive option of sterilization and rely on fertility induction techniques if they desire to have a child. For example, a man may choose to store quantities of his sperm in sperm banks (since it may be stored in a cryopreserved state indefinitely) and then be vasectomized. Should he wish to father a child, he could have his sperm thawed and used in artificial insemination. Although techniques for cryopreservation of ova are not presently as advanced as those for sperm, the future may well provide women with a similar option. That is, a population of ova may be aspirated from a woman's ovaries and stored, and she could then have her Fallopian tubes ligated. At a later date, she could request that one (or more) of her ova be thawed and inseminated in vitro with either fresh or frozen sperm from her spouse or a donor. The blastocyst could then be transferred to her uterus and she could carry the offspring to term. Alternatively, the blastocyst could be transferred to a surrogate. These fertility-enhancing technologies and their various possible uses, however, raise a host of additional moral concerns that, although we cannot take them up here, are increasingly receiving attention in scientific, medical, philosophical, legal, feminist, and popular publications.

Acknowledgment of the rapid development of conception-enhancing technologies alongside the continued development of birth-limiting technologies brings us full circle to the point with which we began in Chapter 1, namely, that it is clear that human beings have always had a crucial interest in controlling when they will and when they will not reproduce. As that interest continues to play itself out in scientific and political arenas, we can surely expect to face new and renewed moral controversies. We hope that this book has contributed to the public understanding of the mechanisms of human reproduction and reproductive control and has provided some insight into how some of the past and present moral controversies surrounding human reproductive control have arisen. And we hope it has gone some way toward showing how such controversies might be sensitively and responsibly resolved.

# References

Aarskog, D. 1971. "Maternal Progestins as a Possible Cause of Hypospadias." *New England Journal of Medicine* 300:75.

Adler, Norman T., ed. 1981. *Neuroendocrinology of Reproduction*. New York: Plenum.

Ahmad, Mohammad M. 1979. "Contraception, Sterilization, and Pregnancy Termination." In *Human Reproduction: Physiology and Pathophysiology*, edited by R. W. Huff and C. J. Pauerstein. New York: Wiley.

Aitken, R. J. 1979. "Contraceptive Research and Development." *British Medical Bulletin* 35:199.

Aitken, R. J., and D. W. Richardson. 1980. "Immunization against Zona Pellucida Antigens." In *Immunological Aspects of Reproduction and Fertility Control*, edited by J. P. Hearn. Baltimore: University Park Press.

Alberman, E., M. Creasey, M. Elliot, and C. Spicer. 1976. "Maternal Factors Associated with Fetal Chromosomal Anomalies in Spontaneous Abortions." *British Journal of Obstetrics and Gynaecology* 83:261.

Albert, A. 1983. "Study of Pregnancies in Women with Intrauterine Devices of Copper." *Reproduction* 7:25.

Alexander, N. J. 1985. "Monoclonal Antibodies Directed against Human Sperm Antigens." In *Future Aspects in Contraception: Male*, edited by B. Runnebaum, T. Rabe, and L. Kiesel. Boston: MTP Press.

Allen, Hilary. 1984. "At the Mercy of Her Hormones: Premenstrual Tension and the Law." *MIF* 9:19.

Ambrus, C. M., K. R. Nisivander, N. G. Courey, and I. B. Mink. 1970. "Effect of Contraceptive Drugs on the Blood Coagulation System." *Hematology Review* 2:163.

American College of Obstetricians and Gynecologists. 1983. *Sterilization by Laparoscopy*. Washington, D.C.: American College of Obstetricians and Gynecologists.

American Medical Association. 1871. *Transactions of the American Medical Association* 22.

Annas, George J. 1982. "Forced Cesareans: The Most Unkindest Cut of All." *Hastings Center Report* 12(3):16.

————. 1986. "Pregnant Women as Fetal Containers." *Hastings Center Report* 16(6):13.

————. 1987. Letters. *Hastings Center Report* 17(3):26.

Application of President and Directors of Georgetown College, 331 F 2d 1000 (D.C. Cir. 1964). Cert den. 337 U.S. 978.

Aref, I., and E. S. E. Hafez. 1977. "Postcoital Contraception: Physiological and Clinical Parameters." *Obstetrics and Gynecology Survey* 32:417.

Associated Press. 1987. "Copper IUD to Become Available in U.S. in 1988." *Lexington Herald Leader*, October 29, p. A4.

Astedt, Birger. 1982. "Oral Contraceptives and Some Debatable Side Effects." *Acta Obstetricia and Gynecologica Scandanavica (Supplement)* 105:17.

Astruc, Johannes. 1738. *De Morbio Venereis*. Paris: n.p.

Avellan, L. 1977. "On Aetiological Factors in Hypospadias." *Scandinavian Journal of Plastic and Reconstructive Surgery* 11:115.

Bahl, Oim P., and Kambadur Muralidhar. 1980. "Current Status of Antifertility Vaccines." In *Immunological Aspects of Infertility and Fertility Regulation*, edited by D. S. Dhindsa and G. F. B. Schumacher. Amsterdam: Elsevier/North Holland.

Bajaj, J. S., and R. Madan. 1983. "New Approaches to Male Fertility Regulation: LHRH Analogs, Steroidal Contraception, and Inhibin." In *Endocrine Mechanisms in Fertility Regulation*, edited by G. Benagiano and E. Diczfalusy. New York: Raven.

Baker, T. G. 1982. "Oogenesis and Ovulation." In *Reproduction in Mammals*, vol. 1, *Germ Cells and Fertilization*, 2d ed., edited by C. R. Austin and R. V. Short. Cambridge: Cambridge University Press.

Barnes, Ann B. 1979. "Menstrual History of Young Women Exposed in Utero to Diethylstilbestrol." *Fertility and Sterility* 32:148.

Barrie, H. 1976. "Congenital Malformation Associated with Intrauterine Contraceptive Device." *British Medical Journal* 1:488.

Baulieu, E. E. 1985. "RU486: An Antiprogestin Steroid with Contragestive Activity in Women." In *The Antiprogestin Steroid RU486 and Human Fertility Control*, edited by E. E. Baulieu and S. J. Segal. New York: Plenum.

———. 1987. "Contragestin by the Progesterone Antagonist RU486: A Novel Approach to Human Fertility Control." *Research in Reproduction* 19:3.

Bayliss, W. M., and E. H. Starling. 1904. "The Clinical Regulation of the Secretory Process." *Proceedings of the Royal Society of London* B73:310.

Beck, L. R., D. R. Cowsar, D. H. Lewis, J. W. Gibson, and C. E. Flowers. 1979. "New Long-acting Injectable Microcapsule Contraceptive System." *American Journal of Obstetrics and Gynecology* 135:419.

Beck, L. R., D. R. Cowsar, and V. Z. Pope. 1980. "Long-acting Steroidal Contraceptive Systems." *Research Frontiers in Fertility Regulation* 1, no. 1.

Beck, L. R. and V. Z. Pope. 1984. "Long-acting Injectable Norethisterone Contraceptive Systems: Review of Clinical Studies." *Research Frontiers in Fertility Regulation* 3, no. 2.

Beck, L. R. and Thomas R. Tice. 1983. "Poly (Lactic Acid) and Poly (Lactic Acid-co-glycolic Acid) Contraceptive Delivery Systems." In *Advances in Human Fertility and Reproductive Endocrinology*, vol. 2, *Long-acting Steroid Contraception*, edited by D. R. Mishell. New York: Raven.

Bedford, J. M. 1975. "Maturation Transport and Fate of Spermatozoa in the Epididymis." In *Handbook of Physiology*, vol. 5, edited by D. W. Hamilton and R. O. Greep. Washington, D.C.: American Physiological Society.

Belenger, A., F. Labrie, A. Lemay, S. Caron, and J. P. Raynaud. 1980. "Inhibitory Effects of a Single Intranasal Administration of (D-Ser (TBU)$^6$des-GLy NH$_2$$^{10}$) LHRH Agonist on Serum Steroid Levels in Normal Adult Men." *Journal of Steroid Biochemistry* 13:123.

Beling, C. G., L. L. Cederqvist, and F. Fuchs. 1976. "Demonstration of Gonadotropin during the Second Half of the Cycle in Women Using Intrauterine Contraception." *American Journal of Obstetrics and Gynecology* 125:855.

Benagiano, G. 1977. "Long-acting Systemic Contraceptives." In *Regulation of Human Fertility*, edited by E. Diczfalusy. Copenhagen: Scriptor.

Benagiano, G., and I. S. Fraser. 1981. "The Depo-Provera Debate: Commentary on the Article Depo-Provera, a Critical Analysis." *Contraception* 24:493.

Benagiano, G., and F. M. Primiero. 1983a. "Long Acting Contraceptives: Present Status." *Drugs* 25:570.

———. 1983b. "Norethindrone Enanthate." In *Advances in Human Fertility and Reproductive Endocrinology*, vol. 2, *Long-acting Steroidal Contraception*, edited by D. R. Mishell. New York: Raven.

Benirschke, Kurt. 1986. "Cytogenetics in Reproduction." In *Reproductive Endocrinology: Physiology, Pathophysiology and Clinical Management*, edited by S. S. C. Yen and R. B. Jaffe. Philadelphia: Saunders.

Benjamin, Martin. 1979. "Moral Agency and Negative Acts in Medicine." In *Medical Responsibility: Paternalism, Informed Consent, and Euthanasia*, edited by Wade Robison and Michael Pritchard. Clifton, N.J.: Humana.

Benn, S. I. 1973. "Abortion, Infanticide, and Respect for Persons." In *The Problem of Abortion*, edited by Joel Feinberg. Belmont, Calif.: Wadsworth. (Reprinted in *The Problem of Abortion*, 2d ed., 1984.)

Bennett, John P. 1974. *Chemical Contraception*. New York: Columbia University Press.

Bennett v. Hymers, 101 N.H. 483, 147 A 2d 108 (1958).

Berger v. Weber, 82 Mich. App. 199, 267 N.W.2d 124 (1978).

Bernstein, E. Lennard. 1940. "Who Was Condom?" *Human Fertility* 5:172.

Berqquist, C., S. J. Nillius, and L. Wide. 1979. "Intranasal Gonadotropin-releasing Hormone Agonist as a Contraceptive Agent." *Lancet* 2:215.

———. 1982. "Long-term Intranasal Luteinizing Hormone-releasing Hormone Agonist Treatment for Contraception in Women." *Fertility and Sterility* 38:190.

Berqquist, C., S. J. Nillius, L. Wide, and A. Lindgren. 1981. "Endometrial Patterns in Women on Chronic Luteinizing Hormone-releasing Hormone Agonist Treatment for Contraception." *Fertility and Sterility* 36:339.

Berry, C. L., ed. 1976. "Human Malformations." *British Medical Bulletin* 32:1.

Bertin, Joan E. 1989. "Reproductive Health Hazards in the Workplace." In *Reproductive Laws for the 1990s*, edited by Sherrill Cohen and Nadine Taub. Clifton, N.J.: Humana.

Besant, Annie. 1879. *The Law of Population: Its Consequences, and Its Bearing upon Human Conduct and Morals*. London: Freethought.

Bhiwandiwala, P. P., S. D. Mumford, and P. J. Feldblum. 1982. "Menstrual Pattern Changes following Laparoscopic Sterilization." *Obstetrics and Gynecology* 27:249.

Biale, Rachel. 1984. *Women and Jewish Law: An Exploration of Women's Issues in Halakhic Sources*. New York: Schocken.

Bibbo, M., W. B. Gill, F. Azizi, R. Blough, V. S. Fang, R. L. Rosenfield, G. R. Schumacker, K. Sleeper, M. G. Sonek, and G. L. Wied. 1977. "Follow-up Study of Male and Female Offspring of DES-exposed Mothers." *Obstetrics and Gynecology* 49:1.

Bibbo, M., W. Haenszel, G. Wied, M. Hubby, and A. Herbst. 1978. "A Twenty-five Year Follow-up of Women Exposed to Diethylstilbestrol." *New England Journal of Medicine* 298:763.

Blatt, Robin J. R. 1987. "To Choose or Refuse Prenatal Testing." *Genewatch* 4:3.

Bloom, W. and D. Fawcett. 1966. *Textbook of Histology*. Philadelphia: Saunders.

Bolton, Martha Brandt. 1979. "Responsible Women and Abortion Decisions." In

*Having Children: Philosophical and Legal Reflections on Parenthood*, edited by Onora O'Neill and William Ruddick. New York: Oxford University Press.

Bonbrest v. Kotz, 65 F. Supp. 138 (DDC. 1946).

Bondeson, William B., H. Tristram Engelhardt, Jr., Stuart F. Spicker, and Daniel H. Winship, eds. 1983. *Abortion and the Status of the Fetus*. Boston: D. Reidel.

Bonte, J., J. M. Decoster, P. Ide, and G. Billiet. 1978. "Hormonoprophylaxis and Hormonotherapy in the Treatment of Endometrial Adenocarcinoma by Means of Medroxyprogesterone Acetate." *Gynecological Oncology* 6:60.

Boorse, Christopher. 1977. "Health as a Theoretical Concept." *Philosophy of Science* 44:542.

Boserup, Ester. 1970. *The Conditions of Agricultural Growth: The Economics of Agrarian Change under Population Pressure*. London: Allen and Unwin.

Boston Women's Health Book Collective. 1984. *The New Our Bodies, Ourselves*. New York: Simon and Schuster.

Boué, A. and J. Boué. 1973. "Actions of Steroid Contraceptives on Genetic Material." *Geburtsh Frauenheilk* 33:77.

Boué, J., A. Boué, and P. Lazar. 1975. "The Epidemiology of Human Spontaneous Abortions with Chromosomal Anomalies." In *Aging Gametes*, edited by R. J. Blandan. Basel: Karger.

Bower v. Hardwick, 92 LE 2d 140 (1986).

Bowes, Watson A., Jr., and Brad Selgestad. 1981. "Fetal versus Maternal Rights: Medical and Legal Perspectives." *Obstetrics and Gynecology* 58:209.

Bracken, M. B., T. R. Holford, C. White, and J. L. Kelsey. 1978. "Role of Oral Contraceptives in Congenital Malformations of Offspring." *International Journal of Epidemiology* 7:309.

Bracken, M. B., and K. Vita. 1983. "Frequency of Non-Hormonal Contraception around Conception and Association with Congenital Malformations in Offspring." *American Journal of Epidemiology* 117:281.

Bradley, D. D., J. Wingerd, D. B. Petitti, R. M. Drauss, and S. Ramcharan. 1978. "Serum High-Density-Lipoprotein Cholesterol in Women Using Oral Contraceptives, Estrogens, and Progestins." *New England Journal of Medicine* 299:17.

Breibart, S., A. M. Bongiovanni, and W. R. Eberlein. 1963. "Progestins and Skeletal Maturation." *New England Journal of Medicine* 268:255.

Brenner, W. E., and D. A. Edelman. 1974. "Dilation and Evacuation at 13 to 15 Weeks' Gestation versus Intra-Amniotic Saline after 15 Weeks' Gestation." *Contraception* 10:171.

———. 1980. "Menstrual Regulation: Risks and Abuses." In *The Safety of Fertility Control*, edited by Louis G. Keith. New York: Springer.

Bromwich, Peter, and Tony Parsons. 1984. *Contraception: The Facts*. Oxford: Oxford University Press.

Brooks, J. R., C. Berman, M. Hichens, R. L. Primka, G. F. Reynolds, and G. H. Rasmusson. 1982. "Biological Activities of a New Steroidal Inhibitor of $A^4$-5$\alpha$-reductase (41309)." *Proceedings of the Society for Experimental Biology and Medicine* 169:67.

Brown, Edward, Chris Hackler, Helga Kuhse, and Colin Thomson. 1987. "The Latest Word." *Hastings Center Report* 17(2):51.

Brown-Woodman, P. D. C., H. Mohri, T. Mohri, D. Suter, and I. G. White. 1978. "Mode of Action of $\alpha$-chlorohydrin as a Male Antifertility Agent: Inhibition of the Metabolism of Ram Spermatozoa by $\alpha$-chlorohydrin and Location of Block in Glycolysis." *Biochemical Journal* 170:23.

Brueschke, E. E., R. A. Kalackas, J. R. Wingfield, T. J. Welsh, and L. J. D. Zaneveld. 1980. "Development of a Reversible Vas Deferens Occlusion Device: VII. Physical and Microscopic Observations after Long-term Implantation of Flexible Prosthetic Devices. *Fertility and Sterility* 33:167.

Brueschke, E. E., L. J. D. Zaneveld, R. Kalackas, and J. R. Wingfield. 1979. "Development of a Reversible Vas Deferens Occlusive Device: VI. Long-term Evaluation of Flexible Prosthetic Devices. *Fertility and Sterility* 31:575.

Buck v. Bell, 274 U.S. 200 (1927).

Burgus, R., M. Butcher, M. Amoss, N. Ling, M. Monshan, J. Rivier, R. Fellows, R. Blackwell, W. Vale, and R. Guillemin. 1972. "Primary Structure of the Ovine Hypothalamic Luteinizing Hormone Releasing Factor (LRF)." *Proceedings of the National Academy of Science USA* 69:278.

Burton, F. G., W. E. Skiens, and G. W. Duncan. 1979. "Low-level, Progestogen-releasing Vaginal Contraceptive Devices." *Contraception* 19:507.

Burton, F. G., W. E. Skiens, N. R. Gordon, J. T. Veal, D. R. Kalkwarf, and G. W. Duncan. 1978. "Fabrication and Testing of Vaginal Contraceptive Devices Designed for Release of Prespecified Dose Levels of Steroids." *Contraception* 17:221.

Calhoun, Arthur W. 1919. *The Social History of the American Family.* Vol. 3. New York: Barnes and Noble.

Callahan, Daniel. 1973. "The WHO Definition of Health." *Hastings Center Studies* 1(3):77.

Callahan, Joan C. 1986a. "The Fetus and Fundamental Rights." *Commonweal* 11(April):203. (Revised and expanded in *Abortion and Catholicism: The American Debate*, edited by Thomas A. Shannon and Patricia B. Jung [New York: Crossroads].)

———. 1986b. "Paternalism and Voluntariness." *Canadian Journal of Philosophy* 16:199.

———. 1986c. "The Silent Scream: A New, Conclusive Argument against Abortion?" *Philosophy Research Archives* 11(1985):181.

———. 1988a. "Acts, Omissions, and Euthanasia." *Public Affairs Quarterly* 2(2):21.

———, ed. 1988b. *Ethical Issues in Professional Life.* New York: Oxford University Press.

Cannon, W. B. 1932. *The Wisdom of the Body.* New York: Norton.

Carlile, Richard. 1826. *Every Woman's Book; or What is Love?* London. (Published previously in Carlile's journal, *The Republican* 11:18 [May 1825].)

Carr, D. H. 1970. "Chromosome Studies in Selected Spontaneous Abortions: 1. Conception after Oral Contraceptives." *Journal of the Canadian Medical Association* 103:343.

Carr-Saunders, A. M. 1922. *The Population Problem.* Oxford: Clarendon Press.

Carson, S. A. and J. L. Simpson. 1983. "Virilization of Female Fetuses following Maternal Ingestion of Progestational and Androgenic Steroids." In *Hirsutism and Virilization*, edited by V. B. Mahesh and R. B. Greenblatt. Boston: John Wright.

Cates, W., Jr. 1982. "Abortion Myths and Realities: Who Is Misleading Whom?" *American Journal of Obstetrics and Gynaecology* 142:954.

Cates, W., Jr., D. A. Grimes, J. C. Smith, and C. W. Tyler, Jr. 1977. "The Risk of Dying from Legal Abortion in the United States, 1972–1975." *International Journal of Gynaecology and Obstetrics* 15:172.

Chang, C. C., and H. J. Tatum. 1973. "Absence of Teratogenicity of Intrauterine Copper Wire in Rats, Hamsters, and Rabbits." *Contraception* 7:413.

Chrisafogeorgis v. Brandenberg, 55 Ill. 2d 368, 304 N.E. 2d 88 (1973).

Christine, G. Maxwell. 1890. "The Medical Profession and Criminal Abortion." In *Transactions of the Homeopathic Medical Society of the State of Pennsylvania* 25(1889):70.

Clark, Colin. 1967. *Population Growth and Land Use.* London: MacMillan.

Clark, Matt, Patricia King, Linda Buckley, and Karen Springen. 1987. "Doctors Grapple with Ethics." *Newsweek*, December 28, p. 62.

Clark, Matt, Karen Springen, and Bruce Alderman. 1986. "An Effective Abortion Pill." *Newsweek*, December 29, p. 62.

Clayton, R. N., and K. J. Catt. 1981. "Gonadotrophin Hormone Releasing Hormone Receptors: Characterization, Physiological Regulation and Relationship to Reproductive Function." *Endocrine Review* 2:186.

Clermont, Y. 1963. "The Cycle of the Seminiferous Epithelium in Man." *American Journal of Anatomy* 112:35.

Clouser, K. Danner, Charles M. Culver, and Bernard Gert. 1981. "Malady: A New Treatment of Disease." *Hastings Center Report* 11(3):29.

Cohen, M. R., G. N. Pandya, and A. Scommegna. 1970. "The Effect of an Intracervical Steroid-releasing Device on the Cervical Mucus." *Fertility and Sterility* 21:715.

Connell, Elizabeth B. 1978. "The Pill: Risks and Benefits." In *Hormonal Contraceptives, Estrogens, and Human Welfare*, edited by M. C. Diamond and C. C. Korenbrat. New York: Academic Press.

Cooke, G. M., and B. Robaire. 1986. "The Effects of Diethyl-4-methyl-3-oxo-4-aza-5α-androstane-17β-carboxamide (4-MA) and (4R)-5,10-seco-19-norpregna-4,5-diene-3,10,20-trione (SECO) on Androgen Biosynthesis in the Rate Testis and Epididymis." *Journal of Steroid Biochemistry* 24:877.

Cordero, J. F., and P. M. Layde. 1983. "Vaginal Spermicides, Chromosomal Abnormalities and Limb Reduction Defects." *Family Planning Perspectives* 15:16.

Corea, Gena. 1985. *The Mother Machine.* New York: Harper & Row.

Council on Environmental Quality. 1981. *Chemical Hazards to Human Reproduction.* Washington: U.S. Government Printing Office.

Coutinho, E. W., and A. R. Da Silva. 1974. "One Year Contraception with Norgestrienone Subdermal Silastic Implants." *Fertility and Sterility* 25:170.

Cramer, Daniel, M. B. Goldman, I. Shiff, S. Belisle, B. Albrecht, B. Stadel, M. Gibson, E. Wilson, R. Stillman, and I. Thompson. 1987. "The Relationship of Tubal Infertility to Barrier Method and Oral Contraceptive Use." *Journal of the American Medical Association* 257:2446.

Cramer, Daniel, I. Shiff, S.C. Schoenbaum, M. Gibson, S. Belisle, B. Albrecht, R. J. Stillman, M. J. Berger, E. Wilson, B. V. Stadel, and M. Seibel. 1985. "Tubal Infertility and the Intrauterine Device." *New England Journal of Medicine* 312:941.

Crist, T., and C. Farrington. 1973. "The Use of Estrogens as a Post-Coital Contraceptive in North Carolina — Trick or Treatment?" *North Carolina Medical Journal* 34:792.

Croll, Elizabeth, Delia Davin, and Penny Kane, eds. 1985. *China's One-Child Family Policy.* New York: St. Martin's.

Cross, B. A. 1972. "The Hypothalamus." In *Reproduction in Mammals,* vol. 3, *Hormones in Reproduction,* edited by C. R. Austin and R. V. Short. Cambridge: Cambridge University Press.

Croxatto, H. B., S. Vera, E. Quinteros, L. Simonette, E. Kaplan, R. Renenet, P. Leixeland, and C. Martinez. 1975. "Clinical Assessment of Subdermal Implants of Megestrol Acetate, d-norgestrel and Norethindrone as a Long Term Contraceptive in Women." *Contraception* 12:615.

Croxatto, H. B., S. Diaz, R. Vera, M. Etchart, and P. Atria. 1969. "Fertility Control in Women with a Progestin Released in Microquantities from Subcutaneous Capsules." *American Journal of Obstetrics and Gynecology* 105:1135.

Csapo, A. I., J. P. Sanvage, and W. G. Weist. 1970. "The Relationship between Progesterone, Uterine Volume, Intrauterine Pressure, and Clinical Progress in Hypertonic Saline-induced Abortions." *American Journal of Obstetrics and Gynecology* 108:950.

Culver, Charles M., and Bernard Gert. 1982. *Philosophy in Medicine: Conceptual and Ethical Issues in Medicine and Psychiatry*. New York: Oxford University Press.

Curlender v. Bio-Science Laboratories and Automated Laboratory Sciences, 165 Calif. Rpt. 477 (1980).

Cziezel, A., J. Toth, and E. Erodi. 1979. "Aetiological Studies of Hypospadias in Hungary." *Human Heredity* 29:166.

Dalton, K. 1964. *The Premenstrual Syndrome*. Springfield, Ill.: Charles C. Thomas.

————. 1970. "Children's Hospital Admission and Mother's Menstruation." *British Medical Journal* 2:27.

————. 1971. *The Menstrual Cycle*. New York: Warner.

————. 1976. "The Curse of Eve." *Occupational Health* 28:129.

————. 1977. *The Premenstrual Syndrome and Progesterone Therapy*. London: William Heinemann Medical Books.

————. 1980. "Criminal Acts in Premenstrual Syndrome." *Lancet* 2:1070.

————. 1984. *The Premenstrual Syndrome and Progesterone Therapy*. Chicago: Yearbook Medical Publishers.

Damon, A. 1974. "Larger Body Size and Earlier Menarche: The End May Be in Sight." *Social Biology* 21:8.

Davis, H. J. 1971. *Intrauterine Devices for Contraception: The IUD*. Baltimore: Williams and Wilkins.

Davis, J. E. 1980. "New Methods of Vas Occlusion." In *Research Frontiers in Fertility Regulation*, edited by G. I. Zatuchni, M. Labbock, and J. J. Sciarria. Hagerstown, Md.: Harper & Row.

Davis, Nancy. 1984. "Abortion and Self Defense." *Philosophy and Public Affairs* 13:175.

DeBoer, C. H. 1972. "Transport of Particulate Matter through the Human Female Genital Tract." *Journal of Reproduction and Fertility* 28:295.

Degler, Carl N. 1980. *At Odds: Women and the Family in America from the Revolution to the Present*. New York: Oxford University Press.

DeLacoste-Utamsing, C., and R. L. Holloway. 1982. "Sexual Dimorphism in the Human Corpus Callosum." *Science* 216:1431.

Delaney, Janice, Mary Jane Lupton, and Emily Toth. 1976. *The Curse: A Cultural History of Menstruation*. New York: Dutton.

Denes, Magda. 1977. *In Necessity and Sorrow*. New York: Penguin.

de Sousa, Ronald. 1985. "Arguments from Nature." In *Morality, Reason, and Truth: New Essays on the Foundations of Ethics*, edited by David Copp and David Zimmerman. Totowa, N.J.: Rowman and Allanheld.

De Stefano, R., H. B. Peterson, and P. M. Layde. 1982. "Risk of Ectopic Pregnancy following Tubal Sterilization." *Obstetrics and Gynecology* 60:326.

Devereux, George. 1976. *A Study of Abortion in Primitive Societies*. Rev. ed. New York: International Universities Press.

Devlin, Patrick. 1959. *The Enforcement of Morals*. Oxford: Oxford University Press.

de Vries, G. J., J. P. de Bruin, H. B. M. Uylings, and M. A. Corner. 1984. *Progress in Brain Research*. Amsterdam: Elsevier.

Diaz, S., M. Paves, P. Miranda, D. N. Robertson, I. Sivin, and H. B. Croxatto. 1982. "A Five-Year Clinical Trial of Levonorgestrel Silastic Implants (Norplant)." *Contraception* 12:615.

Diczfalusy, Egon. 1979. "Gregory Pincus and Steroidal Contraception: A New Departure in the History of Mankind." *Journal of Steroid Biochemistry* 11:3.

_____. 1982. "Gregory Pincus and Steroidal Contraception Revisited." *Acta Obstetricia and Gynecologica Scandanavica (Supplement)* 105:7.

Dietrich v. Inhabitants of Northampton, 138 Mass. 14 (1884).

Dixon, R. L. 1980. "Toxic Responses of the Reproductive System." In *Toxicology: The Basic Science of Poisons*, edited by J. Doull, C. D. Klassen, and M. O. Amdur. New York: Macmillan.

Djerassi, Carl. 1981. *The Politics of Contraception: The Present and the Future*. San Francisco: W. H. Freeman.

Donceel, Joseph F. 1970a. "Immediate Animation and Delayed Hominization." *Theological Studies* 31:76.

_____. 1970b. "A Liberal Catholic's View." In *Abortion in a Changing World*, vol. 1, edited by Robert E. Hall. New York: Columbia University Press.

Dougherty, Charles. 1986. "The Right to Begin Life with Sound Body and Mind: Fetal Patients and Conflicts with Their Mothers." *University of Detroit Law Review* 63(1–2):89.

Dreishpoon, I. H. 1975. "Complications of Pregnancy with an Intrauterine Contraceptive in Place." *American Journal of Obstetrics and Gynecology* 121:412.

Dumontier, A., A. Burdick, B. Ewigman, and M. S. Tahim. 1977. "Effects of Sonication on Mature Rat Testes." *Fertility and Sterility* 28:195.

Duncan, H. C. 1929. *Race and Population Problems*. New York: Longmans.

Dziuk, P. J. and B. Cook. 1966. "Passage of Steroids through Silicone Rubber." *Endocrinology* 78:208.

Edelman, D. A., G. S. Berger, and L. G. Keith. 1980. "Major Complications of Intrauterine Devices." In *The Safety of Fertility Control*, edited by Louis G. Keith. New York: Springer.

Edelman, D. A., W. E. Brenner, and G. S. Berger. 1974. "The Effectiveness and Complications of Abortion by Dilation and Vacuum Aspiration versus Dilation and Rigid Curettage." *American Journal of Obstetrics and Gynecology* 119:473.

Edmonds, D. K., K. S. Lindsay, J. F. Miller, E. Williamson, and P. J. Wood. 1982. "Early Embryonic Mortality in Women." *Fertility and Sterility* 38:447.

Edwards, R. G. 1980. *Conception in the Human Female*. London: Academic Press.

_____, ed. 1988. "Gossypol: Further Studies as a Male Contraceptive." *Research in Reproduction* 20, no. 1.

Eisenstadt v. Baird, 405 U.S. 438 (1972).

Eli, G. E., and M. Newton. 1961. "The Transport of Carbon Particles in the Human Female Reproductive Tract." *Fertility and Sterility* 12:151.

Ellinas, Symeon P. 1980. "Medroxyprogesterone Acetate (Depo-Provera): An Injectable Contraceptive." In *The Safety of Fertility Control*, edited by Louis G. Keith. New York: Springer.

English, Jane. 1975. "Abortion and the Concept of a Person." *Canadian Journal of Philosophy* 5:233.

Fawcett, D. W. 1979. "The Organization of the Seminiferous Epithelium, Its Relevance to Fertility Control." In *Contraception: Science, Technology, and Application*. Washington, D.C.: National Academy of Sciences.

_____. 1982. "Approaches to Fertility Control in the Male." In *Basic Reproductive Medicine*, Vol. 2, *Reproductive Function in Men*, edited by David Hamilton and Frederick Naftolin. Cambridge, Mass.: MIT Press.

Feinberg, Joel. 1970. "Crime, Clutchability, and Individuated Treatment." In *Doing and Deserving: Essays in the Theory of Responsibility*. Princeton: Princeton University Press.

_____, ed. 1973. *The Problem of Abortion*. Belmont, Calif.: Wadsworth.

_____. 1980. "Abortion." In *Matters of Life and Death*, edited by Tom Regan. New York: Random House.

_____. 1984a. *Harm to Others*. New York: Oxford University Press.

_____, ed. 1984b. *The Problem of Abortion*. 2d ed. Belmont, Calif.: Wadsworth.

_____. 1985a. "Comment: Wrongful Conception and the Right Not to Be Harmed." *Harvard Journal of Law and Public Policy* 8:57.

_____. 1985b. *Offense to Others*. New York: Oxford University Press.

_____. 1988. *Harmless Wrongdoing*. New York: Oxford University Press.

Field, Marilyn Jane. 1983. *The Comparative Politics of Birth Control: Determinants of Policy Variation and Change in the Developed Nations*. New York: Praeger.

Finkel, N. C., and B. R. Berliner. 1973. "The Extrapolation of Experimental Findings (Animal to Man): The Dilemma of Systemically Administered Contraceptives." *Bulletin of the Society of Pharmacology and Environmental Pathology* 4:13.

Fitzgerald, P. J. 1967. "Acting and Refraining." *Analysis* 27:133.

Fletcher, Joseph. 1979. *Humanhood: Essays in Biomedical Ethics*. Buffalo, NY: Prometheus.

Fluhmann, C. Frederick. 1939. *Menstrual Disorders: Pathology, Diagnosis and Treatment*. Philadelphia: Saunders.

Foot, Philippa. 1967. "The Problem of Abortion and the Doctrine of Double-Effect." *Oxford Review* 5:5.

Ford, W. C. L., and A. Harrison. 1983. "The Activity of Glyceraldehyde 3-phosphate Dehydrogenase in Spermatozoa from Different Regions of the Epididymis in Laboratory Rodents Treated with $\alpha$-chlorohydrin or 6-chlorodeoxyghicose." *Journal of Reproduction and Fertility* 69:147.

Ford, W. C. L., and G. M. H. Waites. 1982. "Activities of Various 6-chloro-6-deoxy-sugars and (S)-$\alpha$-chlorohydrin in Producing Spermatocoeles in Rats and Paralysis in Mice and in Inhibiting Glucose Metabolism in Bull Spermatozoa." *Journal of Reproduction and Fertility* 65:177.

Forsyth, Adrian. 1986. *A Natural History of Sex*. New York: Scribner.

Fortney, J. A., and L. E. Laufe. 1978. "Menstrual Regulation—Risks and Benefits." In *Risks and Benefits and Controversies in Fertility Control*, edited by J. J. Sciarra, G. I. Zatuchni, and J. J. Speidel. Hagerstown, Md.: Harper & Row.

Fortune, J. E., and D. T. Armstrong. 1978. "Hormonal Control of 17$\beta$-estradiol Biosynthesis in Proestrus Rat Follicles: Estradiol Production by Isolated Theca verses Granulosa." *Endocrinology* 102:227.

Francke, Linda Bird. 1978. *The Ambivalence of Abortion*. New York: Dell.

Frank, R. T. 1931. "The Hormonal Cause of Premenstrual Tension." *Archives of Neurology and Psychiatry* 26:1053.

Franklin, Deborah. 1987. "Brave New Pill." *Hippocrates*, May-June, p. 22.

Fraser, F. C. 1978. "Prevention of Birth Defects: How Are We Doing?" *Teratology* 17:198.

Fraser, I. S. 1981. "Abnormal Uterine Bleeding Due to Hormonal Steroids and Intrauterine Devices." In *Recent Advances in Fertility Regulation,* edited by C. F. Chang, D. Griffin, and A. Wollman. Geneva: World Health Organization.

———. 1982. "Long-acting Injectable Hormonal Contraceptives." *Clinical Reproduction and Fertility* 1:67.

Fraser, I. S., and S. Holck. 1983. "Depot Medroxyprogesterone Acetate." In *Advances in Human Fertility and Reproductive Endocrinology,* vol. 2, *Long-Acting Steroid Contraception,* edited by D. R. Mishell. New York: Raven.

Fraser, I. S., and E. Weisberg. 1981. "A Comprehensive Review of Injectable Contraception with Special Emphasis on Depot Medroxyprogesterone Acetate." *Medical Journal of Australia* (Supplement) 1:1.

Fraser, Laura. 1988. "Pill Politics." *Mother Jones* 12(5):30.

French, F. E., and J. M. Bierman. 1972. "Probability of Fetal Mortality." *Public Health Reports* 77:835.

Frick, J., C. Danner, R. Kohle, and G. Kunit. 1981. "Male Fertility Regulation." In *Research on Fertility and Sterility,* edited by J. Cortes-Prieto, A. Campos da Paz, and M. Neves-e-Castro. Baltimore: University Park Press.

Fryer, Peter. 1965. *The Birth Controllers.* London: Seeker and Warburg.

Furst, A., and R. T. Haro. 1969. "A Survey of Metal Carcinogenesis." *Progress in Experimental Tumor Research* 12:102.

Gal, I., B. Kirman, and J. Stern. 1967. "Hormonal Pregnancy Tests and Neural Tube Defects." *Nature* 216:83.

Gallegos, A. J. 1980. "Vaginal Steroidal Contraception." In *Research Frontiers in Fertility Regulation,* edited by G. I. Zatuchni, M. H. Labbock, and J. J. Sciarra. Hagerstown, Md.: Harper & Row.

Garcia, Celso-Roman. 1987. "Surgical Treatment of Infertility." In *Gynecologic Endocrinology,* 4th ed. edited by J. J. Gold and J. B. Josimovich. New York: Plenum.

Garmendia, F., E. Kesseru, E. Urdanivia, and M. Valencia. 1976. "Luteinizing Hormone and Progesterone in Women under Postcoital Contraception with D-norgestrel." *Fertility and Sterility* 29:275.

Gebhard, Paul, et al. 1958. *Pregnancy, Birth, and Abortion.* New York: Hoeber and Harper.

George, Susan. 1977. *How the Other Half Dies: The Real Reasons for World Hunger.* Montclair, N.J.: Allanheld, Osmun.

Gilman, J. P. W. 1962. "Metal Carcinogenesis: II. A Study on the Carcinogenesis Activity of Cobalt, Copper, Iron, and Nickel Compounds." *Cancer Research* 22:158.

Glantz, Leonard. 1983. "Is the Fetus a Person? A Lawyer's View." In *Abortion and the Status of the Fetus,* edited by William B. Bondeson, H. Tristam Engelhardt, Jr., Stuart F. Spicker, and Daniel H. Winship. Boston: D. Reidel.

Glass, David V. 1940. *Population Policies and Movements in Europe.* Oxford: Clarendon Press.

Glover, Jonathon. 1977. *Causing Death and Saving Lives.* New York: Penguin.

Goldberg, E. 1983. "Current Status of Research on Sperm Antigens: Potential Applications as Contraceptive Vaccines." *Research Frontiers in Fertility Regulation* 2, no. 6.

Goldman, Peter. 1987. "The Face of AIDS." *Newsweek,* August 10, p. 22.

Goldmann, A. S., S. Katsumata, R. Jaffe, and D. L. Gasser. 1977. "Palatal Cytosol Cortisol Binding Protein Associated with Cleft Palate Susceptibility and $H_2$ Genotypes." *Nature* 245:643.

Goldsmith, A., D. A. Edelman, and G. I. Zatuchni. 1985. "Transcutaneous Male Sterilization." *Research Frontiers in Fertility Regulation* 3, no. 4.

Goldzieher, J. W. 1970. "An Assessment of the Hazards and Metabolic Alterations Attributed to Oral Contraceptives." *Contraception* 1:409.

Gorovitz, Samuel. 1982. *Doctors' Dilemmas: Moral Conflict and Medical Care.* New York: Macmillan. (Reissued, New York: Oxford University Press, 1985.)

Gould, K. G., and A. H. Ansari. 1983. "Non-Hormonal Modification of Cervical Mucus." In *Proceedings of the International Symposium on Reproductive Health Care: Contraceptive Delivery Systems,* vol. 3, abstract 40.

Gray, R. H. 1980. "Patterns of Bleeding Associated with Use of Steroidal Contraceptives." In *Endometrial Bleeding and Steroid Contraception,* edited by E. Diczfalusy, I. S. Fraser, and F. T. G. Webb. Bath: Pitman.

———. 1983. "Progestins in Therapy: Teratogenesis." In *Progestogens in Therapy,* edited by G. Benagiano. New York: Raven Press.

Green, J. D., and G. W. Harris. 1947. "The Neurovascular Link between the Neurohypophysis and Adenohypophysis." *Journal of Endocrinology* 5:136.

Green, O. H. 1980. "Killing and Letting Die." *American Philosophical Quarterly* 17:195.

Green, Shirley. 1971. *The Curious History of Contraception.* New York: St. Martin's.

Green, Willard, and Charles Brill. 1987. Letters. *Hastings Center Report* 17(3):25.

Greenberg, G., W. H. W. Inman, J. A. C. Weatherall, A. M. Adelstein, and J. C. Haskey. 1977. "Maternal Drug Histories and Congenital Abnormalities." *British Medical Journal* 2:853.

Greep, R. O. 1974. "History of Research on Anterior Hypophysial Hormones." In *Handbook of Physiology,* Vol. 4, *Endocrinology.* Washington, D.C.: American Physiological Society.

Grimes, D. A., K. E. Schulz, W. Cates, Jr., and C. W. Tyler, Jr. 1980. "The Safety of Midtrimester Abortion." In *The Safety of Fertility Control,* edited by Louis G. Keith. New York: Springer.

Grisez, Germain. 1970. *Abortion: The Myths, the Realities, and the Arguments.* New York: Corpus Books.

Griswold v. Connecticut, 381 U.S. 479 (1965).

Gruhn, John G. 1987. "Historical Introduction to Gonadal Regulation of the Uterus and the Menses. In *Gynecologic Endocrinology,* 4th ed., edited by J. J. Gold and J. B. Josimovich. New York: Plenum.

Grumbach, M. M., J. R. Ducharme, and R. E. Moloshok. 1959. "On the Fetal Masculinizing Action of Certain Oral Progestins." *Journal of Clinical and Endocrinological Metabolism* 19:1369.

Guilleband, J. 1976. "IUD and Congenital Malformations." *British Medical Journal* 1:1016.

Guillemin, R. 1978. "Biochemical and Physiological Correlates of Hypothalamic Peptides: The New Endocrinology of the Neuron." In *The Hypothalamus,* edited by S. Reichlin, R. J. Baldessarini, and J. B. Martin. New York: Raven.

Guttmacher, Alan. 1973. "General Remarks on Medical Aspects of Male and Female Sterilization." In *Eugenic Sterilization,* edited by Jonas Robitscher. Springfield, Ill.: Charles C. Thomas.

Hafez, E. S. E. 1978. *Perspectives in Human Reproduction.* vol. 5, *Human Reproductive Physiology.* Ann Arbor, Mich.: Ann Arbor Science.

Hahn, Do Won, J. L. McGuire, and M. C. Chang. 1980. "Contragestational Agents." In *Research Frontiers in Fertility Regulation,* edited by G. Zatuchni, M. H. Labbock, and J. J. Sciarra. Hagerstown, Md.: Harper & Row.

Hallberg, L., A. Hogdahl, L. Nillson, and G. Rybo. 1966. "Menstrual Blood Loss: A Population Study." *Acta Obstetricia and Gynecologica Scandanavica (Supplement)* 45:320.

Halpern, Sue M. 1987. "RU-486: The Unpregnancy Pill." *Ms.*, April, p. 56.

Harper, M. J. K. 1982. "Sperm and Egg Transport." In *Reproduction in Mammals,* Vol. 1, *Germ Cells and Fertilization,* 2d ed., edited by C. R. Austin and R. V. Short. Cambridge: Cambridge University Press.

——. 1983. *Birth Control Technologies: Prospects by the Year 2000.* Austin: University of Texas Press.

Harris, G. W. 1948. "Electrical Stimulation of the Hypothalamus and the Mechanism of Neural Control of the Adenohypophysis." *Journal of Physiology* (London) 107:418.

Harris, John. 1974. "The Marxist Conception of Violence." *Philosophy and Public Affairs* 3:192.

Harrison, Beverly Wildung. 1983. *Our Right to Choose: Toward a New Ethic of Abortion.* Boston: Beacon.

Hart v. Brown, 29 Conn. Supp. 368, 289 A.2d 386 (Conn. Sup. Ct. 1972).

Hart, H. L. A. 1963. *Law, Liberty, and Morality.* Stanford: Stanford University Press.

Hartmann, Betsy. 1987. *Reproductive Rights and Wrongs: The Global Politics of Population Control and Contraceptive Choice.* New York: Harper & Row.

Haspels, A. A. 1976. "Interception: Postcoital Estrogens in 3016 Women." *Contraception* 14:375.

Haspels, A. A., and R. Andriesse. 1973. "The Effect of Large Doses of Estrogens Post-Coitum in 2000 Women." *European Journal of Obstetrics, Gynaecology, and Reproductive Biology* 3:113.

Hastings Center. 1973. *The Concept of Health.* Hastings Center Studies, vol. 1, no. 3. Hastings-on-Hudson, N.Y.: Hastings Center.

Hatcher, R. A., G. K. Steward, F. Stewart, F. Guest, D. W. Schwartz, and S. A. Jones. 1980. *Contraceptive Technology 1980–1981.* New York: Irvington.

Hayes v. Shelby Memorial Hospital, 726 F 2d 1543 (11th Cir. 1984).

Hayles, A. B., and R. B. Nolan. 1957. "Female Pseudohermaphroditism: Report of Case in an Infant Born of a Mother Receiving Methyltestosterone during Pregnancy." *Mayo Clinic Proceedings* 32:41.

Hearn, J. P. 1978. "Immunological Interference with the Maternal Recognition of Pregnancy in Primates." In *Maternal Recognition of Pregnancy,* Ciba Foundation Symposium no. 64. Amsterdam: Elsevier/North Holland.

——. 1979. "Long Term Suppression of Fertility by Immunization with hCG-subunit and Its Reversibility in Female Marmoset Monkeys." In *Advances in Reproduction and Regulation of Fertility,* edited by G. P. Talivar. Amsterdam: Elsevier/North Holland.

Heinonen, O. P., D. Slone, R. R. Monson, E. B. Hook, and S. Shapiro. 1976. "Cardiovascular Birth Defects in Antenatal Exposure to Female Sex Hormones." *New England Journal of Medicine* 296:67.

Heinonen, O. P., D. Slone, and S. Shapiro. 1977. *Birth Defects and Drugs in Pregnancy.* Littleton, Mass.: Public Sciences Group.

Heller, C. G., and Y. Clermont. 1964. "Kinetics of the Germinal Epithelium in Man." *Recent Progress in Hormone Research* 20:545.

Heller, C. G., B. Y. Flagsolle, and L. J. Matron. 1964. "Histopathology of the Human Testis as Affected by Bis-(dichloroacetyl)-diamines." *Experimental and Molecular Pathology Supplement* 2:107.

Heller, C. G., W. M. Laidlaw, H. T. Harvey, and W. O. Nelson. 1958. "Effects of Progestational Compounds on the Reproductive Process of the Human Male." *Annals of the New York Academy of Science* 71:649.

Henifin, Mary Sue. 1987. "What's Wrong with 'Wrongful Life' Court Cases?" *Genewatch* 4:1.

Henifin, Mary Sue, Ruth Hubbard, and Judy Norsigan. 1989. "Genetic Screening, Therapeutic Abortion, and Reproductive Choice." In *Reproductive Laws for the 1990s.* Clifton, N.J.: Humana.

Henshaw, Stanley. 1987a. "Induced Abortion: A Worldwide Perspective." *International Family Planning Perspectives* 18:250.

———. 1987b. "Abortion Services in the United States, 1984–85." *Family Planning Perspectives* 19:63.

Henzl, Milan R. 1986. "Contraceptive Hormones and Their Clinical Use." In *Reproductive Endocrinology: Physiology, Pathophysiology, and Clinical Management,* 2d ed., edited by S. S. C. Yen and R. B. Jaffe. Philadelphia: Saunders.

Heyner, Susan. 1980. "Antigens of Trophoblast and Early Embryo." In *Immunological Aspects of Infertility and Fertility Regulation,* edited by D. S. Dhindsa and G. F. B. Schumacher. Amsterdam: Elsevier/North Holland.

Heywood, R. 1986. "An Assessment of the Toxicological and Carcinogenic Hazards of Contraceptive Steroids." In *Contraceptive Steroids: Pharmacology and Safety,* edited by A. T. Gregoire and R. P. Blye. New York: Plenum.

Himes, Norman E. 1936. *Medical History of Contraception.* New York: National Committee on Maternal Health. (Reissued, New York: Gamut Press, 1963.)

Hingorani, V. and S. Kumar. 1979. "Anti-hCG Immunization—Phase I Clinical Trials." In *Recent Advances in Reproduction and Regulation of Fertility,* edited by G. P. Talwar. Amsterdam: Elsevier/North Holland.

Hodgen, G. D., H. C. Chen, M. L. Dufau, T. A. Klein, and D. R. Mishell. 1978. "Transitory hCG-like Activity in the Urine of Some IUD Users." *Journal of Clinical Endocrinology and Metabolism* 46:698.

Hoffman, Mark S., ed. 1986. *The World Almanac and Book of Facts, 1987.* New York: Pharos.

Holmes, R. L., and C. A. Fox. 1979. *Control of Human Reproduction.* London: Academic Press.

Hornbuckle v. Plantation Pipe Line, 212 Ga. 504, 93 S.E.2d 727 (1956).

Hrdy, S. B. 1981. *The Woman That Never Evolved.* Cambridge, Mass.: Harvard University Press.

Hsu, C., A. Ferenczy, R. M. Richart, and K. Darabi. 1976. "Endometrial Morphology with Copper-bearing Intrauterine Devices." *Contraception* 14:243.

Huggins, G., M. Vessey, and R. Flavil. 1982. "Vaginal Spermicides and Outcome of Pregnancy: Findings of a Large Cohort Study." *Contraception* 25:219.

Hurst, Jane. 1983. *The History of Abortion in the Catholic Church.* Washington, D.C.: Catholics for a Free Choice.

Husak, Douglas. 1980. "Omissions, Causation, and Liability." *Philosophical Quarterly* 30:318.

Imperato-McGinley, J., L. Guerrero, T. Gautier, and R. E. Peterson. 1974. "Steroid 5α-reductase Deficiency in Man: An Inherited Form of Male Pseudohermaphroditism." *Science* 186:1213.

In re Baby X, 97 Mich. App. 111, 293 N.W.2d 736 (1980).

In re Greene, 52 F. 104 (CCW Ohio 1892).

Insler, V., M. Glexerman, L. Zeidel, D. Berenstein, and N. Misgav. 1980. "Sperm Storage in the Human Cervix: A Quantitative Study." *Fertility and Sterility* 33:288.

Jackson, H. 1970. "Antispermatogenic Agents." *British Medical Bulletin* 26:79.

Jackson, H., and B. Robinson. 1976. "The Antifertility Effects of α-chlorohydrins and Their Steroe-isomers in Male Rats." *Chemico-Biological Interactions* 13:193.

Jacobsen, Glenn D., and Howard P. Krieger. 1977. "Gross Anatomy of the Female Reproductive Tract, Pituitary, and Hypothalamus." In *Obstetrics and Gynecology*, 3d ed., edited by David N. Danforth. Hagerstown Md.: Harper & Row.

Jacobsen, Judith. 1983. *Promoting Population Stabilization: Incentives for Small Families.* Worldwide Paper 54. Washington, D.C.: Worldwatch Institute.

Jaffe, R. B. 1978. "The Endocrinology of Pregnancy." In *Reproductive Physiology*, edited by S. S. C. Yen and R. B. Jaffe. Philadelphia: Saunders.

———. 1986. "Disorders of Sexual Development." In *Reproductive Endocrinology: Physiology, Pathophysiology, and Clinical Management*, 2d ed., edited by Suzanne Boyd. Philadelphia: Saunders.

Janerich, D. T., J. M. Dugan, S. J. Standfast, and L. Strite. 1977. "Congenital Heart Disease and Prenatal Exposure to Exogenous Sex Hormones." *British Medical Journal* 1:1058.

Janerich, D. T., and A. P. Polednak. 1983. "Epidemiology of Birth Defects." *Epidemiologic Review* 5:16.

Janerich, D. T., J. M. Piper, and D. M. Glebatis. 1974. "Oral Contraceptives and Congenital Limb-Reduction Defects." *New England Journal of Medicine* 291:697.

Janowsky, D. S., R. Gorney, and B. Kelley. 1966. "The Curse: Vicissitudes and Variations of the Female Cycle. I. Psychiatric Aspects." *Psychosomatics* 7:242.

Jaszmann, L. J. B. 1976. "Epidemiology of the Climacteric Syndrome." In *The Management of the Menopause and Postmenopausal Years*, edited by S. Campbell. Baltimore: University Park Press.

Jefferson v. Griffin Spalding County Hospital Authority, 247 Ga. 86, 274 S.E.2d 457 (1981).

Jensen, Karen. 1982. *The Human Body: Reproduction: The Cycle of Life.* Washington: U.S. News Books.

Jick, H., A. M. Walder, K. J. Rothman, J. R. Hunter, L. B. Holmes, R. N. Watkins, D. C. D'Ewart, A. Danford, and S. Madsen. 1981. "Vaginal Spermicides and Congenital Disorders." *Journal of the American Medical Association* 245:1329.

Johansson, E. D. B. 1981. "Steroidal Contraceptives: New Modalities." In *Research on Sterility and Fertility*, edited by J. Cortes-Prieto, A. Campos da Paz, and M. Neves-e-Castro. Baltimore: University Park Press.

Johansson, E. D. B., T. Luukkainen, E. Vertianinen, and A. Victor. 1975. "The Effect of Progestin R2323 Released from Vaginal Rings on Ovarian Function." *Contraception* 12:299.

Johansson, E. D. B., and V. Odlind. 1983. "NORPLANT: Biochemical Effects." In *Advances in Human Fertility and Reproductive Endocrinology*, vol. 2, *Long-acting Steroid Contraception*, edited by D. R. Mishell, New York: Raven.

Johnsen, Dawn. 1987. "A New Threat to Pregnant Women's Autonomy." *Hastings Center Report* 17(4):33.

Johnson, P. M., P. J. Brown, and W. P. Faulk. 1980. "Immunobiological Aspects of the Human Placenta." In *Oxford Reviews of Reproductive Biology*, vol. 2, edited by C. A. Finn. Oxford: Oxford University Press.

Jones, A. R. 1978. "The Antifertility Actions of α-chlorohydrin in the Male." *Life Sciences* 23:1625.

———. 1980. "Immunological Factors in Male and Female Infertility." In *Immunological Aspects of Reproduction and Fertility Control,* edited by J. P. Hearn. Baltimore: University Park Press.

Jones, G. S., and A. C. Wentz. 1977. "Adolescence, Menstruation, and Climacteric." In *Obstetrics and Gynecology,* 3d ed., edited by David N. Danforth. Hagerstown, Md.: Harper & Row.

Jones, H. W., Jr., E. J. Cohen, and R. B. Wilson. 1972. *Clinical Aspects of the Menopause.* DHEW Publication no. (NIH) 73. Washington, D.C.: Department of Health, Education and Welfare.

Jost, A. 1970. "Hormonal Factors in the Sex Differentiation of the Mammalian Foetus." *Philosophical Transactions of the Royal Society* B259:119.

Juliano, R. L. 1980. "Controlled Delivery of Drugs: An Overview and Prospectus." In *Drug Delivery Systems,* edited by R. L. Juliano. New York: Oxford University Press.

Karsch, F. J. 1984. "The Hypothalamus and Anterior Pituitary Gland." In *Reproduction in Mammals,* vol. 3, *Hormonal Control of Reproduction,* 2d ed., edited by C. R. Austin and R. V. Short. Cambridge: Cambridge University Press.

Katsh, S. 1959. "Immunology, Fertility, and Infertility: A Historical Survey." *American Journal of Obstetrics and Gynecology* 77:946.

Katz, Z., M. Lancet, J. Skornik, J. Chemke, B. M. Mogilner, and M. Klinberg. 1985. "Teratogenicity of Progestogens Given during the First Trimester of Pregnancy." *Obstetricia and Gynecologica Scandanavica* 55:221.

Katzenellenbogen, B. S. 1986. "Estrogens and Carcinogenicity: An Overview of Information from Studies in Experimental Animal Systems." In *Contraceptive Steroids: Pharmacology and Safety,* edited by A. T. Gregoire and R. P. Blye. New York: Plenum.

Kaufman, D., S. Shapiro, D. Slone, L. Rosenberg, O. S. Miettinen, P. D. Stolley, R. C. Knapp, T. Leavitt, Jr., W. G. Watring, N. B. Rosenshein, J. L. Lewis, Jr., D. Schottenfeld, and R. L. Engle, Jr. 1980. "Decreased Risk of Endometrial Cancer among Oral Contraceptive Users." *New England Journal of Medicine* 303:1045.

Kaufman, R. H., G. I. Binder, P. M. Gray, Jr., and E. Adam. 1977. "Upper Genital Tract Changes Associated with Exposure in Utero to Diethylstilbestrol." *American Journal of Obstetrics and Gynecology* 128:51.

Kearslake, D., and D. Casey. 1967. "Abortion Induced by Means of the Uterine Aspirator." *Obstetrics and Gynecology* 39:35.

Keith, L. G., and G. S. Berger. 1980. "Progestogens, Congenital Defects, and Pregnancy." In *The Safety of Fertility Control,* edited by Louis G. Keith. New York: Springer.

Kesseru-Koos, E., H. Hurtado-Koo, A. Larranaga-Leguia, and H. J. Scharff. 1973. "Fertility Control with Norethindrone Enanthate, a Long-acting Parenteral Progestogen." *Acta European Fertility* 4:203.

Kesseru-Koos, E., A. Larranaga, and J. Parada. 1973. "Post-Coital Contraception with d-norgesterel." *Contraception* 7:367.

Kesseru-Koos, E., P. Noack, and A. Larranaga-Leguia. 1971. "Urinary Pregnanediol during the Use of Different Contraceptive Methods." *Acta Endocrinology Panama* 2:73.

Kirkpatrick, D., J. Schneider, and E. P. Patterson. 1975. "Large Bowel Perforation by Intrauterine Devices." *Obstetrics and Gynecology* 46:610.

Kirton, K. T., R. J. Ericsson, J. A. Ray, and A. D. Forbes. 1970. "Male Antifertility Compounds: Efficacy of U-5897 in Primates (Macaca Mulatta)." Journal of Reproduction and Fertility 21:275.

Kisch, E. H. 1910. The Sexual Life of Woman in Its Physiological, Biological, and Hygienic Aspects. Translated by Paul M. Eden. New York: Rebman.

Knowlton, Charles. 1832. The Fruits of Philosophy. New York.

Koeske, Randi. 1976. "Premenstrual Emotionality: Is Biology Destiny?" Women and Health 1:11.

———. 1983. "Lifting the Curse of Menstruation: Toward a Feminist Perspective on the Menstrual Cycle." Women and Health 8:1.

Koob, G. F., and F. E. Bloom. 1983. "Behavioral Effects of Opioid Peptides." British Medical Bulletin 39:89.

Kovacs, L., B. Resh, J. Szolloso, and J. Herczog. 1970. "The Role of Fetal Death in the Process of Therapeutic Abortion Induced by Intra Amniotic Injection of Hypertonic Saline." Journal of Obstetrics and Gynecology of the British Commonwealth 77:1132.

Kuchera, L. A. 1974. "Postcoital Contraception with Diethylstilbestrol—Updated." Contraception 10:47.

Kullander, S. and B. Kallen. 1976. "A Prospective Study of Drugs and Pregnancy." Acta Obstetricia and Gynecologica Scandanavica 55:221.

Labrie, F., A. Galanger, L. Cusan, C. Sequin, G. Pelletier, P. A. Kelly, J. J. Reeves, F. Lefevre, A. Lemay, Y. Gourdeau, and J. P. Raynand. 1980. "Antifertility Effects of LHRH Agonists in the Male." Journal of Andrology 1:209.

Lammer, E. J., and J. F. Cordero. 1986. "Exogenous Sex Hormone Exposure and the Risk for Major Malformations." Journal of the American Medical Association 255:3128.

Landesman, R., E. M. Coutinho, and B. B. Saxena. 1976. "Detection of Human Chorionic Gonadotropin in Blood of Regularly Bleeding Women Using Copper Intrauterine Contraceptive Devices." Fertility and Sterility 27:1062.

Landing, B. H., A. Goldin, and H. A. Noe. 1949. "Testicular Lesions in Mice following Parenteral Administration of Nitrogen Mustard." Cancer 2:1075.

Langerak, Edward A. 1979. "Abortion: Listening to the Middle." Hastings Center Report 9(5):24.

Lappe, Francis Moore, and Joseph Collins. 1977. Food First: Beyond the Myth of Scarcity. Boston: Houghton Mifflin.

Lauersen, Niels H. 1979. "Investigation of Prostaglandins for Abortion." Acta Obstetricia and Gynecologica Scandanavica (Supplement) 81:1.

———. 1980. "Prostaglandins and Fertility Control." In The Safety of Fertility Control, edited by Louis G. Keith. New York: Springer.

Laurence, M., M. Miller, M. Vowles, K. Evans, and C. Carter. 1971. "Hormonal Pregnancy Tests and Neural Tube Defects." Nature 233:495.

Lauritsen, J. G. 1975. "The Significance of Oral Contraceptives in Causing Chromosome Anomalies in Spontaneous Abortions." Acta Obstetricia and Gynecologica Scandanavica 64:261.

———. 1982. "The Cytogenetics of Spontaneous Abortion." Research in Reproduction 14(3):3.

Layde, P. M., M. F. Goldberg, M. J. Safra, and G. P. Oakley, Jr. 1979. "Failed Intrauterine Device Contraception and Limb Reduction Deformities: A Case Control Study." Fertility and Sterility 31:18.

Lea, O. A., P. Petrus, and F. S. French. 1978. "Purification and Localization of an

Acidic Epididymal Protein (AEG): A Sperm Coating Protein Secreted by the Rat Epididymis." *International Journal of Andrology* (Supplement) 2:592.

Lehfeldt, H. 1973. "Choice of Ethinyl Estradiol as a Postcoital Pill." Letter to the editor. *American Journal of Obstetrics and Gynecology* 116:892.

Lei, H. P., and Z. Y. Hu. 1981. "The Mechanisms of Action of Vacation Pills." In *Recent Advances in Fertility Regulation*, edited by C. F. Chang, D. Griffin, and A. Woolman. Geneva: Atar SA.

Leiberman, J. R., M. Mazor, W. Chaim, and A. Cohen. 1979. "The Fetal Right to Live." *Obstetrics and Gynecology* 53:515.

Leighton, P. C., D. G. Evans, and S. M. Wallis. 1976. "IUD and Congenital Malformations." *British Medical Journal* 1959.

Leiser, Burton M. 1986. *Liberty, Justice, and Morals: Contemporary Value Conflicts.* 3d ed. New York: Macmillan.

Lenow, Jeffrey L. 1983. "The Fetus as Patient: Emerging Legal Rights as a Person?" *American Journal of Law and Medicine* 9:1.

Levi, Don S. 1987. "Hypothetical Cases and Abortion." *Social Theory and Practice* 13:17.

Levy, E. P., A. Cohen, and F. C. Freaser. 1973. "Hormone Treatment during Pregnancy and Congenital Heart Disease." *Lancet* 1:611.

Libbee v. Permanente Clinic, 268 OR 258, 518 P 2d 636. Reh'g den. 268 OR 272, 520 P 2d 361. App dismissed. 269 OR 543, 525 P 2d 1296, (1974).

Linde, R., G. C. Doelle, N. Alexander, F. Kirchner, W. Vale, J. Rivier, and D. Rabin. 1981. "Reversible Inhibition of Testicular Steroidogenesis and Spermatogenesis by a Potent Gonadotropin-releasing Hormone Agonist in Normal Men." *New England Journal of Medicine* 305:663.

Linnet, J., T. Hjort, and P. Fogh-Anderson. 1981. "Association between Failure to Impregnate after Vasovasostomy and Sperm Agglutinins in Semen. *Lancet* 1:117.

Lipsett, M. B. 1977. "Estrogen Use and Cancer Risk." *Journal of the American Medical Association* 237:1112.

————. 1986. "Steroids and Carcinogenesis." In *Contraceptive Steroids: Pharmacology and Safety*, edited by A. T. Gregoire and R. P. Blye. New York: Plenum.

Liu, Z. Q., G. Z. Liu, L. S. Hei, R. A. Zhang, and C. Z. Yu. 1981. "Clinical Trial of Gossypol as a Male Antifertility Agent." In *Recent Advances in Fertility Regulation*, edited by C. F. Chang, D. Griffin, and A. Woolman. Geneva: Atar SA.

Lobl, T. J. 1980. "α-chlorohydrin: Review of a Model Post-Testicular Antifertility Agent." In *Regulation of Male Fertility*, edited by G. R. Cunningham, W. B. Schill, and E. S. E. Hafez. Netherlands: Martinus Nijhoff.

Loebl, Suzanne. 1974. *Conception, Contraception: A New Look.* New York: McGraw-Hill.

Lomansky, Loren E. 1984. "Being a Person—Does It Matter?" *The Problem of Abortion*, 2d ed., edited by Joel Feinberg. Belmont, Calif.: Wadsworth.

Louik, C., A. A. Mitchell, M. M. Werler, J. W. Hanson, and S. Shapiro. 1987. "Maternal Exposure to Spermicides in Relation to Certain Birth Defects." *New England Journal of Medicine* 135:761.

Luker, Kristen. 1984. *Abortion and the Politics of Motherhood.* Berkeley: University of California Press.

McCredie, J., A. Kricker, J. Elliot, and J. Forrest. 1983. "Congenital Limb Defects and the Pill." *Lancet* 2:623.

McCullagh, D. R. 1932. "Dual Endocrine Activity of the Testis." *Science* 76:19.

McDaniel, Ann, George Raine, and Ginny Carroll. 1986. "A Government in the Bedroom: In a Sodomy Case, the High Court Rules against Gays." *Newsweek*, July 14, p. 36.

MacIntyre, Alasdair. 1981. *After Virtue*. Notre Dame, Ind.: University of Notre Dame Press.

Mack, Eric. 1976. "Causing and Failing to Prevent." *Southwest Journal of Philosophy* 7:83.

————. 1980. "Bad Samaritanism and the Causation of Harm." *Philosophy and Public Affairs* 9:230.

Mack, T. M., M. C. Pike, and B. E. Henderson. 1976. "Estrogens and Endometrial Cancer in a Retirement Community." *New England Journal of Medicine* 237:1112.

McKenzie, John L. 1965. *Dictionary of the Bible*. S. v. "Onan." New York: Bruce.

Mackenzie, Thomas B., and Theodore C. Nagel. 1986. "When a Pregnant Woman Endangers Her Fetus: Commentary." *Hastings Center Report* 16(1):24.

Macklin, Ruth. 1972. "Mental Health and Mental Illness: Some Problems of Definition and Concept Formation." *Philosophy of Science* 39:341.

McLaren, Angus. 1983. *Sexuality and the Social Order: The Debate over the Fertility of Women and Workers in France, 1770–1920*. New York: Holmes and Meier.

McLauren, A. 1982. "The Embryo." In *Reproduction in Mammals*, vol. 2, *Embryonic and Fetal Development*, 2d ed., edited by C. R. Austin and R. V. Short. Cambridge: Cambridge University Press.

MacLusky, Neil J., and Frederick Naftolin. 1981. "Sexual Differentiation of the Central Nervous System." *Science* 211:1294.

Marshall, J. 1971. "The Risks of Conception throughout the Menstrual Cycle." *Medical Contrapoint* 3:147.

Marut, Edward L. 1987. "Premenstrual Tension and Idiopathic Edema." In *Gynecologic Endocrinology*. 4th ed., edited by J. J. Gold and J. B. Josimovich. New York: Plenum.

Masters, W. H., V. E. Johnson, and R. C. Kolodny. 1986. *Sex and Human Loving*. Boston: Little, Brown.

Mastroianni, L., Jr., and B. Zausner. 1981. "Transport of Gametes in the Female Reproductive Tract: An Appraisal." In *Research on Fertility and Sterility*, edited by J. Cortes-Prieto, A. Campos da Paz, and M. Neves-e-Castro. Baltimore: University Park Press.

Mathieu, Deborah. 1985. "Respecting Liberty and Preventing Harm." *Harvard Journal of Law and Public Policy* 8:19.

Matsuo, H., Y. Baba, R. M. G. Nair, A. Arimura, and A. V. Schally. 1971. "Structure of the Porcine LH- and FSH-releasing Hormone. I. The Proposed Amino Acid Sequence." *Biochemistry and Biophysics Research Communications* 43:1334.

Mattison, Donald R. 1983. "The Mechanisms of Action of Reproductive Toxins." *American Journal of Industrial Medicine* 4:65.

Mead, Margaret. 1971. *Chemical and Engineering News*, October 21. (Quoted in Carl Djerassi, *The Politics of Contraception: The Present and the Future* [San Francisco: W. H. Freeman, 1981].)

Means, Cyril C. 1968. "The Laws of New York Concerning Abortion and the Status of the Fetus, 1644–1968: A Case of Cessation of Constitutionality." *New York Law Forum* 14:419.

Meek, Ronald L., ed. 1955. *Marx and Engels on Malthus*. London: Lawrence and Wishart. (Quoted in Rosalind Pollack Petchesky, *Abortion and Women's Choice: The State, Sexuality, and Reproductive Freedom* [New York: Longman, 1984].)

Mehrotra, P. K., and K. Srivastava. 1985. "Inflammatory Changes Induced by IUDs in Animal Models." In *Biomedical Aspects of IUDs*, edited by H. Hasson, E. S. E. Hafez, and W. A. van Os. Higham, Mass.: MTP Press.

Mehta, R. R., J. M. Jenco, and R. T. Chatterton. 1981. "Antiestrogenic and Antifertility Actions of Anoudrin." *Steroids* 38:679.

Menge, A. C. 1980. "Clinical Immunologic Infertility: Diagnostic Measures, Incidence of Antisperm Antibodies, Fertility, and Mechanisms." In *Immunologic Aspects of Infertility and Fertility Regulation*, edited by D. A. Dhindsa and G. F. B. Schumacher. New York: Elsevier/North Holland.

_____. 1986. "Sperm Antigens, Immunologic Infertility and Contraception." In *Immunological Approaches to Contraception and Promotion of Fertility*, edited by G. P. Talwar. New York: Plenum.

Menge, A. C., N. E. Medley, C. M. Mangione, and J. W. Dietrick. 1982. "The Incidence and Influence of Antisperm Antibodies in Infertile Human Couples on Sperm–Cervical Mucus Interactions and Subsequent Fertility." *Fertility and Sterility* 38:439.

Meyer-Bahlburg, H. F. L. 1984. "Psychoendocrine Research on Sexual Orientation: Current Status and Future Options." *Progress in Brain Research* 61:375.

Miller, E. G., and R. Kurzrak. 1932. "Biochemical Studies of Human Semen. III Factors Affecting Migration of Sperm through the Cervix." *American Journal of Obstetrics and Gynecology* 24:19.

Mills, J. L., and D. Alexander. 1986. "Teratogens and 'Litogens.'" *New England Journal of Medicine* 315:1234.

_____. 1987. Letter to the editor. *New England Journal of Medicine* 316:1093.

Mills, J. L., E. E. Harley, G. F. Reed, and H. W. Berendes. 1982. "Are Spermicides Teratogenic?" *Journal of the American Medical Association* 248:2148.

Mills, J. L., G. F. Reed, R. P. Nugent, E. E. Harley, and H. W. Berendes. 1985. "Are There Adverse Effects of Periconceptional Spermicide Use?" *Fertility and Sterility* 43:422.

Minkin, S. 1980. "Depo-Provera: A Critical Analysis." *Women's Health* 5:49.

Mischler, T. W., E. Berman, B. Rubio, A. Larranaga, E. Guiloff, and A. V. Moggia. 1974. "Further Experience with Quingestanol Acetate as a Post-Coital Oral Contraceptive." *Contraception* 9:221.

Mishell, D. R., Jr. 1977. "Control of Human Reproduction: Contraception, Induced Abortion, and Sterilization." In *Obstetrics and Gynecology*, 3d ed., edited by D. N. Danforth. Hagerstown, Md.: Harper & Row.

_____. 1979. "Oral Steroids." In *Reproductive Endocrinology, Infertility, and Contraception*, edited by D. R. Mishell, Jr. and Val Davajan. Philadelphia: F. A. Davis.

Mishell, D. R., Jr., M. Lumkin, and T. Jackaniz. 1975. "Initial Clinical Studies of Intra-vaginal Rings Containing Norethindrone and Norgestrel." *Contraception* 12:253.

Mishell, D. R., Jr., M. Lumkin, and S. Stone. 1972. "Inhibition of Ovulation with Cyclic Use of Progestogen-impregnated Intravaginal Devices." *American Journal of Obstetrics and Gynecology* 113:927.

Mishell, D. R., Jr., D. E. Moore, S. Roy, P. F. Brenner, and M. A. Page. 1978. "Clinical Performance and Endocrine Profiles with Contraceptive Vaginal Rings Containing a Combination of Estradiol and D-norgestrel." *American Journal of Obstetrics and Gynecology* 130:55.

Mishell, D. R., Jr., M. Talas, A. F. Parlow, and D. L. Moyer. 1970. "Contraception by Means of a Silastic Vaginal Ring Impregnated with Medroxyprogesterone Acetate." *American Journal of Obstetrics and Gynecology* 107:101.

Moghissi, K. S., F. G. Burton, W. E. Skiens, R. I. Leininger, M. R. Sikov, G. W. Duncan, and L. G. Smith. 1977. "An Intracervical Contraceptive Device. In *Proceedings: Drug Delivery Systems*, edited by H. L. Gabelnick. DHEW Publication no. (NIH) 77-1238. Washington, D.C.: Department of Health, Education and Welfare.

Mohr, James C. 1978. *Abortion in America: The Origins and Evolution of a National Policy, 1800-1900*. New York: Oxford University Press.

Monmaney, Terrence, Mary Hager, Karen Springen, and Lisa Drew. 1987. "A Black Health Crisis." *Newsweek*, July 13, p. 53.

Monteleone, R. N., E. E. Castilla, and J. E. Paz. 1981. "Hypospadias: An Epidemiologic Study in Latin America." *American Journal of Medical Genetics* 10:5.

Montreal Tramways v. Leveille, 4 Dom LR 337 (1933).

Moos, R. H. 1968. "The Development of the Menstrual Distress Questionnaire." *Psychosomatic Medicine* 30:853.

Morley, J. E. 1983. "Review: Effects of Endogenous Opioid Peptides in Human Subjects." *Psychoneuroendocrinology* 8:361.

Morris, J. M., and G. van Wagenen. 1973. "Interception: The Use of Post-Ovulatory Estrogens to Prevent Implantation." *American Journal of Obstetrics and Gynecology* 115:101.

Mosher, W. D. 1980. "Reproductive Impairments among Currently Married Couples: United States, 1976." In *Advanced Data from Vital Statistics and Health Statistics of the National Center for Health Statistics*. Washington, D.C.: Department of Health and Human Services.

Mossman, H. W., and K. L. Duke. 1973. *Comparative Morphology of the Human Ovary*. Madison: University of Wisconsin Press.

Moudgal, N. R. 1981. "A Need for FSH in Maintaining Fertility of Adult Male Subhuman Primates." *Archives of Andrology* 7:117.

Moyer, D. L., and S. T. Shaw, Jr. 1973. "Intrauterine Devices: Biological Action." In *Human Reproduction: Conception and Contraception*, edited by E. S. E. Hafez and T. N. Evans. Hagerstown, Md.: Harper & Row.

Muse, K. N., N. S. Cetel, L. A. Futterman, and S. S. C. Yen. 1984. "The Premenstrual Syndrome: Effects of 'Medical Ovariectomy.'" *New England Journal of Medicine* 311:1345.

Nash, H. 1975. "Depo-Provera: A Review." *Contraception* 12:377.

Nathanson, Bernard. 1985. *The Silent Scream*. Anaheim, Calif.: American Portrait Films. Videotape.

National Academy of Sciences. 1985. *Preventing Low Birthweight*. Prepared by the Committee to Study the Prevention of Low Birthweight, Institute of Medicine. Washington, D.C.: National Academy Press.

National Coordinating Group on Male Antifertility Agents. 1978. "Gossypol: A New Antifertility Agent for Males." *Chinese Medical Journal* 4:417.

Nelson, W. O., and R. G. Bunge. 1957. "Effect of Therapeutic Dosages of Nitrofurantoin (Furadantin) upon Spermatogenesis in Man." *Journal of Urology* 77:275.

Nelson, W. O., and E. Steinberger. 1952. "The Effect of Furadroxyl upon the Testis of the Rat." *Anatomical Record* 112:367.

Neumann, F. 1985. "Steroidal Contraception—Experimental Backgrounds." In *Future Aspects in Contraception: Male*, edited by B. Runnebaum, T. Rabe, and L. Kiesel. Boston: MTP Press.

Newton, J., and J. McEwan. 1977. "Hormone Releasing IUDs—A Proper Perspective Review." *Fertility and Contraception* 1:35.

*New York Times*. 1987. "Excerpts from the Ruling on Baby M." April 1, p. 13.

Nicholson, A. B., and C. Hanley. 1953. "Indices of Physiological Maturity: Derivation and Interrelationships. *Child Development* 24:3.

Nillius, S. J., C. Berqquist, L. Wide. 1978. "Inhibition of Ovulation in Women by Chronic Treatment with a Stimulatory LRH Analogue — A New Approach to Birth Control?" *Contraception* 17:537.

Nishimura, H., C. Uwabe, and R. Semba. 1974. "Examination of Teratogenicity of Progestogens and/or Estrogens by Observation of the Induced Abortuses." *Teratology* 10:93.

Noonan, John T., Jr. 1970. "An Almost Absolute Value in History." In *The Morality of Abortion: Legal and Historical Perspectives*, edited by John T. Noonan, Jr. Cambridge, Mass.: Harvard University Press.

Nora, A. H., and J. J. Nora. 1975. "A Syndrome of Multiple Congenital Anomalies Associated with Teratogenic Exposure." *Archives of Environmental Health* 30:17.

Nora, J. J., and A. H. Nora. 1973. "Preliminary Evidence for a Possible Association between Oral Contraceptives and Birth Defects." *Teratology* 7:A24.

North Central Bronx Hospital v. Headley, No. 1992–85 (N.Y. Sup. Ct. January 6, 1986).

North, Douglas C., and Robert P. Thomas. 1973. *The Rise of the Western World: A New Economic History*. Cambridge: Cambridge University Press.

Noyes, John Humphrey. 1849. *First Annual Report of the Oneida Community*. Oneida, N.Y.: n.p.

———. 1870. *Oneida Circular, VIII*. Oneida, N.Y.: n.p.

Oakley, G. P., J. W. Flynt, and A. Falek. 1973. "Hormonal Pregnancy Tests and Congenital Malformations." *Lancet* 2:256.

O'Connor, Sandra Day. 1983. Akron v. Akron Center for Reproductive Health. Dissenting opinion. 462 US 416.

Ohno, S. Y., Y. Nagai, S. Ciccarese, and H. Iwata. 1979. "Testis-organizing H-Y Antigen and the Primary Sex-determining Mechanism of Mammals." *Recent Progress in Hormone Research* 35:449.

O'Rand, M. G. 1980. "Antigens of Spermatozoa and Their Environment." In *Immunological Aspects of Infertility and Fertility Regulation*, edited by D. S. Dhindsa and G. F. B. Schumacher. New York: Elsevier/North Holland.

Organski, Katherine, and A. F. K. Organski. 1961. *Population and World Power*. New York: Knopf.

Orgebin-Crist, M. C., B. J. Danzo, and J. Davies. 1975. "Endocrine Control of the Development and Maintenance of Sperm Fertilizing Ability in the Epididymis." In *Handbook of Physiology*, vol. 5, edited by D. W. Hamilton and R. O. Greep. Washington: D.C.: American Physiological Society.

Ory, H. W. 1977. "Association between Oral Contraceptives and Myocardial Infarction." *Journal of the American Medical Association* 237:2619.

Overall, Christine. 1987. *Ethics and Human Reproduction: A Feminist Analysis*. Boston: Allen and Unwin.

Owen, Robert Dale. 1831. *Moral Physiology; or a Brief and Plain Treatise on the Population Question*. New York: Wright and Owen.

Palmer, J. H. 1875. *Individual, Family and National Poverty*. London: Truelove.

Pardthaison, T., R. H. Gray, and E. B. McDaniel. 1980. "Return of Fertility after Discontinuation of Depot Medroxyprogesterone Acetate and Intrauterine Devices in Northern Thailand." *Lancet* 1:509.

Parness, Jeffrey A. 1983. "The Duty to Prevent Handicaps: Laws Promoting the Prevention of Handicaps to Newborns." *Western New England Law Review* 5:431.

———. 1985. "Crimes against the Unborn: Protecting and Respecting the Potentiality of Human Life." *Harvard Journal on Legislation* 22:97.

———. 1986. "The Abuse and Neglect of the Human Unborn." *Family Law Quarterly* 20:197.

———. 1987. Letters. *Hastings Center Report* 17(3):26.

Parness, Jeffrey A., and Susan K. Pritchard. 1982. "To Be or Not to Be: Protecting the Unborn's Potentiality of Life." *University of Cincinnati Law Review* 51:257.

Patanelli, D. J., and W. L. Nelson. 1964. "A Quantitative Study of Inhibition and Recovery of Spermatogenesis." *Recent Progress in Hormone Research* 20:491.

Paul, Julius. 1973. "State Eugenic Sterilization History: A Brief Overview." In *Eugenic Sterilization*, edited by Jonas Robitscher. Springfield, Ill.: Charles C. Thomas.

People v. Estergard, 457 P.2d 698 (CO S. Ct. 1969).

People v. Stewart, No. M508197, San Diego Mun. Ct. (February 23, 1987).

Perelman, Michael. 1977. *Farming for Profits in a Hungry World: Capital and the Crisis in Agriculture*. Montclair, N.J.: Allanheld, Osmun.

Peschel, E. R., and R. E. Peschel. 1987. "Medical Insights into the Castrati in Opera." *American Scientist* 75 (November-December):578.

Petchesky, Rosalind Pollack. 1984. *Abortion and Women's Choice: The State, Sexuality, and Reproductive Freedom*. New York: Longman. (Reissued, Northeastern Series in Feminist Theory [Boston: Northeastern University Press, 1985].)

Philibert, D., M. Moguilewsky, I. Mary, D. Lecaque, C. Tournemine, J. Secchi, and R. Deraedt. 1985. "Pharmacological Profile of RU486 in Animals." In *The Antiprogestin Steroid RU486 and Human Fertility Control*, edited by E. E. Baulieu and S. J. Segal. New York: Plenum.

Phillips v. United States, 508 F. Supp. 537 (DSC. 1980).

Piotrow, P. T., W. Rinehart, and J. C. Schmidt. 1979. "IUDs—Update on Safety, Effectiveness and Research." *Population Research*, series B, no. 3.

Planned Parenthood Federation of America. 1985. *Ways to Chart Your Fertility Pattern*. New York: Planned Parenthood Federation of America.

———. 1986. *Basics of Birth Control*. New York: Planned Parenthood Federation of America.

Poland, B. 1970. "Conception Control and Embryonic Development." *American Journal of Obstetrics and Gynecology* 106:365.

Polednak, A. P., D. T. Janerich, and D. M. Glebatis. 1982. "Birth Weight and Birth Defects in Relation to Maternal Spermicide Use." *Teratology* 26:27.

Popa, G. T., and U. Fielding. 1930. "A Portal Circulation from the Pituitary to the Hypothalamic Region." *Journal of Anatomy* 65:88.

———. 1933. "Hypophysis-Portal Vessels and Their Colloid Accompaniment." *Journal of Anatomy* 67:227.

Population Institute. 1987. *A Blueprint for World Population Stabilization*. Washington, D.C.: Population Institute.

Porter, C. W., Jr., R. S. Waife, and H. R. Haltrop. 1983. *Contraception: The Health Provider's Guide*. New York: Grune & Stratton.

Potts, M., P. Diggory, and J. Peel. 1977. *Abortion*. Cambridge: Cambridge University Press.

Potts, D. M., and P. Diggory. 1973. "Termination of Pregnancy." In *Human Reproduction: Conception and Contraception*, edited by E. S. E. Hafez and T. N. Evans. Hagerstown, Md.: Harper & Row.

Prema, K., T. L. Gayathry, B. A. Ramalakshmi, R. Madhavapeddi, and F. S. Philips.

1981. "Low Dose Injectable Contraceptive Norethisterone Enanthate 20 mg Monthly. I. Clinical Trials." *Contraception* 23:11.

Quay, Eugene. 1960–61. "Justifiable Abortion: Medical and Legal Foundations." Parts 1, 2. *Georgetown Law Journal* 49:173, 295.

Rabe, T., L. Kiesel, and B. Runnebaum. 1985. "Future Aspects in Contraception: An Overview." In *Future Aspects in Contraception: Male*, edited by B. Runnebaum, T. Rabe, and L. Kiesel. Boston: MTP Press.

Rabin, D., R. Linde, G. Doelle, and N. Alexander. 1981. "Experience with a Potent Gonadotrophin Releasing Hormone Agonist in Normal Men: An Approach to the Development of a Male Contraceptive." In *LHRH Peptides as Female and Male Contraceptives*, edited by G. I. Zatuchni, J. D. Shelton, and J. J. Sciarra. Philadelphia: Harper & Row.

Rachels, James. 1975. "Active and Passive Euthanasia." *New England Journal of Medicine* 292:78.

Rainey v. Horn, 222 Miss. 269, 72 S.2d 434 (1954).

Raleigh Fitkin-Paul Morgan Memorial Hospital v. Anderson, 42 N.J. 421, 201 A.2d 337 (N.J. S. Ct. 1964).

Ratnam, S. S., and R. N. V. Prasad. 1980. "Recent Developments in Steroidal Contraception." *Singapore Journal of Obstetrics and Gynaecology* 3:7.

―――――. 1984. "New Approaches to Female Fertility Regulation: An Overview." In *Fertility and Sterility*, edited by R. F. Harrison, J. Bonnar, and W. Thompson. Boston: MTP Press.

Reddy, P. R. K., and J. M. Rao. 1972. "Reversible Antifertility Action of Testosterone Propionate in Human Males." *Contraception* 5:295.

Regnier, Mathurin. 1609. "Les Satyrs." In *Oeuvres Completes*. Paris: n.p., 1958.

Reid, R. L., and S. S. C. Yen. 1981. "Premenstrual Syndrome." *American Journal of Obstetrics and Gynecology* 139:85.

Reijonen, K., M. Kormano, and R. J. Ericsson. 1975. "Studies on the Rat Epididymal Blood Vessels following Alpha-chlorohydrin Administration." *Biology of Reproduction* 12:483.

Reilly, W. A., F. Hiniman, D. E. Pickering, and J. T. Crane. 1958. "Phallic Urethra in Female Pseudohermaphroditism." *American Journal of Diseases of Children* 95:9.

Renfree, M. B. 1982. "Implantation and Placentation." In *Reproduction in Mammals*, vol. 2, *Embryonic and Fetal Development*, 2d ed., edited by C. R. Austin and R. V. Short. Cambridge: Cambridge University Press.

Renslow v. Mennonite Hospital. 67 IL 2d 348, 369 NE 2d 1250 (1977).

Reuter, E. B. 1923. *Population Problems*. Philadelphia: Lippincott.

*Revised Statutes of New York, 1828–1835 Inclusive*. 1836. vol. 1. Albany.

Rhoden, Nancy K. 1986. "The Judge in the Delivery Room: The Emergence of Court-ordered Cesareans." *California Law Review* 74:1951.

Rivera, R., J. R. Gaitan, M. Ortega, C. Flores, and A. Hernandez. 1984. "The Use of Biodegradable Norethisterone Implants as a 6-Month Contraceptive System." *Fertility and Sterility* 42:228.

Robaire, B., and L. Hermo. 1988. "Efferent Ducts, Epididymis, and Vas Deferens: Structure, Functions, and Their Regulation." In *The Physiology of Reproduction*, edited by E. Knobil and J. D. Neill. New York: Raven.

Robaire, B., D. F. Convey, C. H. Robinson, and L. L. Ewing. 1977. "Selective Inhibition of Rate Epididymal Steroid 4-5α-reductase by Conjugated Allenic 3-oxo-5,10-secosteroids." *Journal of Steroid Biochemistry* 8:307.

Robaire, B., J. Duron, and T. J. Lobl. 1986. "Inhibition of Epididymal 4-ene-5α-reductase (5α-R) and 3α-hydroxysteroid dehydrogenase (3α-HSD) by 17-substituted Chloroformate Androgen Analogs." *Journal of Andrology* 7:20P.

Robertson, Dale N. 1983. "Norgestrel-releasing Silastic Rods: Clinical Effects, Biochemical Effects, and In Vivo Release Rates." In *Advances in Human Fertility and Reproductive Endocrinology*, vol. 2, *Long-acting Steroid Contraception*, edited by D. R. Mishell. New York: Raven.

Robertson, John A. 1982. "The Right to Procreate and In Utero Fetal Therapy." *Journal of Legal Medicine* 3:333.

———. 1985. "Legal Issues in Fetal Therapy." *Seminars in Perinatology* 9:136.

———. 1986. "Legal Issues in Prenatal Therapy." *Clinical Obstetrics and Gynecology* 29:603.

Robertson, John A., and Joseph D. Schulman. 1987. "Pregnancy and Prenatal Harm to Offspring: The Case of Mothers with PKU." *Hastings Center Report* 17(4):23.

Robitscher, Jonas. 1973a. "Eugenic Sterilization: A Biomedical Intervention." In *Eugenic Sterilization*, edited by Jonas Robitscher. Springfield, Ill.: Charles C. Thomas.

———, ed. 1973b. *Eugenic Sterilization*. Springfield, Ill.: Charles C. Thomas.

Roe v. Wade, 410 U.S. 113 (1973).

Rolleston, H. D. 1936. *The Endocrine Glands in Health and Disease with an Historical Review*. London: Oxford University Press.

Rome, Ester. 1986. "Premenstrual Syndrome Examined through a Feminist Lens." In *Culture, Society, and Menstruation*, edited by V. L. Olesen and N. F. Woods. Washington, D.C.: Hemisphere.

Rooks, J. B., and W. Cates, Jr. 1977. "Emotional Impact of D and E vs. Instillation." *Family Planning Perspectives* 9:276.

Rosenberg, L., S. Shapiro, D. Slone, D. W. Kaufman, S. P. Helmrich, O. S. Mieltinen, P. D. Stolley, N. B. Rosenshein, D. Schottenfeld, and R. L. Engle, Jr. 1982. "Epithelial Ovarian Cancer and Combination Oral Contraceptives." *Journal of the American Medical Association* 247:3210.

Rothman, Barbara Katz. 1986. "When a Pregnant Woman Endangers Her Fetus: Commentary." *Hastings Center Report* 16(1):25.

Rothman, K. J. 1982. "Spermicide Use and Down's Syndrome." *American Journal of Public Health* 72:399.

Rowe, P. J. 1981. "The Intrauterine Device: A Review of Recent Advances and Controversies." In *Oxford Reviews of Reproductive Biology*, vol. 3., edited by C. A. Finn. Oxford: Clarendon Press.

Roy, S., J. Wilkins, and D. Mishell. 1981. "The Effect of a Contraceptive Vaginal Ring and Oral Contraceptives on the Vaginal Flora." *Contraception* 24:481.

Royal College of General Practitioners. 1976. "The Outcome of Pregnancy in Former Oral Contraceptive Users." *British Journal of Obstetrics and Gynaecology* 83:608.

Rozier, J. C., and P. B. Underwood. 1974. "Use of Progestational Agents in Endometrial Adenocarcinoma." *Obstetrics and Gynecology* 44:60.

Ruddick, William, and William Wilcox. 1982. "Operating on the Fetus." *Hastings Center Report* 12(5):10.

Sacco, A. G., E. C. Yurewing, M. G. Subramanian, and F. J. DeMayo. 1981. "Zona Pellucida Composition: Species Cross Reactivity and Contraceptive Potential of Antiserum to a Purified Pig Zona Antigen (PPZA)." *Biology of Reproduction* 25:997.

Salazar v. St. Vincent Hospital, 95 N.M. 150, 619 P.2d 826 (N.M. Ct. App. 1980).

Salomon, D. S., and R. M. Pratt. 1976. "Glucocorticoid Receptors in Murine Embryonic Facial Mesenchyme Cells." *Nature* 264:174.

Sanger, Margaret. 1919. "Why Not Birth Control in America?" *Birth Control Review*, May, p. 10.

_____. 1922. *The Pivot of Civilization*. New York: Brentano.

_____. 1932. "My Way to Peace." Speech to the New York History Society, January 17. In Sanger Manuscripts. Sophia Smith Collection, Smith College, Northampton, Mass.

_____. 1938. *An Autobiography*. New York: Norton. (Reissued, New York: Dover, 1971.)

Saxton, Marsha. 1987. "Prenatal Screening and Discriminatory Attitudes about Disability." *Genewatch* 4:8.

Schally, A. V. 1978. "Aspects of Hypothalamic Regulation of the Pituitary Gland: Its Implications for the Control of the Reproductive Processes." *Science* 202:18.

Schally, A. V., D. H. Coy, and A. Arimura. 1980. "LH-RH Agonists and Antagonists." *International Journal of Gynaecology and Obstetrics* 18:318.

Schearer, S. B. 1978. "Current Efforts to Develop Male Hormonal Contraception." *Studies in Family Planning* 9:229.

Schearer, S. B., F. Alvarez-Sanchez, J. Anselmo, P. Brenner, E. Coutinho, A. Latham-Faundes, J. Frick, B. Heinild, and E. D. B. Johansson. 1978. "Hormonal Contraception for Men." *International Journal of Andrology Supplement* 2:680.

Schijf, C. P. T., C. M. G. Thomas, P. N. M. Demacker, W. H. Doesburg, and R. Rolland. 1984. "The Influence of the Triphasic Pill and a Desogestrel-containing Combination Pill on some Physical, Biochemical and Hormonal Parameters: A Preliminary Report." In *Fertility and Sterility*, edited by R. F. Harrison, J. Bonnar, and W. Thompson. Higham, Mass.: MTP Press.

Schmidt-Gollwitzer, M., W. Hardt, K. Schmidt-Gollwitzer, and J. Nevinny-Stickel. 1981. "Influence of the LH-RH Analogue Buserelin on Cyclic Ovarian Function and on Endometrium: A New Approach to Fertility Control?" *Contraception* 23:187.

Schindler, A. E., S. Ladanyi, R. Coser, and E. Keller. 1980. "Postcoital Contraception with an Injectable Estrogen Preparation." *Contraception* 22:165.

Schumacher, M., J. J. Legros, and J. Balthazart. 1987. "Steroid Hormones, Behavior and Sexual Dimorphism in Animals and Men: The Nature-Nurture Controversy." *Experimental and Clinical Endocrinology* 90:129.

Schwallie, P. C. 1974. "Experience with Depo-Provera as an Injectable Contraceptive." *Journal of Reproductive Medicine* 13:113.

Segal, S. J., ed. 1985. *Gossypol: A Potential Contraceptive for Man*. New York: Plenum.

Seigel, I. 1963. "Conception Control by Long-acting Progestagens: Preliminary Report." *Obstetrics and Gynecology* 21:666.

Sen, Amartya. 1981. *Poverty and Famines: An Essay on Entitlement and Deprivation*. Oxford: Clarendon Press.

Setchell, B. P. 1978. *The Mammalian Testis*. Ithaca, N.Y.: Cornell University Press.

Settlage, D. S. F., M. Motoshima, and D. R. Tredway. 1973. "Sperm Transport from the External Cervical Os to the Fallopian Tube in Women: A Time and Quantitation Study." *Fertility and Sterility* 24:655.

Shapiro, S., D. H. Slone, O. P. Heinonen, D. W. Kaufman, L. Rosenberg, A. A. Mitchell, and S. P. Helmrich. 1982. "Birth Defects and Vaginal Spermicides." *Journal of the American Medical Association* 247:2381.

Shapiro, S., D. H. Slone, L. Rosenberg, and D. W. Kaufman. 1979. "Oral-Contraceptive Use in Relation to Myocardial Infarction." *Lancet* 1:743.

Shaw, Margery W. 1983. "The Destiny of the Fetus." In *Abortion and the Status of the Fetus,* edited by William B. Bondeson, H. Tristram Engelhardt, Jr., Stuart F. Spicker, and Daniel H. Winship. Boston: D. Reidel.

Shivers, C. Alex, and Phillip M. Sieg. 1980. "Antigens of Oocytes and Their Environment." In *Immunological Aspects of Infertility and Fertility Regulation,* edited by D. A. Dhindsa and G. F. B. Schumacher. Amsterdam: Elsevier.

Short, R. V. 1984. "Oestrous and Menstrual Cycles." In *Reproduction in Mammals,* vol. 3, *Hormonal Control of Reproduction,* 2d ed., edited by C. R. Austin and R. V. Short. Cambridge: Cambridge University Press.

Shriner, Thomas L. 1979. "Maternal versus Fetal Rights — A Clinical Dilemma." *Obstetrics and Gynecology* 53:518.

Silber, S. J. 1980. "Reversal of Vasectomy and the Treatment of Male Infertility." *Journal of Andrology* 1:261.

Silberner, Joanne. 1986. "Spermicides and Birth Defects." *Science Digest* 130:399.

Simcock, B. W. 1985. "IUD Complications." In *Biomedical Aspects of IUDs,* edited by H. Hasson, E. S. E. Hafez, and W. A. van Os. Higham, Mass.: MTP Press.

Simon, Julian. 1981. *The Ultimate Resource.* Princeton, N.J.: Princeton University Press.

Simpson, J. L. 1984. "Mutagenicity and Teratogenicity of Injectable and Implantable Progestins: Probable Lack of Effect." In *Long-acting Contraceptive Delivery Systems,* edited by G. I. Zatuchni, A. Goldsmith, J. D. Shelton, and J. J. Sciarra. Philadelphia: Harper & Row.

————. 1985a. "Relationship between Congenital Anomalies and Contraception." *Advances in Contraception* 1:3.

————. 1985b. "Do Contraceptive Methods Pose Fetal Risks?" *Research Frontiers in Fertility Regulation* 3, no. 6.

————. 1987. "Ovarian Dysgenesis and Related Genetic Disorders." In *Gynecologic Endocrinology,* 4th ed., edited by J. J. Gold and J. B. Josimovich. New York: Plenum.

Sivin, Irving. 1983. "Clinical Effects of NORPLANT Subdermal Implants for contraception." In *Advances in Human Fertility and Reproductive Endocrinology,* vol. 2, *Long-acting Steroid Contraception,* edited by D. R. Mishell. New York: Raven.

Sivin, I., F. Alvarez-Sanchez, S. Diaz, E. Coutinho, O. McDonald, D. N. Robertson, and J. Stern. 1983. "Three-Year Experience with Norplant Subdermal-Contraception." *Fertility and Sterility* 35:799.

Sloane, Ethel. 1980. *Biology of Women.* New York: Wiley.

Smith, Adam. 1776. *An Inquiry into the Nature and Causes of the Wealth of Nations.*

Smith, Anthony. 1985. *The Body.* New York: Viking Penguin.

Smith, D. C., R. Printice, D. J. Thompson, and W. L. Herrmann. 1975. "Association of Exogenous Estrogen and Endometrial Carcinoma." *New England Journal of Medicine* 293:1164.

Smith, Holly M. 1983. "Intercourse and Responsibility for the Fetus." In *Abortion and the Status of the Fetus,* edited by William B. Bondeson, H. T. Engelhardt, Jr., Stuart F. Spicker, and Daniel H. Winship. Boston: D. Reidel.

Smith v. Brennan, 31 NJ 353, 157 A 2d 497 (1960).

Snowden, R. 1976. "IUD and Congenital Malformation." *British Medical Journal* 1:770.

Sobel, S. 1986. "A Twenty Year Summary of FDA Animal Safety Testing of Contraceptive Steroids." In *Contraceptive Steroids: Pharmacology and Safety*, edited by A. T. Gregoire and R. P. Blye. New York: Plenum.

Sobrero, A. J., and J. McLeod. 1962. "The Immediate Post Coital Test." *Fertility and Sterility* 13:184.

Soderstrom, Richard M. 1980. "Ten Questions Regarding IUDs, Salpingitis, and Ectopic Pregnancy." In *The Safety of Fertility Control*, edited by Louis G. Keith. New York: Springer.

Solomon, Robert C. 1983. "Reflections on the Meaning of (Fetal) Life." In *Abortion and the Status of the Fetus*, edited by William B. Bondeson, H. T. Engelhardt, Jr., Stuart F. Spicker, and Daniel H. Winship. Boston: D. Reidel.

Spallone, Patricia, and Deborah Lynn Steinberg. 1987. *Made to Order: The Myth of Reproductive and Genetic Progress*. New York: Pergamon.

Speck v. Finegold, 268 Pa. Sup. 342, 408 A.2d 496 (1979).

Stadel, Bruce. 1986. "Oral Contraceptives and the Occurrence of Disease." In *Contraceptive Steroids: Pharmacology and Safety*, edited by A. T. Gregoire and R. P. Blye. New York: Plenum.

Stanczyk, F. Z., M. Hiroi, U. Goebelsmann, P. F. Brenner, M. E. Lumkin, and D. R. Mishell, Jr. 1975. "Radioimmunoassay of Serum d-norgestrel in Women following Oral and Intravaginal Administration." *Contraception* 12:279.

Stanworth, Michelle, ed. 1987. *Reproductive Techniques: Gender, Motherhood, and Medicine*. Minneapolis: University of Minnesota Press.

Steinberger, A., and D. N. Ward. 1988. "Inhibin." In *The Physiology of Reproduction*, edited by E. Knobil and J. D. Neill. New York: Raven.

Steinberger, Emil. 1980. "Current Status of Research on Hormonal Contraception in the Male." *Research Frontiers in Fertility Regulation* 1, no. 2.

Stern, E. 1977. "Steroid Contraceptive Use and Cervical Dysplasia: Increase in the Risk of Progression." *Science* 1966:1460.

Stevens, J. D., and I. S. Fraser. 1974. "The Outcome of Pregnancy after Failure of an Intrauterine Contraceptive Device." *British Journal of Obstetrics and Gynaecology* 81:282.

Stevens, V. C. 1980. "The Current Status of Anti-pregnancy Vaccines Based on Synthetic Fractions of HCG." In *Immunological Aspects of Reproduction and Fertility Control*, edited by J. P. Hearn. Baltimore: University Park Press.

Steward, Morse. 1867. "Criminal Abortion." *Detroit Review of Medicine and Pharmacy* 2:7.

Storer, Horatio R., and Franklin Fiske Heard. 1868. *Criminal Abortion: Its Nature, Its Evidence and Its Law*. Cambridge, Mass.: n.p.

Stroh, G., and A. R. Hinman. 1976. "Reported Live Births following Induced Abortion: Two and One-half Years' Experience in Upstate New York." *American Journal of Obstetrics and Gynecology* 126:83.

Strunk v. Strunk, 445 S.W.2d 145 (Ky. Ct. App. 1969).

Sumner, L. W. 1981. *Abortion and Moral Theory*. Princeton: Princeton University Press, chap. 4. (A revised version of this chapter appears as "A Third Way" in *The Problem of Abortion*, 2d ed., edited by Joel Feinberg [Belmont, Calif.: Wadsworth].)

Sumner, W. G., A. G. Keller, and M. Davie. 1927. *The Science of Society*. New Haven: Yale University Press.

Sussman, N. 1976. "Sex and Sexuality in History." In *The Sexual Experience*, edited by B. J. Saddock, H. I. Kaplan, and A. M. Freedman. Baltimore: Williams and Wilkins.

Swaab, D. F., and E. Fliers. 1985. "A Sexually Dimorphic Nucleus in the Human Brain." *Science* 228:1112.

Sweet, R. A., H. G. Schroat, R. Kurland, and O. S. Cupl. 1974. "Study of the Incidence of Hypospadias in Rochester, Minnesota, 1940–1970, and a Case-Control Comparison of Possible Etiologic Factors." *Mayo Clinic Proceedings* 49:52.

Sylvestrini, B., S. Burberi, B. Catanese, U. Cioli, F. Coulston, R. Lisciani, and P. Scorza. 1975. "Antispermatogenic Activity of 1-p-chlorobenzyl-1H-indazol-3-carbosylic Acid (AF-1312/TS) in Rats." *Experimental and Molecular Pathology* 23:288.

Taft v. Taft, 338 Mass. 331, 446 N.E.2d 395 (1983).

Talwar, G. P. 1980. "Vaccines Based upon the Beta-subunit of hCG." In *Immunological Aspects of Reproduction and Fertility Control*, edited by J. P. Hearn. Baltimore: University Park Press.

Tatum, H. J. 1977. "Intrauterine Contraception." In *Frontiers in Reproduction and Fertility Control*, edited by R. O. Greep and M. A. Koblinsky. Cambridge, Mass.: MIT Press.

Tatum, H. J., F. H. Schmidt, and A. K. Jain. 1976. "Management and Outcome of Pregnancies Associated with the Copper T Intrauterine Contraceptive Device." *American Journal of Obstetrics and Gynecology* 126:869.

Tatum, H., F. H. Schmidt, D. Phillips, M. McCarty, and W. M. O'Leary. 1975. "The Dalkon Shield Controversy: Structural and Bacteriological Studies of IUD Tails." *Journal of the American Medical Association* 231:711.

Tejuja, S. 1970. "Use of Subcutaneous Silastic Capsules for Long-term Steroid Contraception." *American Journal of Obstetrics and Gynecology* 197:954.

Thanavala, Y. M., J. P. Hearn, F. C. Hay, and M. Hulme. 1979. "Characterization of the Immunological Response in Marmoset Monkeys Immunized against hCG-subunit and Its Relationship with their Subsequent Fertility. *Journal of Reproductive Immunology* 1:263.

Theurer, R., and J. J. Vitale. 1977. "Drug and Nutrient Interactions." In *Nutritional Support of Medical Practice*, edited by H. Schneider, C. E. Anderson, and D. B. Coursin. Hagerstown, Md.: Harper & Row.

Thompson, W. S. 1935. *Population Problems*. Rev. ed. New York: McGraw-Hill.

Thomson, Judith Jarvis. 1971. "A Defense of Abortion." *Philosophy and Public Affairs* 1:173.

Tietze, C. 1960. "Probability of Pregnancy Resulting from a Single Unprotected Coitus." *Fertility and Sterility* 11:485.

———. 1973. "Intrauterine Devices: Clinical Aspects." In *Human Reproduction: Conception and Contraception*, edited by E. S. E. Hafez, and T. N. Evans. Hagerstown, Md.: Harper & Row.

———. 1981. *Induced Abortion: A World Review, 1981*. New York: The Population Council.

Tietze, C., and Lewit, S. 1970. "Evaluation of Intrauterine Devices: Ninth Progress Report of the Cooperative Statistical Program." *Studies in Family Planning* 55:1.

———. 1972. "Joint Program for the Study of Abortion (JPSA): Early Medical Complications of Legal Abortion." *Studies in Family Planning* 3:97.

Tooley, Michael. 1972. "Abortion and Infanticide." *Philosophy and Public Affairs* 2:37.

———. 1983. *Abortion and Infanticide*. New York: Oxford University Press.

———. 1984. "A Defense of Abortion and Infanticide." In *The Problem of Abortion*, edited by Joel Feinberg. Belmont, Calif.: Wadsworth.

Tortora, Gerald J., and Ronald L. Evans. 1986. *Principles of Human Physiology*. 2d edition. New York: Harper & Row.

Tuchmann-Duplessis, H. 1983. "The Teratogenic Risk." *American Journal of Industrial Medicine* 4:245.

Turner, David. 1717. *Syphilis: A Practical Treatise on the Venereal Disease.* London: n.p.

Tyrer, Louise B. 1980. "The Risks and Benefits of Intrauterine Devices." In *The Safety of Fertility Control,* edited by Louis G. Keith. New York: Springer.

United States Centers for Disease Control. 1988a. *AIDS Weekley Surveillance Report.* Atlanta: United States Centers for Disease Control.

United States Centers for Disease Control. 1988b. *AIDS Surveillance Slide Series.* Code L-178, slide #2, October. Atlanta: United States Centers for Disease Control.

United States Environmental Protection Agency. 1980. "Availability of TSCA: Revised Inventory." *Federal Register* 45:50544.

Union Pacific R. Co. v. Botsford, 141 U.S. 250 (1891).

Vaillancourt v. Medical Center Hospital of Vermont, 139 Vt. 138, 425 A.2d 92 (1980).

Van der Vlugt, P. 1973. *Uterine Aspiration Techniques.* Population Report F(3). Washington, D.C.: George Washington University.

Van de Warker, Ely. 1872. *The Detection of Criminal Abortion and a Study of Foeticidal Drugs.* Boston: James Campbell.

Verkennes v. Corniea, 229 Minn. 365, 38 N.W.2d 838 (1949).

Vessey, M. P. 1979. "Risk of Ectopic Pregnancy and Duration of Use of an Intrauterine Device." *Lancet* 2:501.

Vessey, M. P., R. Doll, R. Peto, B. Johnson, and P. Wiggins. 1976. "A Long-term Follow-up Study of Women Using Different Methods of Contraception: An Interim Report." *Journal of Biosocial Science* 8:373.

Victor, A., L. E. Edqvist, P. Lindberg, K. Elamsson, and E. D. B. Johansson. 1975. "Peripheral Plasma Levels of d-norgestrel in Women after Oral Administration of d-norgestrel and When Using Intravaginal Rings Impregnated with d-norgestrel." *Contraception* 12:261.

Victor, A., and E. D. B. Johansson. 1977. "Contraceptive Rings: Self-administered Treatment Governed by Bleeding." *Contraception* 16:137.

Viinikka, L., A. Victor, O. Janne, and J. P. Raynaud. 1975. "The Plasma Concentration of a Synthetic Progestin, R2323, Released from Polysilastic Vaginal Rings." *Contraception* 12:309.

Wachtel, S. S. 1977. "H-Y Antigen: Genetics and Serology." *Immunology Review* 33:33.

―――. 1979. "Immunogenetic Aspects of Abnormal Sexual Differentiation." *Cell* 16:691.

Wachtel, S. S., and S. Ohno. 1979. "The Immunogenetics of Sexual Development." In *Progress in Medical Genetics,* vol. 3, edited by A. G. Steinberg. Philadelphia: Saunders.

Wade, N. 1981. *The Nobel Duel.* New York: Doubleday.

Warburton, D., R. H. Neugut, A. Lustenberger, A. G. Nicholas, and J. Kline. 1987. "Lack of Association between Spermicide Use and Trisomy." *New England Journal of Medicine* 317:478.

Warren, Mary Anne. 1973. "On the Moral and Legal Status of Abortion." *Monist* 57:120.

―――. 1975. "On the Moral and Legal Status of Abortion, Postscript on Infanticide." In *Today's Moral Problems,* edited by Richard A. Wasserstrom. New York: Macmillan.

―――. 1985. *Gendercide: The Implications of Sex Selection.* Totowa, N.J.: Rowman and Allanheld.

Warwick, Donald. 1982. *Bitter Pills: Population Policies and Their Implications in Eight Developing Countries.* Cambridge: Cambridge University Press.

Weideger, Paula. 1976. *Menstruation and Menopause, the Physiology and Psychology, the Myth and the Reality.* New York: Knopf.

Weiss, R. 1987. "Caveat Laden, the Copper IUD Returns." *Science News* 132:318.

Wells v. Ortho Pharmaceutical Corporation, 788F.2d 741 (11th Cir. 1986).

Wertheimer, Roger. 1971. "Understanding the Abortion Argument." *Philosophy and Public Affairs* 1:67.

Westoff, C. F., and E. F. Jones. 1977. "Contraception and Sterilization in the United States: Methods of Fertility Control 1955, 1960 and 1965." *Studies in Family Planning* 17:1.

Wheat, T. E., and E. Goldberg. 1983. "Sperm-specific Lactate Dehydrogenase $C_4$: Antigenic Structure and Immunosuppression of Fertility." *Isozymes: Current Topics in Biology and Medical Research* 7:113.

Whitbeck, Caroline. 1976. "Theories of Sex Difference." In *Women and Philosophy: Toward a Theory of Liberation*, edited by Carol C. Gould and Marx W. Wartofsky. New York: Putnam.

———. 1983. "The Moral Implications of Regarding Women as People." In *Abortion and the Status of the Fetus*, edited by William B. Bondeson, H. Tristram Engelhardt, Jr., Stuart F. Spicker, and Daniel H. Winship. Boston: D. Reidel.

White, Byron R. 1973. Roe v. Wade. Dissenting opinion. 410 US 113.

Whitby, R. M., R. D. Gordon, and B. R. Blair. 1979. "The Endocrine Effects of Vasectomy: A Prospective Five-Year Study." *Fertility and Sterility* 31:518.

WHO Task Force on Prostaglandins for Fertility Regulation. 1981. "Vaginal Administration of 15-methyl-$PGF_{2\alpha}$ Methyl Ester for Preoperative Cervical Dilation." *Contraception* 21:251.

Wickings, E. J., and E. Nieschlag. 1983. "Immunological Approach to Male Fertility Control." In *Endocrine Mechanisms in Fertility Regulation*, edited by G. Benagiano and E. Diczfalusy. New York: Raven.

Wilbur, Amy E. 1986. "The Contraceptive Crisis." *Science Digest*, September, p. 54.

Wilkins, L., H. W. Jones, G. H. Holman, and R. S. Stempfel. 1985. "Masculinization of the Female Fetus Associated with Administration of Oral and Intramuscular Progestins during Gestation: Non-Adrenal Female Pseudohermaphroditism." *Journal of Clinical and Endocrinological Metabolism* 18:559.

Williams, G. 1958. *The Sanctity of Life and the Criminal Law.* London: Faber.

Wilson, J. G. 1977. "Current Status of Teratology. General Principles and Mechanisms Derived from Animal Studies." In *Handbook of Teratology*, vol. 1, edited by J. G. Wilson and F. C. Fraser. New York: Plenum.

Wilson, J. G., and R. L. Brent. 1981. "Are Female Sex Hormones Teratogenic?" *American Journal of Obstetrics and Gynecology* 141:567.

Wiseman, R. A., and I. C. Dodds-Smith. 1984. "Cardiovascular Birth Defects and Antenatal Exposure to Female Sex Hormones: A Reevaluation of Some Base Data." *Teratology* 30:359.

Wislocki, G. B., and L. S. King. 1936. "The Permeability of the Hypophysis and the Hypothalamus to Vital Dyes, with a Study of the Hypophysial Vascular Supply." *American Journal of Anatomy* 58:421.

Womack v. Buckhorn, 384 Mich. 718, 187 N.W.2d 218 (1976).

Women's Global Network on Reproductive Rights. 1986a. "All But One IUD Withdrawn from USA Market." *Newsletter*, January-March, p. 19.

———. 1986b. "The Dalkon Shield: The Latest." *Newsletter*, April-June, p. 15.

_____. 1986c. "Why Searle Took Copper IUDs Off USA Market." *Newsletter*, April-June, p. 19.

_____. 1986d. "Norplant Trials Stopped in Brazil." *Newsletter*, July-September, p. 4.

_____. 1987a. "Fifth International Women and Health Meeting." *Newsletter*, May p. 5.

_____. 1987b. "Intrauterine Devices: Benefits and Risks." *Newsletter*, May p. 21.

_____. 1988. "RU-486 Becomes Political Football." *Newsletter*, September-December, 24.

Wong, P. Y. D., C. L. Au, and H. K. Ngai. 1980. "Effects of 6-chloro-6-deoxyglucose on Electrolyte and Water Transport in the Epididymis and Fertility of Male Rats." *International Journal of Andrology* 3:82.

Wong, P. Y. D., C. H. Yeung, and H. K. Ngai. 1977. "Effect of α-chlorohydrin on Transport Processes in Perfused Rat Cauda Epididymides." *Contraception* 16:637.

Wood, Clive, and Beryl Suitters. 1970. *The Fight for Acceptance: A History of Contraception.* Aylesbury: Medical and Technical Publishing Co.

Wood, D. M., C. Liu, and B. S. Dunbar. 1981. "Effect of Alloimmunization and Heteroimmunization with Zonae Pellucidae on Fertility in Rabbits." *Biology of Reproduction* 25:439.

Woodburne, R. T. 1965. *Essentials of Human Anatomy.* New York: Oxford University Press.

World Bank. 1984. *World Development Report 1984.* Oxford: Oxford University Press.

World Health Organization. 1958. "Preamble to the Constitution of the World Health Organization." In *The First Ten Years of the World Health Organization.* Geneva: World Health Organization.

_____. 1978. *Seventh Annual Report: Special Programme of Research, Development and Research Training in Human Reproduction.* Geneva: World Health Organization.

_____. 1979. *Eighth Annual Report: Special Programme of Research, Development and Research Training in Human Reproduction.* Geneva: World Health Organization.

_____. 1980. *Ninth Annual Report: Special Programme of Research, Development and Research Training in Human Reproduction.* Geneva: World Health Organization.

_____. 1981. *The Effect of Female Sex Hormones on Fetal Development and Infant Health.* World Health Organization Technical Report Series 657. Geneva: World Health Organization.

_____. 1982. *Injectable Hormonal Contraceptives: Technical and Safety Aspects.* WHO Offset Publication no. 65. Geneva: World Health Organization.

_____. 1985. "Facts about an Implantable Contraceptive." *Bulletin of the World Health Organization* 63:3.

Wright v. Olin Corporation, 697 F.2d 1172 (4th Cir. 1982).

Wrigley, E. A. 1969. *Population and History.* New York: McGraw-Hill.

Wyshak, G., and R. E. Frisch. 1982. "Evidence for a Secular Trend in Age of Menarche." *New England Journal of Medicine* 306:1033.

Yen, S. S. C. 1986. "The Human Menstrual Cycle." In *Reproductive Endocrinology: Physiology, Pathophysiology, and Clinical Management*, 2d ed., edited by S. S. C. Yen, and R. B. Jaffe. Philadelphia: Saunders.

Yuzpe, A. Albert. 1980. "Postcoital Contraception." In *The Safety of Fertility Control*, edited by Louis G. Keith. New York: Springer.

Zacharias, L., W. M. Rand, and R. J. Wurtman. 1976. "A Prospective Study of Sexual Development in American Girls: The Statistics of Menarche." *Obstetrics and Gynecology Survey* 31:325.

Zacharias, L., R. J. Wurtman, and S. Schatzoff. 1970. "Sexual Maturation in Contemporary American Girls." *American Journal of Obstetrics and Gynecology* 108:833.

Zanartu, J., and C. Navarro. 1968. "Fertility Inhibition by an Injectable Progestogen Acting for 3 Months: A Clinical Survey of 130 Fertile Women Treated with Norethisterone Enanthate." *Obstetrics and Gynecology* 31:627.

Zatuchni, Gerald I., ed. 1985. "Immunologic Methods of Fertility Regulation: Report of a Workshop." *Research Frontiers in Fertility Reproduction* 3(3):1.

Zatuchni, G. I., J. J. Sciarra, and J. J. Spiedel. 1979. *Pregnancy Termination: Procedures, Safety and New Developments*. Hagerstown, Md.: Harper & Row.

Ziel, H. K., and W. D. Finkle. 1975. "Increased Risk of Endometrial Carcinoma among Users of Conjugated Estrogens." *New England Journal of Medicine* 293:1187.

Zilbergeld, B. 1978. *Male Sexuality: A Guide to Sexual Fulfillment*. Boston: Little, Brown.

Zipper, J., M. Medel, and R. Prager. 1969. "Suppression of Fertility by Intrauterine Copper and Zinc in Rabbits: A New Approach to Intrauterine Contraception." *American Journal of Obstetrics and Gynecology* 105:529.

Zita, Jacquelyn N. 1988. "The Premenstrual Syndrome: 'Dis-easing' the Female Cycle." *Hypatia* 3(1):77.

Zuniga v. Kleberg County Hospital, 692 F.2d 986 (5th Cir. 1982).

# Index